Student Work Manual for
INTRODUCTORY MEDICAL - SURGICAL NURSING
Second Edition

Student Work Manual for
INTRODUCTORY MEDICAL - SURGICAL NURSING
Second Edition

Jeanne C. Scherer, R.N., M.S.
Assistant Director and
Medical-Surgical Coordinator
Sisters of Charity Hospital
School of Nursing, Buffalo, N.Y.

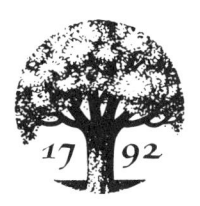

J. B. Lippincott Company
Philadelphia
NEW YORK SAN JOSE TORONTO

Copyright © 1977 by J. B. Lippincott Company

This book is fully protected by copyright and, with the exception of brief excerpts for review, no part of it may be reproduced in any form by print, photoprint, microfilm, or by any other means without the written permission of the publishers.

Distributed in Great Britain by
Blackwell Scientific Publications
London   Oxford   Edinburgh

ISBN 0-397-54206-2

Printed in the United States of America

4 6 8 9 7 5

PREFACE

This Student Work Manual has been designed to accompany the textbook, *Introductory Medical-Surgical Nursing*. Its purpose is to provide a means of reviewing the material covered in the text and reinforcing the learning of important content. The manual has been aimed primarily at the major areas covered in the textbook and various questioning methods have been employed to test the reader's general comprehension of the material. The manual is correlated chapter-by-chapter with *Introductory Medical-Surgical Nursing* and the questions are based entirely upon its content.

The questions are written with the aim of assisting the student in the learning process. The manual contains a composite of true or false, multiple choice, matching, and completion questions stressing a knowledge of general facts and clinical nursing. Essay questions found at the end of most chapters may be answered in the manual or on a separate sheet of paper, or used as topics for discussion in seminars, clinical conferences, or the classroom. Some essay questions will require individual judgment or opinion and are included to allow students to explore their personal feelings on various topics of concern to nurses and to help them to become more aware of some of the problems which may confront patients and their families.

With the exception of some personal opinion essays, the answer to each question in the manual is provided in the Appendix. In addition to the answer, page references to the textbook are provided in parentheses to enable the student to review the material as needed. Both the source of the question and the answer will be found in the text on the indicated pages.

All pages of the manual are perforated, providing students and instructors with various options for use. The instructor may wish to remove the Appendix before the student uses the manual, returning the answer pages after each chapter of the manual has been used for self-testing. Each page is also punched so that, once removed from the book, the student may file it in a notebook and refer to it for future study.

Jeanne C. Scherer
March 1977

To the memory of Diane Goodspeed,
a member of the class of 1978,
who left us all too soon.

CONTENTS

Preface v

UNIT ONE
Concepts basic to the care of patients 1
1 Care of adults throughout the life cycle 3
2 Nurse-patient relationships 7
3 Fundamental processes of health and illness 10
4 The interaction of body and mind 14
5 The patient in pain 16
6 Dependence on and abuse of alcohol, drugs, and tobacco 18
7 Care of the dying patient 22
8 Nursing in emergencies 25
9 The surgical patient 29

UNIT TWO
Oncologic nursing 35
10 Care of the patient with cancer 37
11 Nursing management in radiotherapy 41

UNIT THREE
Disturbances of body supportive structures and locomotion 45
12 The patient with a fracture 47
13 The patient with a disease of the bones and joints 56
14 The patient with an amputation 62

vii

UNIT FOUR
Disorders of cognitive, sensory, or psychomotor function 67
15 The patient with neurological disturbance 69
16 The patient with cerebrovascular disease 79
17 The patient with spinal cord impairment 84
18 The patient with visual and hearing impairment 89

UNIT FIVE
Threats to adequate respiration 99
19 The patient with a disease of the nose or the throat 101
20 The patient with acute respiratory disorder 106
21 The patient with chronic respiratory disorder 111

UNIT SIX
Insults to cardiovascular integrity 119
22 The patient with a blood or lymph disorder 121
23 The patient with heart disease: anatomy; diagnostic tests 127
24 The patient with heart disease 130
25 The patient with inflammatory or valvular disease of the heart 134
26 The patient with cardiovascular disease: coronary artery disease; functional heart disease; hypertension 137
27 The patient with peripheral vascular disease: thrombosis and embolism 142

UNIT SEVEN
Disturbances of ingestion, digestion, absorption and elimination 151
28 Introduction, diagnostic tests, functional disorders 153
29 The patient with ulcerative colitis, peptic ulcer 158
30 The patient with cancer of the gastrointestinal tract 163
31 The patient with an ileostomy or a colostomy 169
32 The patient with an intestinal or a rectal disorder 174
33 The patient with a disorder of the liver, gallbladder, or pancreas 180
34 The urologic patient 187

UNIT EIGHT
Problems resulting from endocrine imbalance 197
35 The patient with an endocrine disorder 199
36 The patient with diabetes mellitus 207

UNIT NINE
Disturbances of sexual structures or reproductive function 213
37 Introduction: the female reproductive pattern 215
38 The woman with a disorder of the reproductive system 219
39 The man with a disorder of the reproductive system 225
40 The patient with breast disease 230
41 The patient with venereal infection 234

UNIT TEN
Common problems involving disfigurement 239
42 The patient with a dermatological condition 241
43 The patient undergoing plastic surgery 245

UNIT ELEVEN
Intensive care nursing 247

44 and **45** Introduction to intensive care nursing and the patient in shock 249

46 Respiratory insufficiency and failure 252

47 The patient with heart disease: cardiac arrhythmias 256

48 The patient with acute myocardial infarction 261

49 Cardiac surgical nursing 266

50 The patient in renal failure 269

51 The burned patient 273

52 The patient with neurological disease 278

Appendix 283

UNIT ONE
Concepts basic to the care of patients

CHAPTER—1

Care of adults throughout the life cycle

The aging process occurs at different rates in different individuals. Thus, the nurse may note that one individual at the age of 63 is mentally and physically unable to care for himself while another is actively employed and self-supporting. It is important to understand the developmental pattern of the adult so that normal changes are not confused with the changes of disease.

The following questions deal with the contents of Chapter 1.

I. True or false.

Read each statement carefully and place your answer in the space provided.

___ 1. The aging process occurs at different rates in different individuals.
___ 2. Not all societies place identical emphasis on working, making money, and getting ahead.
___ 3. The patient in the later years of life is as physically resilient as a young adult.
___ 4. The young patient might accept suggestions from the nurse that he wouldn't accept from his parents or other relatives.
___ 5. The young adult who is still developing a concept of his physical self is usually able to accept illness.
___ 6. The middle years are a time when productivity is decreased.
___ 7. Height tends to remain constant until old age at which time the individual may become shorter.
___ 8. Presbyopia may be defined as the inability to see distant objects.
___ 9. There is a tendency for individuals to lose weight during the later years.
___ 10. Chronic constipation is a frequent problem of the elderly.

II. Multiple choice questions.

Select the most appropriate answer and place it in the space provided.

1. Developmental tasks may be defined as ___.
   a. all the activities performed throughout life
   b. learned physical activities primarily occurring in the middle years
   c. things to be learned and changes to be accomplished
   d. all actions taken when confronted with specific problems

CLINICAL SITUATION

Jim, age 18, is admitted to the hospital for an emergency appendectomy. It is 5 days since his surgery, he is ambulating, and will probably be discharged from the hospital in the next few days. The following 2 questions apply to this patient.

2. Jim has many visitors, but during nonvisiting hours he seems lonely and frightened. Jim's feelings might be explained by the fact that ____.
   a. relationships with friends may be superficial
   b. young adults are often moody and resentful
   c. young adults always have difficulty adjusting to new situations
   d. young adults usually resent being left alone for even short periods of time

3. Jim persists in turning up the volume of his television set and breaking other hospital rules. This may be Jim's way of ____.
   a. trying to forget his illness
   b. showing his friends that he can accept illness
   c. trying to force his ideas on other patients
   d. showing dissatisfaction with authority and hospital rules

4. A slow and barely perceptible decline in physical ability begins ____.
   a. around age 18 to 20
   b. at age 40
   c. in the mid-50s
   d. at age 65

5. The nurse can improve communication with a hard of hearing patient by ____.
   a. speaking very loudly
   b. speaking slowly and clearly
   c. gesturing with the hands
   d. being as pleasant and brief as possible

6. The elderly may have difficulty in adjusting to temperature extremes. It is harder for the elderly patient to adjust to a cool or cold temperature because his ____.
   a. clothes fit more loosely and therefore do not conserve body heat
   b. metabolism is slower
   c. food intake is less
   d. awareness of the change in temperature is decreased

7. One problem with the use of bath oil in tub baths is the ____.
   a. oil can cause swelling and peeling of the skin
   b. oil prevents removal of dirt, crusts, and dried skin
   c. danger of the patient slipping in the tub
   d. possibility of plugging the pores of the skin

8. Hearing is usually most acute at the age of ____.
   a. 14
   b. 25
   c. 40
   d. 60

9. Though it may vary considerably with different individuals, menopause usually occurs between the ages of ____ and ____.
   a. 35 and 45
   b. 45 and 55
   c. 55 and 65
   d. 65 and 70

10. The loss of hearing which occurs as a result of age is called ____.
    a. mastoiditis
    b. presbyopia
    c. presbycusis

III. Fill-in and discussion questions.

Read each question carefully and place your answer in the space provided.

1. Older people often have the mistaken notion that they are no longer capable of learning. Discuss some of the measures that may help the nurse to teach older patients.

_____
_____
_____
_____

2. Below are some common areas where noticeable changes occur during the aging process. It should be noted that what is observed in one or two individuals may not be generally true of the majority of members of a certain age group. The first line has been completed to show how the remainder of the question is to be answered.

	ADULT YEARS 18 TO 35	MIDDLE YEARS 35 TO 65	LATE YEARS 65 AND OVER
Skin	smooth, acne may be present	begins to show lines and/or wrinkles	skin dry, lines and wrinkles more prominent
Teeth			
Height and weight			
Speed of reaction			
Vision			
Hair (color)			
Hearing			
Physical growth and strength			
Eating habits			

3. Children often find it extremely difficult to place an aged parent in a nursing home. Briefly explain how you might feel if you were forced to make this decision within the next few weeks. _____
_____
_____
_____
_____

4. A major problem confronting the individual who becomes ill during middle life is the change from independence and productivity to dependence and a curtailment of productivity. Thinking in terms of your parents or anyone you know in the middle years, briefly discuss the implications of a serious illness on an individual—male or female—in this age group. _____
_____
_____
_____
_____
_____

5. List some of the reasons that might prevent an adult from visiting his aged parent in a nursing home. _____
_____
_____
_____
_____
_____

6. Elderly patients may be confused in the unfamiliar surroundings of a hospital, especially during the evening and night hours. List ways in which the evening or night nurse may reduce episodes of confusion in these patients. _____
_____
_____
_____
_____
_____

CHAPTER—2

Nurse-patient relationships

Caring for medical-surgical patients requires a high degree of ability. Listening is a very important part of nursing and is one way in which the nurse-patient relationship is established. By listening, the nurse begins to understand the patient, and the patient learns that the nurse is concerned with his welfare.

The establishment of a good nurse-patient relationship helps the nurse to deal with the patient's problems—both physical and emotional. The nurse who concentrates on the patient and his feelings, recognizes his needs, establishes physical contact, performs technical skills with competence, is supportive, and understands the patient's physical and emotional needs will most likely create a therapeutic atmosphere.

The following questions deal with the contents of Chapter 2.

I. True or false.

Read each statement carefully and place your answer in the space provided.

_____ 1. Emotional stress can aggravate illness.
_____ 2. Anxiety is the same as fear.
_____ 3. Anxiety can be defined as an emotional response.
_____ 4. Providing the patient with the opportunity to talk may open the way to understanding.
_____ 5. Anxiety may range from the mild to the panic level.
_____ 6. Crying is an inappropriate response to grief.
_____ 7. The patient's reaction to a loss may be determined by the magnitude of other serious losses in his life.
_____ 8. The nurse is usually not required to observe the patient's response during diagnostic procedures.
_____ 9. Patients who speak of suicide rarely commit the act.
_____ 10. The nurse is bound to be affected by unpleasant sights and odors.
_____ 11. When a patient appears to be unconscious, the nurse need not fear that he may hear what is being said.

II. Multiple choice questions.

Select the most appropriate answer and place it in the space provided.

1. The cause of anxiety is _____.
   a. easy to identify
   b. not easy to identify
   c. not important when planning nursing care
   d. important to know but need not be identified

7

2. Patients usually ____.
   a. are not aware of the cause(s) of their anxiety
   b. know what is causing their anxiety
   c. like to talk about their anxieties
   d. expect the nurse to point out the causes of their anxiety

3. When a person is very anxious, he ____.
   1. is unable to see all aspects of a problem
   2. sees each aspect of a problem clearly
   3. tends to magnify one or two details of daily living
   4. tends to overlook details of daily living

   a. 1 and 3
   b. 2 and 4
   c. 1 and 4
   d. 2 and 3

4. When a patient has a life-threatening physical need and is also terrified, attention is first given to ____.
   a. finding out what is causing the patient's terror
   b. helping the patient understand his fears
   c. whatever care the patient asks for
   d. the patient's physical need

5. Nurses can experience anxiety which in turn can lead to errors in nursing practice. Two insurances against anxiety are ____.
   a. understanding and a calm attitude
   b. empathy and ability to listen
   c. energy and the desire to help others
   d. knowledge and competence

6. If the nurse experiences anxiety about a situation, she should ____.
   a. ask if someone else can do the work while she takes a rest period
   b. stop what she is doing (except in an emergency) and think the situation through
   c. ignore the feeling as it will probably go away
   d. keep working as this will occupy her mind

7. When an individual sets a goal but some barrier prevents its fulfillment, the result is ____.
   a. indecision
   b. expectation
   c. fear
   d. frustration

8. Conflict can be described as ____.
   a. feeling torn between 2 alternatives or goals
   b. being faced with 2 alternatives—one good and one bad
   c. feeling sad about the alternative that must be selected

9. Mrs. Wagner has been depressed and now talks about suicide. Besides reporting this to her physician and charting all the facts, the nurse should plan to ____.
   a. place the patient in the day room or any area where there are other patients or visitors
   b. stay with the patient until she is seen by a physician
   c. call her family and ask them to come and stay with the patient
   d. check to see if any sedation or tranquilizers have been ordered

10. Nurses should remember that an unconscious patient ____.
    a. rarely recovers from his illness
    b. may hear what is being said
    c. only requires one nurse to give care
    d. usually requires only minimal nursing care

III. Fill-in and discussion questions.

Read each question carefully and place your answer in the space provided.

1. Grief is an intense sadness. Many patients experience this emotion for various reasons, such as disfiguring surgery. In your own words, explain how you might feel at this time if you were faced with a loss such as an amputation of an arm or leg, a disfiguring accident such as severe burns, or a serious disease such as cancer. _____

   _____
   _____
   _____
   _____
   _____
   _____
   _____

2. The contact between the nurse and the patient is not always a long-term one, but the nurse-patient relationship is still important. List 3 measures which may help the nurse to develop a supportive relationship with a patient during a brief period of time.

   1. _____

   2. _____

   3. _____

CHAPTER—3

Fundamental processes of health and illness

Nursing, as one of the health professions, is concerned with helping people obtain and maintain optimal health as well as with preventing disease and caring for those who are ill.

The body attempts to remain in a dynamic state of equilibrium by constantly adapting to the external and internal environment. The nurse, by understanding the process of equilibrium, is able to deal with stress and situations which place stress on the patient.

The following questions deal with the contents of Chapter 3.

I. True or false.

Read each statement carefully and place your answer in the space provided.

_____ 1. Stress can be created by fear, rage, or severe illness.
_____ 2. Most people cannot adapt to stressful situations for more than a short time.
_____ 3. Terminal usually means a stage preceding death.
_____ 4. The term *trauma* is used only in reference to physical injury.
_____ 5. *Ischemia* may be defined as an increase in blood supply to an area.
_____ 6. *Benign tumors* typically stay within their capsules and do not spread to other sites.
_____ 7. The term *metastasize* means to stay in one area.
_____ 8. A *pathogenic organism* is one capable of causing harm.
_____ 9. The term *idiopathic* means of unknown origin.
_____ 10. The human body consists of 10 percent water.
_____ 11. Ordinarily, a healthy person consumes more water and electrolytes than the body needs.
_____ 12. All the fluid removed from the bloodstream by the kidneys is excreted from the body.
_____ 13. Blood transfusion reactions only occur when the wrong blood is given to the wrong patient.
_____ 14. When *epinephrine* is released into the bloodstream, the body becomes rested and quiet.
_____ 15. A pocket of pus is called an *abscess*.
_____ 16. The use of antiseptics and specialized techniques in hospitals makes special precautions against pathogenic organisms unnecessary.
_____ 17. An *antitoxin* is a substance formed after exposure to a bacteria or virus.
_____ 18. Allergies are only seen in the young and rarely occur in individuals over age 20.
_____ 19. Even a minute amount of a drug to which an individual is sensitive can cause allergic symptoms.
_____ 20. There are 2 methods of skin testing—the scratch test and the intradermal injection.

II. Multiple choice questions.

Select the most appropriate answer and place it in the space provided.

1. Homeostasis may be defined as a ____.
    a. condition where opposing forces create an imbalance
    b. state of inequality
    c. method of keeping the body in a neutral state
    d. state of the body when it is in a dynamic state of equilibrium

2. Management of the external environment is often necessary to promote rest. Nursing activities which promote rest include ____.
    1. controlling or eliminating noise when possible
    2. giving a blanket to the patient who is cold
    3. spacing nursing activities for the benefit of the patient rather than the convenience of the nurse
    4. offering between-meal feedings
    5. keeping the patient out of bed as much as possible so he will sleep well at night
        a. 1, 2, 3
        b. 1, 2, 4
        c. 3, 4, 5
        d. all of these

3. A disease that is *acute* ____.
    a. has a poor prognosis
    b. is always a serious illness
    c. has a rapid onset and progress
    d. is followed by a chronic state

4. When a disease is described as *primary* it is assumed to have ____.
    a. occurred first
    b. no known cause
    c. developed independently of any other disease
    d. caused all other diseases the patient may have

5. A statement issued by the health department included the following: "the flu epidemic affected 50 people in a town of 5,000." This rate of illness is an example of a(n) ____.
    a. morbidity rate
    b. mortality rate
    c. illness rate
    d. none of the above

6. The term *neoplasm* may be defined as the ____.
    a. growth of a malignant tumor
    b. new formation of abnormal tissue
    c. development of a localized growth
    d. beginning of cell formation

7. An infarction may be defined as a(n) ____.
    a. heart attack
    b. development of a tumor or tumorlike growth
    c. tissue deprived of its blood supply long enough to become necrotic
    d. increase of blood supply to an organ or structure

8. Mrs. Wilson had a biopsy of a tumor and it was found to be malignant. This means the tumor ____.
    a. will tend to stay in one place but may later spread if not removed
    b. should be biopsied again to be sure of the diagnosis
    c. will cause death in a short time
    d. can invade, crowd, or weaken normal body structures

9. Insensible fluid loss is that which is ____.
    a. lost at night rather than during the day
    b. lost during a severe illness
    c. not replaced
    d. not measurable except by use of special equipment

11

10. The primary cause of insensible fluid loss is ____.
    a. vomiting
    b. diarrhea
    c. perspiration
    d. an increased fluid intake

11. Intravenous fluid therapy may be used to replace ____.
    1. fluid
    2. electrolytes
    3. glucose
    4. blood
    5. dextran
    a. 1, 3, 5
    b. 1, 2, 4
    c. 2, 3, 4
    d. all of these

12. Injecting medication into intravenous tubing will ____.
    a. give a more concentrated dose of the medication
    b. give a less concentrated dose of the medication
    c. have no effect upon the dosage of the medication

13. Blood transfusion reactions may occur ____.
    1. before the transfusion
    2. during the transfusion
    3. soon after the transfusion
    4. weeks after the transfusion
    a. 1 only
    b. 1, 3, 4
    c. 2, 4
    d. 2, 3

14. Inflammation is the body's response to ____.
    a. a release of epinephrine
    b. the ingestion of drugs
    c. the damage of cells
    d. an emergency

15. When there is a break in tissue, such as a surgical incision, the cells bordering the tissue break ____.
    a. begin to multiply and fill in the defect
    b. die and are carried away by the bloodstream
    c. shift and form new tissue
    d. are not replaced

16. Ideal healing is ____.
    a. the formation of scar or granulation tissue
    b. seen only when epithelium grows over a scar
    c. healing by first intention
    d. healing by second intention

17. An infection that has not spread is said to be ____.
    a. stagnant
    b. localized
    c. stationary
    d. limited

18. The lymphatic system is a defense against ____.
    a. inflammation
    b. resistance
    c. healing
    d. infection

19. One method of treating an allergy is ____.
    a. giving a vaccine
    b. the administration of histamine
    c. the avoidance of the allergen
    d. the administration of a scratch test

20. When a person is allergic to a substance the physician may use desensitization to help the patient develop a tolerance to the substance. Desensitization is accomplished by ____.
    a. giving small doses of the antigen subcutaneously
    b. prescribing antihistamines until the worse stage is over
    c. having the patient move to a dry climate and then giving a vaccine
    d. total avoidance of the antigen

III. Fill-in and discussion questions.

Read each question carefully and place your answer in the space provided.

1. The patient may lose fluids and electrolytes through body fluid loss. List 4 body fluids through which electrolytes as well as fluids may leave the body.

    1. _____   3. _____
    2. _____   4. _____

2. List 3 signs that might indicate the patient is having a blood transfusion reaction.

    1. _____   3. _____
    2. _____

3. One way in which the body maintains homeostasis is by protection. The following are sources of body protection. After each, list *what* or *how* the organ or structure protects the body.

    1. Skin _____   3. Skull _____
    _____   _____

    2. Rib cage _____ 4. Autonomic nervous system _____
    _____   _____

4. List the 4 cardinal symptoms of inflammation.

    1. _____   3. _____
    2. _____   4. _____

5. Briefly describe or define each of the following types of immunity.

    1. Actively acquired immunity _____
    _____

    2. Artifically acquired immunity _____
    _____

    3. Passive immunity _____
    _____

6. While you are administering medications to the patients assigned to your care, you give Mr. Allen, who was admitted to the hospital several hours ago, his medication. He asks if the "white pill" is penicillin and you reply that it is. He then tells you that he is allergic to penicillin. What would you do? _____
    _____
    _____

7. Anaphylactic shock is a term used to describe a sudden, severe allergic reaction. Below are areas which will show a change if this phenomenon occurs. Describe the change in the blank provided.

    1. Skin _____   3. Pulse _____
    2. Blood pressure _____   4. Conscious state _____

CHAPTER—4

The interaction of body and mind

The mind and the body are not separate; what affects one very often affects the other. The effect of the mind on the body and the illnesses that may be produced because of the mind's influence are not fully understood.

The following questions deal with the contents of Chapter 4.

I. True or false.

Read each statement carefully and place your answer in the space provided.

_____ 1. Psychosomatic illness may be defined as the occurrence of physical symptoms that have no known cause.

_____ 2. Certain diseases, such as eczema and colitis, have been considered as possibly psychosomatic in origin.

_____ 3. An individual may subconsciously develop an illness as a way of handling a desperate need.

_____ 4. A malingerer is one who deliberately fakes an illness in order to achieve money or some other gain.

_____ 5. A psychosomatic illness is easily cured.

_____ 6. An illusion is a sensory experience in which the patient sees an object that is really not present in the environment.

_____ 7. A hallucination is a sensory experience that occurs without stimulation from the environment.

_____ 8. Most hospitals require a physician's order for the application of physical restraints.

II. Multiple choice questions.

Select the most appropriate answer and place it in the space provided.

1. The first step in treating psychomatic illness is _____.
   a. helping the patient to accept and acknowledge his illness
   b. suggesting the patient seek psychiatric help
   c. letting the patient talk about his problems
   d. seeing that the patient is not left alone

2. In order to understand the patient with a psychosomatic illness, the nurse should remember that these patients are _____.
   a. best left alone and do not like to talk about their illness
   b. malingerers
   c. able to snap out of it if they really want to
   d. not pretending or imagining their symptoms

3. Delirium is ____.
   1. usually temporary and reversible
   2. usually permanent once it develops
   3. a state of disorientation and confusion
   4. an inability to think clearly

   a. 1, 3
   b. 1, 4
   c. 2, 3
   d. 2, 4

4. The delirious patient should not be scolded for his actions because ____.
   a. he cannot hear you
   b. it is impossible to get his attention
   c. he cannot control his behavior
   d. it will be of no value because he does not want to follow directions

III. Fill-in and discussion questions.

Read each question carefully and place your answer in the space provided.

1. Nursing management of the patient who is delirious includes keeping sensory stimuli to a minimum. Below are some ordinary objects or events in a hospital area. Describe the specific nursing action warranted to reduce sensory stimuli.

   1. lights _____
   2. noise _____
   3. tone of voice _____
   4. explanations to patient _____

2. The patient with a phychosomatic illness is often neglected by nursing personnel. Briefly give 2 reasons why nurses may avoid contact with these patients.

   1. _____
   _____
   2. _____
   _____

CHAPTER—5

The patient in pain

Pain is often difficult to evaluate and there is no method the nurse can use to determine the actual amount of pain experienced by a patient. The only information the nurse has is that given by the patient—his description of the pain and how he feels, his facial expression and/or body movements. Thus, if the patient says he has pain—*he has pain!*
The following questions deal with the contents of Chapter 5.

I. True or false.
Read each statement carefully and place your answer in the space provided.

_____ 1. Not everyone reacts to pain in the same manner.
_____ 2. Response to pain or discomfort may be culturally learned.
_____ 3. Pain experienced in the past has no influence on pain experienced in the present or future.
_____ 4. Pain can deepen shock.
_____ 5. The patient's description of his pain is often inaccurate as patients have a tendency to exaggerate their problems.

II. Multiple choice questions.
Select the most appropriate answer and place it in the space provided.

1. When a patient has pain, the nurse should first _____.
   a. call the patient's physician
   b. check the patient's chart to see what has been ordered for his pain
   c. give an analgesic
   d. evaluate the patient's pain before nursing measures are instituted or drugs given

2. Sudden and severe pain _____.
   a. can cause shock
   b. should not be treated with narcotics because the patient will become addicted
   c. is rarely seen in the usual hospital setting
   d. usually goes away in a short time

3. Intractable pain may be defined as pain that _____.
   a. is not real but imagined
   b. cannot be controlled by analgesics and good nursing management
   c. is always treated with narcotic analgesics
   d. is seen in those with psychosomatic illnesses

4. A cordotomy is ____.
   a. a transverse sectioning of the spinal cord
   b. an interruption of pain pathways in the spinal cord
   c. an interruption of motor and sensory pathways in the spinal cord
   d. an injury to the spinal cord
5. Surgical measures such as a cordotomy or rhizotomy may be employed to control intractable pain. If the patient complains of pain in the same area during the immediate postoperative period, the nurse knows that ____.
   a. it may take several days before relief is noted
   b. the surgery was not successful
   c. the patient is upset and can't think clearly
   d. it is best not to discuss the surgery with the patient

III. Fill-in and discussion questions.
Read each question carefully and place your answer in the space provided.
1. List some of the descriptive terms a patient might use in describing his pain.

_____
_____
_____
_____
_____

2. Mr. Kloss has terminal lung cancer and has a great deal of pain. Give 5 nursing measures that might be used to relieve some or most of his pain.
   1. _____
   2. _____
   3. _____
   4. _____
   5. _____

CHAPTER—6

Dependence on and abuse of alcohol, drugs, and tobacco

Drug dependence and addiction is a complex subject. Repeated use of some drugs can lead to dependence—a complicated interaction between physical craving and psychological longing.

The following questions deal with the contents of Chapter 6.

I. True or false.

Read each statement carefully and place your answer in the space provided.

_____ 1. When an individual is addicted to a drug such as heroin, he has a tendency to increase the dose of the drug as he continues its use.

_____ 2. The use of alcohol among teenagers and young adults appears to be decreasing.

_____ 3. Personal problems often lead to excessive drinking as the use of alcohol is one way of relieving anxiety.

_____ 4. It is possible to become addicted to alcohol.

_____ 5. Most alcoholics live in economically deprived areas.

_____ 6. Alcohol is a central nervous system stimulant.

_____ 7. The onset of delirium tremens (DT's) is usually sudden.

_____ 8. Alcoholics Anonymous (AA) is an organization run by psychiatrists, social workers, and other medical personnel equipped to handle the alcoholic's problems.

_____ 9. Amphetamines are central nervous system stimulants.

_____ 10. Death from an overdose of amphetamines may occur in the chronic user, especially when the drug is administered intravenously.

_____ 11. LSD always produces the same effects in an individual, providing the same dosage is used.

_____ 12. Use of LSD has been known to produce prolonged psychotic reactions.

_____ 13. Marihuana is a drug capable of causing addiction.

_____ 14. The use of marihuana almost always leads to use of other harmful drugs.

_____ 15. Heroin is a legal narcotic.

_____ 16. Intravenous self-administration of heroin can result in infections such as septicemia and hepatitis.

_____ 17. Addicts usually require smaller doses of preoperative medication and anesthesia for surgery.

_____ 18. Individuals addicted to heroin and other opiates may be weaned from these drugs with methadone.

_____ 19. The risk of lung cancer increases with the number of cigarettes smoked per day.

II. Multiple choice questions.

Select the most appropriate answer and place it in the space provided.

1. The length of time required to develop drug dependence _____.
   a. depends on the type of drug used
   b. varies with the drug or drugs used and the individual
   c. depends on the reason for use of the drug

2. When drug tolerance develops _____.
   a. an increased dose of the drug is necessary to obtain the desired effect
   b. the individual can no longer take the drug
   c. the individual begins to take less of the drug to obtain the desired effect
   d. signs of drug allergy become apparent

3. After the ingestion of alcohol the body function first affected is the _____.
   a. heart rate
   b. respiratory rate
   c. muscular functions
   d. higher intellectual functions

4. Characteristics of delirium tremens (DT's) are _____.
   1. hallucinations
   2. a desire to increase the dosage of the drug
   3. extreme anxiety
   4. tremors
   5. drowsiness
   a. 1, 2, 3
   b. 1, 3, 4
   c. 2, 4, 5
   d. 2, 3, 4

5. The patient, when deprived of his supply of alcohol, usually develops signs of delirium tremens (DT's) in _____.
   a. 2 to 3 hours
   b. 6 to 12 hours
   c. 2 to 3 days
   d. 5 to 7 days

6. Prolonged use of medically prescribed tranquilizers is contraindicated in the alcoholic because the patient may _____.
   a. have periods of increased anxiety when taking these drugs
   b. have difficulty substituting tranquilizers for alcohol
   c. become dependent on the tranquilizers
   d. experience delirium tremens

7. If disulfiram (Antabuse) is given to an alcoholic as part of a rehabilitation program, the patient _____.
   a. should be aware of the symptoms that will occur if he takes a drink
   b. should not be told the effects of the drug as it may encourage him to stop taking the drug and return to alcohol
   c. should not be told the effects of the drug as he may imagine the side effects

8. LSD (lysergic acid diethylamide) is capable of producing a mental state said to be similar to _____.
   a. chronic alcoholism
   b. states observed in some psychoses
   c. a state similar to that experienced by the marihuana user
   d. a deep sleep

9. Simultaneous use of alcohol *and* sedatives such as tranquilizers and barbiturates, usually results in ____.
    a. the alcohol potentiating the effects of the tranquilizer or barbiturate
    b. hypertension and coma
    c. a quicker than normal addiction to alcohol
    d. extreme anxiety and apprehension

10. Use of heroin normally results in ____.
    1. an LSD-like trip
    2. an intense euphoria or "high"
    3. drug tolerance
    4. an inability to tolerate other drugs
    5. dependence
        a. 1, 2, 5
        b. 1, 3, 4
        c. 2, 3, 4
        d. 2, 3, 5

11. Use of tobacco is ____.
    a. addicting
    b. habituating

III. Fill-in and discussion questions.

Read each question carefully and place your answer in the space provided.

1. List at least 5 symptoms of alcoholism.

    1. _____
    2. _____
    3. _____
    4. _____
    5. _____

2. Give 3 effects of alcoholism on the family with regard to family unity and the problems experienced by the family when one member is an alcoholic.

    1. _____
    2. _____
    3. _____

3. List 3 or more reasons why people misuse drugs.

    1. _____
    2. _____
    3. _____

4. Give 4 signs of narcotic (opiate) drug withdrawal.

    1. _____   3. _____
    2. _____   4. _____

5. Give 3 of the possible harmful *physical* effects that may result from the use of tobacco.

   1. _____   3. _____
   2. _____

6. Give 3 symptoms that may occur when an individual stops smoking.

   1. _____   3. _____
   2. _____

CHAPTER—7

Care of the dying patient

The role of health professionals in supporting the dying patient and his loved ones is often deemphasized while stress is usually placed on details of therapy and life-prolonging techniques. Because of the nature of their work, nurses have the opportunity to be involved with patients and their families at the time of death. It is the concern and thoughtfulness of the nurse that often makes this difficult time easier for the family and as comfortable as possible for the patient.

The following questions deal with the contents of Chapter 7.

I. True or false.

Read each statement carefully and place your answer in the space provided.

_____ 1. In the hospital environment death is usually viewed as a natural and universal experience.

_____ 2. It is important to the dying patient's mental attitude that those who provide his care appear to be as cheerful as possible at all times.

_____ 3. An individual's personal philosophy of death is usually fully developed by the time he reaches adulthood and is unlikely to be changed.

_____ 4. Patients may not always follow Dr. Elisabeth Kübler-Ross's 5 stages of the dying process in an orderly fashion and may even exhibit characteristics of 2 or more stages at the same time.

_____ 5. It is not unusual for the patient to wish to be left alone during the acceptance stage.

_____ 6. The patient will usually mourn the loss of money, a change in body image, or the loss of employment during the first stage of the dying process.

_____ 7. Since dying patients tend to become isolated from others, it is often important for the nurse to spend time with them beyond that which is required for their physical care.

_____ 8. One problem among the family members of a dying patient may be their inability to communicate frankly with the patient.

II. Multiple choice questions.

Select the most appropriate answer and place it in the space provided.

1. Members of the health professions often avoid dying patients and their families because _____.
    1. they do not wish to confront their own anxieties about death

2. providing support for the patients and their families is more appropriately the duty of the clergy and other trained professionals
3. the death of the patient may signify their failure as healers
4. most families have had experiences with death before and are usually prepared to cope with the situation in their own way
   a. 1, 3
   b. 2, 3
   c. 2, 4
   d. all of these

2. According to Dr. Elisabeth Kübler-Ross's definition of the 5 stages of the dying process, the patient's full awareness of the truth of his situation will usually occur in the stage of _____.
   a. denial
   b. anger
   c. depression
   d. acceptance

3. The stage in which the patient is most likely to ask the question, "Why me?" is the _____.
   a. denial stage
   b. anger stage
   c. bargaining stage
   d. depression stage

4. Family members of a dying patient may tend to _____.
   1. withdraw emotionally from the patient
   2. draw closer to the patient, expressing greater tenderness
   3. express anger that the patient is about to leave them
   4. appear to be very cheerful
   5. burden the patient with their own grief

   a. 1, 3, 4
   b. 1, 3, 5
   c. 2, 4, 5
   d. all of these

III. Fill-in and discussion questions.

Read each question carefully and place your answer in the space provided.

1. Two years ago Mrs. King, 31 years old, was admitted to the hospital for a biopsy of a lump on her right breast. The biopsy showed a malignancy, and a right radical mastectomy (removal of the breast) was performed. Despite surgery and chemotherapy, the tumor has now spread. Mrs. King is now terminally ill.

   According to Dr. Elisabeth Kübler-Ross, Mrs. King has gone through, or will go through, 5 stages prior to death. These stages are listed below.

   Explain or describe how Mrs. King *might* act or think as she progresses through these stages.

   1. Denial _____

   2. Anger _____

   3. Bargaining _____

   4. Depression _____

   5. Acceptance _____

23

2. Give ways in which the nurse can help the family of a dying patient with regard to physical and mental comfort and support. _____

_____

_____

_____

_____

_____

CHAPTER—8

Nursing in emergencies

Many illnesses are of an emergency nature both in and out of the hospital. First aid consists of measures that keep the patient alive and prevent further damage until definitive medical treatment can be initiated. The nurse must be prepared to administer first aid, either alone or as a member of the health team. In addition, the nurse must also be prepared to meet emergencies occurring in the hospital by recognition of the problem and knowledge of the nursing measures required to meet the emergency.

The following questions deal with the contents of Chapter 8.

I. True or false.

Read each statement carefully and place your answer in the space provided.

_____ 1. It is safe to assume that injured patients can be moved as long as there are no signs of active bleeding.

_____ 2. It is safe to give an injured patient water as long as he appears to be able to swallow.

_____ 3. Losing a quart or more of blood leads to hemorrhagic shock.

_____ 4. If bleeding cannot be controlled by the application of pressure and elevation of the injured extremity, a tourniquet may be necessary.

_____ 5. A blood pressure cuff should never be used as a tourniquet.

_____ 6. The treatment for ventricular fibrillation resulting from a severe electric shock is defibrillation.

_____ 7. If an individual has been bitten by a poisonous snake, it is not necessary to identify the snake as long as the venom has been removed from the wound.

_____ 8. Tetanus immunization is given following a bite from a warm-blooded animal only if the animal is proven to be rabid.

_____ 9. Vomiting should be induced in all cases of poison ingestion.

_____ 10. Administration of an antidote for drug poisoning often depends upon the correct identification of the drug or poison that has been ingested.

_____ 11. In heat stroke (sunstroke), the body's normal responses to increasing temperature are not functioning.

_____ 12. In frostbite, there is ischemia of the involved tissues.

_____ 13. When an individual is bitten by a tick, he should first pull the tick off the skin and then remove the pincers.

_____ 14. Patients admitted to the emergency department of a hospital should have their valuables sent home with a relative or deposited in the hospital safe.

II. Multiple choice questions.

Select the most appropriate answer and place it in the space provided.

1. The most accepted position for the patient in shock is _____.
    a. flat with the feet elevated 8 to 12 inches higher than the head
    b. placement of the head lower than the trunk
    c. turning the patient on his side with the knees flexed
    d. a prone position with the legs slightly elevated
2. The patient in shock should be kept warm but not hot because excessive heat results in _____.
    a. vasoconstriction
    b. hypertension
    c. bradycardia
    d. vasodilatation
3. The organism causing botulism—*clostridium botulinum*—is most often found in _____.
    a. infected wounds
    b. contaminated soil
    c. food left standing overnight in a warm room
    d. foods that have been improperly canned
4. Syrup of ipecac _____.
    1. is a drug that does not require a prescription
    2. is never given to children
    3. may be used to induce vomiting after poison ingestion
    4. is used when chemicals, such as an alkali, are ingested
        a. 1, 4
        b. 1, 3
        c. 2, 3
        d. 2, 4
5. If an individual is suspected of being poisoned by gas in his home, the first thing you would do is _____.
    a. get the individual out of the room
    b. immediately open the window and remove the person from the room
    c. open the window, see if the person can stand, and walk him around the room
    d. open the window and have the person stand in front of the window and take deep breaths
6. The *immediate* first aid treatment of a patient with heat stroke is to _____.
    a. give fluids to replace lost electrolytes
    b. cover the patient with a lotion to prevent blistering and loss of body water
    c. cool the patient
7. The presently accepted treatment for frostbite is _____.
    a. placing the patient in a warm room
    b. rubbing the affected area with snow or ice
    c. wrapping the affected area in cool dressings and slowly increasing the temperature of the dressings
    d. bathing the affected part in comfortably warm water for 10 minutes
8. Fainting is _____.
    a. a momentary deficiency in cerebral oxygenation
    b. caused by an increase in pressure in cerebral blood vessels
    c. a lapse of consciousness in which the victim may or may not fall to the ground
    d. caused by a sudden increase and then a decrease in blood pressure

III. Fill-in and discussion questions.

Read each question carefully and place your answer in the space provided.

1. Emergency nursing involves establishing priorities of care, especially when there is more than one seriously ill or injured patient. Highest priority is given to those with

the most severe illness or injury. List 5 conditions or illnesses that would receive the highest priority in an emergency.

1. _____
2. _____
3. _____
4. _____
5. _____

2. The following are emergency situations which the nurse might encounter and in which she might be required to give initial care. After each situation give the appropriate *nursing* actions to be taken.

   1. Hemorrhage: at the site of an automobile accident— _____
   _____
   _____
   _____
   _____

   2. Shock: a patient on arrival in the emergency department— _____
   _____
   _____
   _____
   _____

   3. Wounds, small: an individual outside of the hospital— _____
   _____
   _____
   _____
   _____

   4. Poisonous snakebite: a camp counselor immediately after the incident— _____
   _____
   _____
   _____
   _____

   5. Drug/chemical poisoning: what drug can be given to induce vomiting? _____
   _____
   _____
   _____
   _____

6. Heat stroke: the individual involved is still on the golf course— _____
   _____
   _____
   _____
   _____

7. Frostbite: occurring at a winter ski resort— _____
   _____
   _____
   _____
   _____

8. Fainting: the individual faints at home— _____
   _____
   _____
   _____
   _____

9. Bite by tick: the individual is camping— _____
   _____
   _____
   _____
   _____

10. Sting by a hornet, bee, or wasp: the individual is in his backyard— _____
    _____
    _____
    _____
    _____

CHAPTER 9

The surgical patient

The immediate preoperative preparation of the surgical patient usually takes place on the nursing unit. Thus, it is the nurse who is responsible for the preparation and education of the patient during the preoperative period. Postoperative management involves intensive nursing care designed to help the patient through the postoperative period.

The following questions deal with the contents of Chapter 9.

I. True or false.

Read each statement carefully and place your answer in the space provided.

__T__ 1. The possibility of a diagnosis of cancer may arouse fears of pain and death.
__F__ 2. Preparation for surgery should not begin until the night before surgery.
__T__ 3. Use of simple, factual explanations that are adjusted to the patient's ability and need are an essential part of preoperative teaching.
__T__ 4. Tranquilizers may be prescribed during the preoperative period to relieve tension and anxiety.
__T__ 5. Choice of preoperative medication(s) is based on the patient, the surgery, and the type of anesthetic to be administered to the patient.
__F__ 6. Only abdominal surgery requires the patient to void before going to the operating room.
__F__ 7. Only patients having surgery on the bowel require an enema the evening before surgery.
__T__ 8. The needs of each patient are more important than the routine of a nursing unit.
__T__ 9. Intense pain can also cause shock.
__F__ 10. The most severe pain resulting from surgery occurs immediately after the patient awakens from anesthesia and disappears within approximately 24 hours.
__T__ 11. Narcotics should not be administered to the patient in shock unless the patient has first been evaluated by a physician.
__F__ 12. Narcotics have few side effects.
__T__ 13. Minutes seem like hours to the patient in severe pain.
__T__ 14. Oral fluids, when first introduced to the postoperative patient, should be given slowly and in small amounts.
__F__ 15. Patients with catheters cannot be ambulated until the catheter is removed.
__F__ 16. Dark brownish blood indicates fresh bleeding from a vein and bright red, fresh bleeding from an artery.
__F__ 17. The subcutaneous route of drug administration is usually used when the patient is in shock.

_T_ 18. Patients who have had abdominal surgery often have difficulty voiding after surgery.

_T_ 19. Catheterization entails the risk of bladder infection.

_T_ 20. One of the first symptoms of the development of a wound infection may be increasing pain in the area of the incision.

II. Multiple choice questions.

Select the most appropriate answer and place it in the space provided.

1. Patients who are extremely frightened during the preoperative period __B__.
   a. must be heavily sedated prior to surgery
   b. are prone to complications such as cardiac arrest and irreversible shock
   c. require less than normal amount of anesthesia
   d. should not be given a preoperative medication

2. Preoperative preparation of the patient __C__.
   a. usually begins the morning of surgery
   b. should include an explanation of the surgery only if the patient asks questions
   c. may extend over a period of several days and include tests, x-ray studies, and patient education
   d. should be as brief as possible

3. The purpose of skin preparation prior to surgery is to __A__.
   a. make the skin as free of microorganisms as possible
   b. condition the skin so that healing will be more rapid
   c. decrease the amount of superficial bleeding during surgery
   d. sterilize the skin

4. Patients who have had spinal anesthesia may complain of numbness and a heavy feeling in their legs as the anesthesia wears off. At this time the nurse could tell the patient that __B__.
   a. the symptoms will disappear in 12 to 16 hours
   b. the numbness and heavy feeling are normal and will disappear in a short time
   c. a medication will be given that will counteract the numbness
   d. if he moves his legs the numbness will be gone by the following day

5. Most postoperative patients require the *frequent* administration of a narcotic analgesic for __B__.
   a. the first 12 hours after surgery
   b. approximately 3 days after surgery
   c. 1 week after surgery
   d. 2 weeks after surgery

6. Unless ordered otherwise, postoperative patients should begin to move their legs __A__.
   a. as soon as they have recovered from the anesthesia and are awake
   b. after the first 12 hours
   c. after the first 24 hours
   d. as soon as they have less pain

7. The primary purpose of early ambulation is to __D__.
   a. encourage an improved mental outlook after surgery
   b. lessen postoperative pain
   c. decrease the patient's need for narcotics
   d. prevent postoperative complications

8. Internal hemorrhage is a possible complication during the postoperative period and may be manifested by __D__.
   a. the appearance of blood on the surgical dressing
   b. complaints of severe chills and fever
   c. fall in blood pressure, slowing of the pulse, restlessness
   d. pallor, fall in blood pressure, tachycardia

9. During the *immediate* postoperative period, the surgical dressing may become soiled with blood or drainage. At this time the nurse should __B__.
   a. change the dressing
   b. reinforce the dressing
   c. turn the patient on his side to facilitate drainage
   d. elevate the head of the bed to prevent further drainage

10. An oropharnygeal airway is used to __D__.
    a. enable the nurse to suction the patient
    b. keep secretions out of the esophagus
    c. prevent the swallowing of secretions
    d. prevent the tongue from blocking the air passages

11. Paralytic ileus is a postoperative complication in which there is a(n) __BC__.
    a. increase in peristalsis plus abdominal distention
    b. interruption in the movement of food or fluid through the large bowel
    c. paralysis of the intestines and absence of peristalsis
    d. regurgitation of small amounts of fluid and the abdomen appears distended

12. The nurse may help prevent thrombophlebitis by __AD__.
    1. encouraging the patient to drink large quantities of fluids
    2. encouraging leg exercises
    3. preventing the patient from resting on his side
    4. avoiding prolonged pressure on the patient's legs
        a. 1, 2
        b. 1, 3
        c. 2, 3
        d. 2, 4

III. Fill-in and discussion questions.

Read each question carefully and place your answer in the space provided.

1. VOCABULARY. Define the following terms.

   a. atelectasis: *a collapse of the lung which may involve a small or large area*

   b. dehiscence: *separation of all layers of a wound or surgical incision*

   c. embolus: *a solid, liquid, or gaseous mass carried by the blood stream or a lymphatic vessel*

   d. evisceration: *separation of wound edges c protrusion of internal organs*

   e. flatus: *gas*

   f. hypostatic pneumonia: *pneumonia due to the lying in one position for prolonged periods of time*

   g. hypoxia: *Lack of adequate amount of oxygen*

h. phlebothrombosis: _a clot in a vein_

i. thrombophlebitis: _inflammation of a vein_

2. Below are three nursing actions usually performed during the immediate *pre*operative period. In the column at the right give the rationale for these nursing actions.

NURSING ACTIONS	RATIONALE
1. Having the patient void before surgery	Decrease bladder size therefore reduce possibility of damage to the bladder.
2. Removal of plastic or metal objects from the patient's hair	To protect pt. from harming themself if they become restless
3. Removal of makeup and nail polish	Color of face, lips & nailbeds are observed by anesthesist

3. Mrs. Long, age 37, was admitted to the hospital 5 days ago with a chief complaint of pain in the right upper abdomen. After a series of tests and x-ray studies, she was found to have stones in her gallbladder (cholelithiasis) and a cholecystectomy (removal of the gallbladder) was performed yesterday. The following 3 questions concern the postoperative nursing management of Mrs. Long.

   1. The physician's order reads "out of bed in chair B.I.D. starting today." As Mrs. Long appears to be uncomfortable, what can the nurse do with regard to the timing of the administration of the narcotic and getting the patient out of bed?

   Give the narcotic before getting pt out of bed, about 1 hr before.

   2. Sometimes pain in the operative site is intensified because of minor physical discomforts. *Along with* the administration of a narcotic, the nurse can use simple comfort measures to try and relieve Mrs. Long's pain and discomfort. Briefly describe 3 comfort measures that may reduce some of Mrs. Long's discomfort.

      1. _Change position_
      2. _Use small pillow to support back & shoulders_
      3. _Massage areas subject to pressure_

3. List 2 nursing measures that can be used to prevent the development of pneumonia in Mrs. Long.

    1. ① Change position frequently ② Cough, turn, deep breath
    2. Suction mucouse from nose & throat while she is unconscious.

4. Mr. Billings had an inguinal herniorrhaphy (repair of a hernia) 3 days ago. At present he is complaining of abdominal discomfort; his abdomen is distended. Mr. Billings' surgeon states that the discomfort is due to gas. If Mr. Billings is allowed out of bed and can have a soft diet, what *nursing* measures may be used to relieve his discomfort?

    Ambulate
    Take to bathroom
    Offer hot or warm fluids

5. Patients usually ask for water shortly after waking from anesthesia. If the physician's orders read "nothing by mouth," what 2 *nursing* measures might relieve this discomfort?

    1. Offer mouth rinse
    2. Place cool wet cloth or ice chips on lips

6. Coughing and deep-breathing exercises are essential if postoperative pulmonary complications are to be prevented. Coughing will usually place a strain on the incision, especially if the surgery was in the chest or abdomen. List 2 nursing actions that may eliminate some of the discomfort the patient experiences when coughing and deep breathing.

    1. Use of pillow or nurses hand to support incision
    2. Give narcotic approx 45-60 min before coughing & deep breathing exercises.

UNIT TWO
Oncologic nursing

CHAPTER—10

Care of the patient with cancer

Certain body cells sometimes undergo changes in structure and appearance and begin to multiply, giving rise to a colony of cancer cells. These cells may occur in any part of the body, at any time and from any cell that can proliferate. Cancer cells multiply rapidly, invading and destroying surrounding normal tissues by pressure and competing with normal cells for nutrients and oxygen.

It is sometimes difficult to halt the growth and spread of cancer cells. Some patients enter the hospital terminally ill; others respond to various methods of therapy and the cancer is cured or arrested.

The following questions deal with the contents of Chapter 10.

I. True or false.

Read each statement carefully and place your answer in the space provided.

_____ 1. Tumors are usually named after the types of tissues from which they arise.

_____ 2. A complete, regular physical examination is the first weapon in the struggle to discover cancer in its early stages.

_____ 3. Radiation is the ability of a substance to emit a ray called a gamma ray.

_____ 4. Many drugs used in the treatment of cancer have an effect on normal cells as well as cancer cells.

_____ 5. Most drugs used in the treatment of cancer have few side effects.

_____ 6. Most physicians and nurses feel that patients should not be told if a biopsy, surgery, or examination confirms the diagnosis of cancer.

_____ 7. Cancer patients usually require very little physical care but do need much emotional support.

_____ 8. Public education has been most instrumental in encouraging awareness of the warning signals of cancer.

_____ 9. Nurses should try to avoid a patient's questions about his treatment or disease.

_____ 10. Early detection of most cancers increases the chance of curing the disease.

II. Multiple choice questions.

Select the most appropriate answer and place it in the space provided.

1. Benign tumors _____.
   a. may spread to other areas but do so slowly
   b. are usually found in the young rather than elderly patient

37

    c. have the same characteristics as malignant tumors
    d. remain at the original site of their development

2. A pathologist is a physician specializing in the ____.
   a. identification of tissue changes
   b. diagnosis of cancer
   c. treatment of cancer
   d. surgical management of acute diseases

3. Radiation is one method used in the treatment of cancer and is effective in many cases because ____.
   a. radiation affects cancer cells while leaving normal healthy cells unharmed
   b. it is able to penetrate the body and dissolve cancer cells and tumor masses
   c. the concentration of radiation is harmful to living cells including normal *and* malignant cells

4. Common side effects of drugs used in the treatment of cancer are related to the ____.
   a. skin and related structures
   b. gastrointestinal tract and bone marrow
   c. bone and cartilage
   d. red blood cells and nervous system

5. A profound decrease in the manufacture of blood components by the bone marrow can result in ____.
   1. anemia
   2. an increase in red blood cells
   3. bleeding tendencies
   4. blood clots
   5. leukopenia
       a. 1, 2, 3
       b. 1, 3, 5
       c. 2, 3, 4
       d. 2, 4, 5

6. John is 19 years old and has leukemia. If the drugs being used to treat his disease depress the bone marrow, John must be observed for early signs of infection which may be manifested by ____.
   a. chills, fever, sore throat
   b. fatigue, easy bruising, headache
   c. cough, fever, alopecia
   d. aching muscles, increased nasal secretions, bleeding tendency

7. Certain hormones such as estrogen (a female hormone) are of value in treating some types of cancer as these drugs ____.
   a. shrink tumors and destroy cancer cells
   b. prevent tumor cells from metastasizing
   c. provide a less favorable environment for the growth of cancer cells
   d. decrease the size of the cancer cell

8. Corticosteroids are used in the treatment of ____.
   a. all cancers
   b. only bone cancers
   c. patients with cancer who are allergic to all other drugs
   d. various forms of leukemia

9. The nursing needs of the patient with cancer often depend upon ____.
   1. his and his family's reaction to the diagnosis
   2. the location of the cancer
   3. the stage of the disease
   4. the prognosis
   5. the impairment of body functions as a result of the disease
       a. 1, 2, 4
       b. 2, 3, 4
       c. 1, 3, 5
       d. all of these

10. Mr. Evans has lung cancer and asks you about the treatment he is receiving. As a nurse you know that ____.
    a. you need not answer this question but should help him find the appropriate answer, referring him to the appropriate person such as a physician

b. it is best if Mr. Evans is told that nurses are not allowed to answer this type of question and it is best if he asks a doctor or someone else who is permitted to discuss this information

11. Though Mrs. Lee is terminally ill, she remains physically able to care for herself. Knowing this the nurse should ____.
    a. encourage her to let the nurses assume the responsibility for her care
    b. allow her to do as much for herself as she wishes
    c. talk to the family and suggest they supervise her care
    d. have a talk with her and explain why she shouldn't exert herself

III. Fill-in and discussion questions.

Read each question carefully and place your answer in the space provided.

1. VOCABULARY. Define the following terms.

    a. alopecia: _____

    b. antineoplastic: _____

    c. chemotherapy: _____

    d. isotope: _____

    e. leukemia: _____

    f. leukopenia: _____

    g. leukoplakia: _____

    h. metastasis: _____

    i. radioactivity: _____

    j. stoma: _____

    k. stomatitis: _____

2. List 3 ways in which malignant tumors differ from benign tumors.

    1. _____

2. _____

3. _____

3. The cause of cancer is unknown; however, there are some factors that are thought to be related to the occurrence of cancer. Give 4 factors or activities that might be related to the development of cancer in some individuals.

   1. _____
   2. _____
   3. _____
   4. _____

4. Give any 3 of the 7 warning signals of cancer as listed by the American Cancer Society.

   1. _____
   _____

   2. _____
   _____

   3. _____
   _____

5. Name 3 diagnostic tests that may be used to diagnose cancer.

   1. _____
   2. _____
   3. _____

6. Name the 3 basic methods that may be employed in the treatment of cancer.

   1. _____
   2. _____
   3. _____

7. Briefly comment on whether you would wish to be told if a biopsy was positive for cancer. Include reasons why you would or would not wish to know this information.

   _____
   _____
   _____
   _____

CHAPTER—11

Nursing management in radiotherapy

The term "radiotherapy" refers to the therapeutic application of ionizing radiation from x-ray machines or radioactive materials. Radiotherapy is frequently employed in the treatment of cancer to destroy malignant, rapidly dividing cells while leaving the rest of the body well (or able to recover) and able to eliminate the dead cancer cells.

Nursing management of the patient before, during, and after the course of therapy will include physical care as well as emotional support and patient/family teaching.

The following questions deal with the contents of Chapter 11.

I. True or false.

Read each statement carefully and place your answer in the space provided.

_____ 1. The aim of radiotherapy is an orderly destruction of malignant, rapidly dividing cells.

_____ 2. Use of technical terms should be avoided when explaining a treatment to a patient.

_____ 3. Cells that divide slowly are more sensitive to radiation than cells that divide rapidly.

_____ 4. If radiation reactions such as nausea and vomiting become severe, the therapist may halt treatments to give the body a chance to recover.

_____ 5. Skin markings are to be removed after each radiation treatment followed by reapplication the following morning.

_____ 6. The degree of possible radiation hazard to individuals involved in the care of patients receiving therapy depends on the type and amount of radioactive materials used.

_____ 7. Precautions to be taken when caring for patients with internal radiotherapy are stated by the radiation safety officer or radiologist.

_____ 8. It is good nursing practice not to explain what will be done when the patient has internal radiotherapy as this will usually upset the patient and may interfere with therapy.

_____ 9. A sign depicting the radiation symbol is attached to the door of the patient's room when the patient is receiving daily external x-ray therapy.

_____ 10. All nursing personnel and workers in radiotherapy should be made aware that radiation materials are being used in the area.

II. Multiple choice questions.

Select the most appropriate answer and place it in the space provided.

1. In the treatment of cancer, radioisotopes are used for _____.
   a. diagnostic procedures
   b. therapeutic procedures
   c. both a and b
   d. b only

2. Radiotherapy attempts to kill cancer cells by _____.
   a. ionizing radiation
   b. dissolving the protoplasm of the cell
   c. altering the pattern of cell division
   d. affecting normal cells around the cancer cells

3. The amount of radiation sickness experienced by any one patient usually depends on the _____.
   1. dose of radiation
   2. site being radiated
   3. type of x-ray machine used
   4. size of the area radiated
   5. type of cancer
      a. 1, 3, 5
      b. 1, 2, 4
      c. 2, 3, 4
      d. 2, 4, 5

4. Patients receiving radiotherapy may develop varying degrees of bone marrow depression. To detect beginning bone marrow depression the physician orders _____.
   a. serum electrolyte studies
   b. serum enzyme studies
   c. bone marrow aspiration studies
   d. complete blood counts

5. Side effects of radiotherapy _____.
   a. can occur after the course of treatment is terminated
   b. only occur during the time of treatment
   c. are seen most often in the elderly
   d. are usually mild and cause no problem

6. Radioactive iodine (^{131}I) is primarily used to treat cancer of the _____.
   a. bone
   b. gastrointestinal tract
   c. thyroid gland
   d. lung

7. Skin markings are used as guides by the radiologist and are necessary _____.
   a. to compare with normal skin for detecting the type of skin reaction occurring during treatment
   b. for setting and adjusting of the x-ray machine over the area to be radiated
   c. as a guide in determining the number of treatments to be given
   d. in patients having allergic skin reactions

III. Fill-in and discussion questions.

Read each question carefully and place your answer in the space provided.

1. VOCABULARY. Define the following terms:

   a. antiemetic: _____

   b. radioisotope: _____

   c. radiologist: _____

   d. radiotherapy: _____

2. Briefly explain what the nurse should do if an internal radiotherapy applicator became dislodged from its area of insertion. _____
_____
_____
_____
_____

3. Patients undergoing radiotherapy usually experience skin changes over the area radiated. Give the general points of skin care and the precautions exercised when the patient is undergoing radiotherapy. _____
_____
_____
_____
_____
_____

4. Below are the 3 safety principles to be observed when giving nursing care to patients receiving therapy with radioactive materials. In the spaces provided, explain the meaning of the safety principle or why observance of the principle makes the handling of these materials reasonably safe.

   1. Time

   2. Distance

   3. Shielding

5. In the spaces provided below, give *examples* of how the nurse should observe the 3 principles of safety when giving nursing care to patients receiving internal radiotherapy.

SAFETY PRINCIPLE	EXAMPLE OF OBSERVANCE
Time	
Distance	
Shielding	

43

UNIT THREE
Disturbances of body supportive structures and locomotion

CHAPTER—12

The patient with a fracture

Most accidents occur in the home and on the highway. One common accidental injury is a fracture of the bone. Some fractures require extensive surgical intervention and many weeks or months in the hospital. Others may be managed in the emergency department of the hospital with the patient discharged shortly after immobilization of the injured extremity. Nursing management of the patient with a fracture ranges from giving instructions to the patient and his family regarding care of a newly applied cast to extensive nursing management encompassing short- and long-term goals.

The following questions deal with the contents of Chapter 12.

I. True or false.

Read each statement carefully and place your answer in the space provided.

_____ 1. A fracture may be defined as a break in the continuity of a bone.

_____ 2. If a patient has a compound fracture, the bone has broken through the skin and there is an increased danger of infection.

_____ 3. Pathological fractures usually occur in children because their bones have not fully developed.

_____ 4. About a year of healing must take place before a fractured bone regains its former strength.

_____ 5. "Splint them where they lie" is no longer considered a safe maneuver in the first aid treatment of a fracture.

_____ 6. Immobilization of a fracture is necessary for the healing of the bone, but this maneuver also increases the pain that follows this type of injury.

_____ 7. A cast holds the bone in place until healing occurs.

_____ 8. When handling or moving a wet cast, support the cast with the palm of the hand.

_____ 9. Although casts are durable they can break.

_____ 10. Compression of a nerve or blood vessel located underneath the cast can result in permanent damage to these structures.

_____ 11. If a cast is applied after an open reduction and there is bleeding from the surgical wound, blood will quickly seep through the plaster.

_____ 12. Exercises are an important part of rehabilitation after a cast has been applied, but it is only necessary to exercise the part that has been casted.

_____ 13. The mattress on the bed of a patient in traction should be soft to prevent pressure on exposed parts and bony prominences.

_____ 14. Russell traction is a form of skin traction.

_____ 15. Traction is used to realign and immobilize a fractured bone.

_____ 16. Buck's extension may be used to temporarily align bone ends while

the patient awaits internal fixation.
___ 17. Patients in traction must use a regular bed pan as the hips should be elevated to maintain traction alignment.
___ 18. The sacral area is a common site of skin breakdown and decubitus ulcer formation.
___ 19. Hip fractures are usually treated by closed reduction.
___ 20. The hip is a ball-and-socket-type joint.
___ 21. A fractured clavicle may be immobilized with a figure-of-8 bandage.

II. Multiple choice questions.

Select the most appropriate answer and place it in the space provided.

1. After a fracture, the muscles surrounding the bone go into spasm causing ___.
   a. increased deformity and interference with the vascular and lymphatic circulation
   b. a second fracture
   c. relief from the pain that occurred at the time of the fracture
   d. decreased deformity and increased interference with circulation

2. Nursing measures that promote adequate circulation in the fracture area encourage ___.
   a. interference with the deposit of calcium in the bone
   b. loss of calcium from the bone, which is necessary in the healing of the fracture
   c. healing of the bone

3. The administration of correct first aid after a fracture is extremely important. Control of bleeding from the wound of an open fracture is initially accomplished by ___.
   a. application of a tourniquet above and below the area of injury
   b. alignment of the extremity and application of pressure with the palm of the hand above the area of injury
   c. direct pressure applied to the bleeding wound with a sterile dressing and a pressure bandage
   d. application of a dry sterile dressing

4. Before a patient is moved from the scene of an accident, the affected part must be ___.
   a. cleaned of dirt and other debris
   b. immobilized
   c. straightened and placed in proper alignment
   d. placed in a plaster cast

5. Skin traction ___.
   a. is a type of traction using wires, pins, ropes, and weights
   b. utilizes pullon tapes or traction strips attached to the skin
   c. is only used for fractures of the arm
   d. utilizes braces and slings to provide pull in the opposite direction

6. Skeletal traction ___.
   a. uses a wire or pin inserted in the bone with pull applied to the pin or wire
   b. is only used on the lower extremity
   c. is only used for simple and greenstick fractures
   d. uses tapes or traction strips attached to ropes to provide pull in the opposite direction

7. A principle of traction, that is traction and countertraction, means ___.
   a. a force applied against another force
   b. two forces pulling away from a center
   c. a pulling force alternating with a release of force
   d. the application and release of weights

8. A complication of prolonged bed rest *and* limited fluid intake is ____.
   a. edema
   b. kidney stones
   c. poor circulation
   d. decubitus ulcers

9. The patient with a fracture of the spine is usually placed in a position of ____.
   a. abduction
   b. adduction
   c. hyperextension
   d. hypoextension

10. In crutch walking, the weight is carried on the hands, not the axillae. The patient who carries weight on his axilla rather than his hands may ____.
    a. place an extra strain on the muscles of his arms
    b. not be able to use a swing-through crutch gait
    c. develop abrasions on his hands
    d. injure the brachial plexus

Clinical Situations

Mr. Hall, age 37, fell off a ladder while painting his garage. He was admitted to the emergency department where an x-ray examination revealed a compound fracture of his left ankle. He also had minor abrasions and contusions and one small laceration on his right palm that required 4 sutures. Treatment included an open reduction of the fractured ankle.

11. Skin preparation for an open reduction of Mr. Hall's fracture may include ____.
    1. shaving the area
    2. applying an antiseptic to the skin
    3. scrubbing the skin with a cleansing agent
    4. wrapping the extremity in a sterile covering
       a. 1, 2, 3
       b. 1, 3, 4
       c. 2, 4
       d. all of these

12. When Mr. Hall returns from surgery his left leg should be ____.
    a. maintained in a parallel alignment with his right leg
    b. kept flat
    c. placed in an adducted position
    d. elevated to prevent edema

13. Three days after surgery, the physician cuts a window in Mr. Hall's cast. A cast window is a(n) ____.
    a. opening in the cast over the area of discomfort permitting direct visualization of the area
    b. enlargement of the opening normally found in all casts to permit drainage of blood and serum
    c. plastic device inserted into the plaster when the cast is first applied

14. After Mr. Hall's cast had been on 9 weeks, his physician decided to bivalve the cast. A bivalve cast is one that ____.
    a. is split along both sides of the cast
    b. is removed from the affected extremity and saved for future use
    c. is split over the area of the surgical incision
    d. has 2 or more cast windows

Mary, age 16, fell and injured her right arm while playing tennis. Her father brought her to the emergency department of the hospital and an x-ray examination showed a simple fracture of the radius. The physician decides to apply a plaster cast to Mary's lower arm and wrist. After the cast has set, Mary will be allowed to go home.

15. After application of a cast, an x-ray is usually taken to ____.
    a. determine if the swelling has been controlled
    b. check bone alignment
    c. check the clearance between the cast and the skin
    d. determine if bleeding has occurred

16. The physician suggests a sling be given to Mary's father with directions for applying it to her arm once the cast is dry. The sling will be used to support Mary's arm and prevent edema of her fingers and hand. Mary's father should be shown how to adjust the sling so that the fingers are ____.
    a. lower than her elbow
    b. completely protected by a section of the sling
    c. kept close to her body
    d. higher than her elbow

17. Two days after the application of Mary's cast her father brings her back to the emergency department because several rough edges on her cast have caused irritation of her skin. Her physician will be delayed ½ hour due to an emergency elsewhere. In the meantime to make Mary comfortable the nurse could ____.
    a. use a file to smooth the rough edges on the top of the cast
    b. insert cotton between the arm and cast and down into the cast to protect Mary's skin until the physician arrives
    c. elevate the arm to prevent edema and wait until the physician arrives
    d. temporarily cover the edges of the cast with a gauze dressing and anchor the dressing with adhesive tape

18. Eight weeks later Mary is scheduled to have her cast removed. Casts are removed by a mechanical cutter which is noisy and often frightening. Mary should be told that ____.
    a. the machine is safe, provided that she doesn't move
    b. if she takes deep breaths the noise will not be disturbing
    c. the cast cutter will not cut her skin
    d. the physician can tell when the cutting blade is too close to the skin by the type of noise made by the blade

Mr. Brown, age 61, is in Russell traction for a fracture of his right femur—a bone in the upper leg. The traction was applied 3 days ago and he has been cooperative in assisting the nurses with his care. He is able to use a trapeze bar suspended over his bed as an aid in moving.

19. When checking Mr. Brown's traction the nurse must check the weights which should ____.
    a. be supported on a chair
    b. only be lowered every 2 hours
    c. be taped to the pulley and anchored to the bed frame
    d. hang free and not touch the bed

20. Mr. Brown asks if the head of his bed can be raised as high as possible because he wants to write letters. In this instance you would ____.
    a. raise the head of the bed to the position requested by Mr. Brown
    b. not raise the head of the bed as the bed is always kept flat
    c. check the physician's orders to see how high the head of the bed can be elevated
    d. call Mr. Brown's physician and ask what should be done

21. Mr. Brown's physician has ordered range-of-motion (ROM) exercises to be taught by the physical therapist. After Mr. Brown has learned how to do these exercises, the nurse should check to be sure he is exercising. These exercises are ordered for the ____.
    a. affected and unaffected extremities
    b. right leg only
    c. arms only as both legs must remain immobile
    d. left leg only

22. To prevent pneumonia and other lung complications, Mr. Brown should practice deep-breathing exercises ____.
    a. every 4 hours
    b. before and after each meal
    c. every 1 to 2 hours while awake
    d. 4 times a day

23. Mr. Brown asks if he can have an extra container of water kept at his bedside. The nurse's response to this request will be based on the fact that ____.
    a. unless the physician orders otherwise, an increased amount of fluid should be taken by patients who are immobile for long periods
    b. fluids are limited when the patient has a fracture because of the danger of edema in the involved extremity

24. Mr. Brown is to be removed from the Russell traction. The adhesive tape on his leg is best removed with ____.
    a. soap and water
    b. alcohol or benzoin
    c. oil and water
    d. ether or acetone

Mrs. Willard, age 79, slipped on a small rug and fell, injuring her right hip. Her son found her several hours after the incident and called her physician who ordered an ambulance to transport her to the hospital.

25. On arrival in the emergency room, Mrs. Willard was examined by a physician who determined that she probably had a fracture of her right hip. Signs of a hip fracture include ____.
    a. pain in the area and difficulty in walking
    b. weakness on the affected side and internal rotation of the leg
    c. shortening of the leg and external rotation of the leg and foot
    d. muscle spasm and a lengthening of the affected leg

26. Mrs. Willard required surgery with internal fixation of the fracture. The postoperative orders include turning her every 2 hours. To turn Mrs. Willard correctly ____.
    a. place a pillow lengthwise between her legs, keep the affected leg straight and turn the entire body in one movement
    b. elevate the head of the bed, raise the side rails and use pillows to support the patient while turning
    c. keep the bed flat, flex the affected leg and turn the patient onto the unaffected side
    d. place pillows under both hips, a small pillow under the knee of the operated leg, and turn the patient on either side

27. Mrs. Willard is to be ambulated on the fifth day after surgery. When first getting her out of bed, weight-bearing on the operated leg is ____.
    a. avoided
    b. encouraged

28. A complication of the internal fixation procedure is necrosis of the femur. If Mrs. Willard were to develop this complication, early recognition would be important. Early signs of necrosis of the femur are ____.
    1. pain
    2. paralysis
    3. swelling of the entire leg
    4. muscle spasm
    5. a limp while ambulating
        a. 1, 2, 3
        b. 1, 4, 5
        c. 2, 3, 4
        d. 2, 4, 5

Mrs. Lane, age 48, has had severe arthritis of her left hip for 6 years. Due to severe arthritic degeneration, disabling pain, and severe limitation of movement in the hip joint, her physician has decided to perform a total hip replacement.

29. Following surgery the physician orders Mrs. Lane's leg to be kept in an *abducted* position at all times. Which drawing illustrates an abducted position of the left (L) leg? ____.
    a. | |
        R L
    b. | \
        R L

30. It is extremely important that the physician's order be followed. If the leg is not kept in the abducted position, the _____.
    a. femur may refracture
    b. patient may experience more than an average amount of postoperative pain
    c. prosthetic femoral head may dislocate from the acetabulum
    d. leg may shorten

31. While each patient is different, patients who have a total hip replacement usually begin ambulation 1 week after surgery. Prior to ambulation, Mrs. Lane will begin exercising the affected limb. Since the exercises will be painful _____.
    a. Mrs. Lane should be told that after she has performed the exercises a narcotic will be given
    b. they are best done ½ to 1 hour after the administration of an analgesic
    c. the nurse should prepare the analgesic ordered by the physician and keep it at Mrs. Lane's bedside in case the pain becomes too severe

III. Fill-in and discussion questions.

Read each question carefully and place your answer in the space provided.

1. VOCABULARY. Define the following terms.

   a. abduction: _____

   b. adduction: _____

   c. acetabulum: _____

   d. axilla: _____

   e. blanching: _____

   f. brachial plexus: _____

   g. clavicle: _____

   h. closed reduction: _____

   i. dislocation: _____

   j. ecchymotic: _____

   k. femur: _____

l. mandible: _____

m. necrosis: _____

n. open reduction: _____

o. osteomyelitis: _____

p. sprain: _____

2. Many accidents occur in the home. List some of the hazards found in the average home that might cause an accident. _____

3. Mrs. Bell fractured her right wrist when she slipped on a small throw rug in her home. Name 4 symptoms or signs that were most likely experienced shortly after the accident.

   1. _____   3. _____
   2. _____   4. _____

4. Name 2 materials or appliances used to immobilize a fractured extremity before the patient is transported to the hospital.

   1. _____   2. _____

5. Briefly discuss the care of a plaster cast during the drying (setting) stage with regard to the handling of the cast by the nurse and the positioning of the extremity.

   _____

6. List 4 nursing observations or actions to be taken if a patient has recently had a plaster cast applied to an extremity.

   1. _____
   2. _____

53

3. _____

4. _____

7. Eight days ago, Mr. Tremont incurred multiple injuries in an automobile accident. A cast was applied to his right forearm for a fracture of the ulna. He now tells the nurse that he has throbbing pain in his right arm and asks for something for his pain. The physician's orders include an oral analgesic for pain. What should the nurse do? Give a reason for your answer. _____

8. Mr. Grant had a cast applied after an open reduction for a fracture of the tibia, a bone in the lower leg. The nurse notes a small red spot on the upper surface of the newly applied cast. What might the nurse do to determine if any further enlargement of the spot has occurred since the time the discoloration was first noted? _____

9. Areas underneath a cast often itch, especially during hot weather. Patients are tempted to use an object such as a knitting needle or a small stick to reach the annoying areas. Give a reason why such objects should *not* be inserted into a cast. _____

10. Bob had a plaster cast applied in the emergency department to his right forearm for a simple fracture of the radius. His physician says he can go home in 1 hour. Patients going home with a newly applied cast should be given instructions regarding cast care and general care of the injured extremity. Give at least 3 instructions Bob should receive before going home.

    1. _____

    2. _____

    3. _____

11. Any patient immobilized for a long period of time requires special skin care as decubitus ulcers can form in a very short time. Give 3 early signs of decubitus ulcer formation.

    1. _____
    2. _____
    3. _____

12. Although elderly patients in traction often develop decubitus ulcers, this problem is not limited to the elderly and may be seen in all age groups. List 3 measures that can be used at the first sign of skin breakdown to prevent further skin breakdown.

    1. _____
    2. _____
    3. _____

13. Patients in traction may develop an impairment in the circulation of the affected extremity. Signs of circulatory impairment are:

    1. _____.
    2. _____.
    3. _____.

14. A patient with a fracture of the spine may have to remain relatively immobile for 6 or more weeks. For this patient, good skin care is essential. If the patient cannot turn on his side and must remain on his back, how may the nurse give this patient back care? _____
    _____
    _____

15. List areas or parts of the body that are prone to decubitus ulcer formation. _____
    _____
    _____
    _____

16. MATCHING. In column B place the number identifying the type of fracture named in column A.

    COLUMN A
    1. open (compound)
    2. closed (simple)
    3. displaced
    4. greenstick
    5. comminuted
    6. impacted
    7. pathological

    COLUMN B
    ____ one portion of the bone is driven into another
    ____ bone ends are separated at the fracture line
    ____ bone breaks through the skin
    ____ bone breaks without sufficient trauma to fracture a normal bone
    ____ any fracture that is not open
    ____ bone is splintered into many small fragments, bone ends are separated and misaligned
    ____ bone bends and splits but does not break clear through

CHAPTER—13

The patient with a disease of the bones and joints

Diseases of the bones and joints, particularly the many forms of arthritis, are common medical disorders affecting a large portion of the population. For many, bone and joint disease results in physical, economic, and social disability. While corrective surgery and drugs have helped some, others require an alteration of life style and acceptance of their limitations.

The following questions deal with the contents of Chapter 13.

I. True or false.

Read each statement carefully and place your answer in the space provided.

_____ 1. Direct trauma, such as a sharp blow or sudden twist, can eventually result in arthritis.

_____ 2. Rheumatoid arthritis is a systemic disorder of unknown etiology.

_____ 3. With proper treatment, almost all cases of rheumatoid arthritis are cured.

_____ 4. Salicylates are often used in the treatment of various forms of arthritis and have anti-inflammatory as well as analgesic action.

_____ 5. Patients on high doses of aspirin should be instructed to watch for evidence of gastrointestinal bleeding.

_____ 6. If a patient is taking aspirin in the dosage recommended by his physician, he can substitute an enteric-coated or a buffered aspirin if he develops gastric distress.

_____ 7. Fat emboli are a common complication in fractures of or surgery on the long bones.

_____ 8. Emotional factors play a great part in the management of rheumatoid arthritis.

_____ 9. Heat may be used to ease the pain and discomfort of arthritis, but it is more of a comfort than a curative measure.

_____ 10. Ankylosing spondylitis is a disease of the long bones of the body.

_____ 11. Degenerative joint disease is similar to rheumatoid arthritis in that it has periods of remission when the patient looks and feels better.

_____ 12. Gout is due to overeating as well as the eating of the wrong type of foods.

_____ 13. The serum alkaline phosphatase may be elevated if the patient has a malignant bone tumor.

_____ 14. Metastatic bone tumors are usually considered inoperable but may be controlled with radiation, antineoplastic drugs, and hormone therapy.

___ 15. Acute, localized osteomyelitis is usually caused by direct contamination of the bone, such as the wound contamination seen in a compound fracture.

II. Multiple choice questions.

Select the most appropriate answer and place it in the space provided.

1. The onset of rheumatoid arthritis usually occurs over a period of time. Early signs of this disease include ___.
    1. immobility of a joint
    2. swelling and pain in the joints that come and go
    3. morning stiffness
    4. hypertension
    5. joint soreness
        a. 1, 2, 3
        b. 1, 3, 5
        c. 2, 4, 5
        d. 2, 3, 5

2. Treatment of rheumatoid arthritis is aimed at ___.
    1. preventing or correcting deformities
    2. curing the disease as quickly as possible
    3. making the patient more comfortable
    4. destroying the organism causing the disease
        a. 1, 2
        b. 1, 3
        c. 2, 3
        d. 2, 4

3. Patients with rheumatoid arthritis or any chronic disease should ___.
    a. be told of the probable course of the disease so they can plan a future
    b. not be told of the effects of the disease as only a small percentage of patients develop deformities
    c. not be told of the progress of the disease until signs of crippling deformities are apparent

4. Braces, bivalve casts, or splints may be applied to joints that are painful or in spasm to help prevent ___.
    a. inflammation and swelling
    b. dislocations and deformities
    c. pain and fractures around the joint
    d. contractures and joint sprains

CLINICAL SITUATIONS

Mrs. Todd, a 59-year-old housewife, has had a right hip arthroplasty for an arthritic deformity. Prior to surgery, she had limited motion of the joint, along with moderate to severe discomfort when walking. Following surgery, she was placed in a balanced suspension traction. It is now her second postoperative day.

5. The surgeon orders a trochanter roll for Mrs. Todd's unoperated leg to prevent ___.
    a. internal rotation
    b. external rotation
    c. hyperextension of her left knee
    d. footdrop

6. If a pillow is placed between Mrs. Todd's knees, it will prevent ___.
    a. accidental adduction
    b. accidental abduction
    c. external rotation of the leg
    d. hyperextension of the knee and ankle

7. A nursing assistant tells you that Mrs. Todd has asked to have the head of her bed raised. Your decision is to tell the nursing assistant ___.
    a. to raise the head of the bed
    b. to tell Mrs. Todd that you will call her physician later for an order to raise the head of her bed
    c. that you will explain to Mrs. Todd that, because of her surgery, the head of the bed will need to remain flat until her physician permits it to be raised

8. One of the other nurses states that she is not familiar with the nursing management of a patient with a hip arthroplasty and asks how long Mrs. Todd will remain in traction. Your answer is _____.
   a. 24 to 72 hours
   b. approximately 4 to 6 weeks
   c. usually 7 days
   d. approximately 3 weeks

Sandy, age 26, developed rheumatoid arthritis at 18. At present she has extensive damage to most of her joints, but particularly to her hands, wrists, hips, and knees.

9. Sandy asks if she could take a buffered aspirin product as the plain aspirin has been causing nausea. Your response will be based on the knowledge that _____.
   a. only the physician can answer any question concerning her drugs
   b. aspirins are all alike and one can be substituted for another
   c. buffered aspirin contains an alkali and in high doses could cause an electrolyte imbalance

10. Sandy tells you that she is getting tired of taking drugs, is feeling better, and, therefore, is going to stop taking all medications. Your response is based on the knowledge that _____.
    a. relief of symptoms is a sign that the disease is improving and drug therapy should be discontinued
    b. consistent medical supervision and drug therapy is important even though the patient may feel good and have relief from pain and stiffness
    c. other drugs will probably be necessary but the aspirin should be continued until the physician has time to order other drugs

11. Sandy tells you that she has decided to take long, slow walks to keep her muscles and joints free from stiffness. Your response to this statement is based on the knowledge that _____.
    a. rest and exercise are important, but the physician's advice must be followed since too much or too little of each can be harmful
    b. exercise is necessary for all patients with rheumatoid arthritis, but all exercise must be done slowly
    c. walking is considered one of the best forms of exercise and will reduce the possibility of joint stiffness and deformity

Mrs. Carroll, age 63, has osteoarthritis—a degenerative joint disease. Although admitted to the hospital for other reasons, her arthritis has begun to cause discomfort.

12. Mrs. Carroll's osteoarthritis is _____.
    a. rarely seen under the age of 65
    b. more common in women
    c. frequently due to an earlier infectious process
    d. a reflection of the generalized aging process

13. Mrs. Carroll asks if her arthritis can either be cured or at least stopped from getting worse. Although this is a question a physician will answer, the nurse should know that osteoarthritis is _____.
    a. curable only if diagnosed early
    b. best treated with hot baths to prevent joint degeneration
    c. easily controlled with medications
    d. a progressive disease

14. Mrs. Carroll complains of stiffness and soreness, especially in the morning hours. To help Mrs. Carroll, the nurse should plan to _____.
    a. help her with exercises to loosen up her joints when she first gets out of bed
    b. allow her to complete her morning care at her own rate

c. encourage her to do all her own care as this will prevent joint stiffness the next day
   d. tell her to stay in bed until the afternoon hours

15. Mrs. Carroll brought bedroom slippers to the hospital but did not bring shoes. To promote better foot and leg support the nurse should ____.
    a. suggest that Mrs. Carroll's family bring her shoes to the hospital
    b. tell Mrs. Carroll that she should not go barefoot and wear her slippers when out of bed
    c. suggest that her family purchase orthopedic arch supports for her slippers
    d. tell Mrs. Carroll to walk slowly and plant each foot firmly on the ground

Mr. Lewis, 56 years of age, has had gout for many years. Because he fails to adhere to the medication and dietary regimen prescribed by his physician, he occasionally has acute attacks of gout.

16. Purines are the end-products in the digestion of ____.
    a. fats
    b. carbohydrates
    c. certain types of proteins

17. The physician may diagnose Mr. Lewis' gout by ____.
    1. blood tests, particularly serum uric acid levels
    2. biopsy of the tissue around the joint(s)
    3. physical examination of the affected joint(s)
    4. x-ray examination of the affected joint(s)
    5. stool samples
       a. 1, 2, 5
       b. 1, 3, 4
       c. 2, 3, 4
       d. 2, 4, 5

18. Mr. Lewis has an acute attack of gout and his physician prescribes colchicine to be given hourly until ____.
    a. his joints are less stiff and he can move without pain
    b. his temperature returns to normal
    c. pain, redness, and joint enlargement have disappeared
    d. pain subsides or nausea, vomiting, diarrhea, or intestinal cramping occur

19. Although Mr. Lewis has not adhered to treatment in the past, he now states that the pain during this last attack was so severe he intends to follow his physician's orders. Future treatment will be aimed at ____.
    a. raising Mr. Lewis' serum uric acid level
    b. making Mr. Lewis adhere to a medication schedule
    c. preventing future attacks and permanent joint damage
    d. curing the disease through intensive drug therapy

20. Mr. Lewis will be taking allopurinol (Zyloprim) once the acute phase of his attack has subsided. When this, as well as other drugs for gout, is taken, it is recommended that the patient increase his fluid intake to ____.
    a. dissolve any stones that may form in the urinary tract
    b. reduce the possibility of urate stone formation in the kidney
    c. wash out any stones that may form

III. Fill-in and discussion questions.

Read each question carefully and place your answer in the space provided.

1. VOCABULARY. Define the following terms.

   a. arthritis: _____

b. arthroplasty: _____

c. fibrous ankylosis: _____

d. hyperuricemia: _____

e. osseous ankylosis: _____

f. ossify: _____

g. osteotomy: _____

h. salicylism: _____

i. synovectomy: _____

j. synovitis: _____

k. tinnitus: _____

l. tophi: _____

2. One danger of open orthopedic injuries or orthopedic surgery is osteomyelitis. Symptoms usually occur suddenly and must be reported to the physician immediately. Give 3 symptoms that might be indicative of osteomyelitis.

   1. _____   3. _____
   2. _____

3. Mr. Burns has osteomyelitis which apparently is due to a direct contamination of the bone following a fracture of his left ankle. Nursing management will need to include devices to prevent deformities and skin breakdown. Name 4 devices that may be utilized to prevent these problems while Mr. Burns is on total bed rest for treatment of the infection.

   1. _____   3. _____
   2. _____   4. _____

4. Many patients with arthritis are told to take a salicylate such as aspirin. Often high doses are prescribed and the patient may develop symptoms of salicylism. Name 4 signs or symptoms of salicylism.

   1. _____   3. _____
   2. _____   4. _____

5. Orthopedic surgeries carry some risk. Two serious complications are infection and thrombophlebitis. Give 3 signs or symptoms that may indicate the occurrence of thrombophlebitis.

   1. _____
   2. _____
   3. _____

6. Primary malignant tumors of the bone require amputation of the extremity. Often, the patient with a primary bone tumor is young and will need to face a serious alteration in his body image. An important part of nursing is understanding how or why the patient feels as he does. If you were faced with this drastic but necessary surgery, what problems might you face and how do you think you would feel the night before surgery?

   _____
   _____
   _____
   _____
   _____
   _____

CHAPTER—14

The patient with an amputation

The loss of an extremity is psychologically damaging. The patient may be able to accept the amputation with the realization that it was necessary surgery to benefit his general physical health. On the other hand, he may consent to the surgery but have great difficulty accepting the change in his body image.

The loss of an extremity creates physical, mental, and socioeconomic problems with the patient requiring intensive nursing care during the immediate pre- and postoperative periods as well as long-range plans involving the use of a prosthesis and ultimate rehabilitation.

The following questions deal with the contents of Chapter 14.

I. True or false.

Read each statement carefully and place your answer in the space provided.

_____ 1. The patient's response to an amputation is highly individual, with some patients able to accept the loss of an extremity better than others.

_____ 2. The amount of grief experienced by a patient after an amputation is thought to be proportional to the symbolic significance of the part lost.

_____ 3. Only patients who have had below-the-knee amputations can be fitted with a prosthesis.

_____ 4. In some cases of amputation, a prosthesis may be attached immediately after surgery.

_____ 5. If skin flaps cover the bone end, this is called a "closed" or "flap" amputation.

_____ 6. Closed amputations are usually covered with pressure dressings.

_____ 7. It is unusual to see drainage or oozing around an incision after an amputation.

_____ 8. When a patient has had an amputation, it is important to start physical therapy early in the postoperative period.

_____ 9. Family attitude appears to have little bearing on how the patient will accept his surgery and cooperate in his postoperative care and rehabilitation.

_____ 10. Most patients with an upper extremity amputation cannot be fitted with a prosthesis.

_____ 11. If a patient complains of pain in his stump late in the postoperative period, the pain could be due to a stump neuroma.

_____ 12. A prosthesis is designed to replace the lost limb and will function as well as the lost limb.

II. Multiple choice questions.

Select the most appropriate answer and place it in the space provided.

Clinical Situations

Six months ago, Joe, age 16, fell down an embankment and severely injured his left leg. After several operations and a constant battle with infections and poor circulation in the lower part of the leg, it has become necessary to amputate the leg below the knee. Joe has had time to prepare himself for the surgery and understands what will be done and what type of prosthesis will be used.

1. Before Joe returns from the operating room his bed should _____.
    a. be placed on blocks with the head of the bed higher than the foot
    b. fitted with a bed board and firm mattress
    c. be moved to an area where Joe is with people his own age
    d. have all frames and boards removed

2. A footboard is placed on the bed to _____.
    a. provide a place to anchor the top sheet
    b. support the foot of the unoperated extremity
    c. give the lower half of the mattress firm support
    d. support a bed frame and trapeze bar

3. On return from surgery, the physician gives orders that Joe's stump is to be elevated on a pillow to _____.
    a. prevent hemorrhage
    b. reduce pain
    c. relax the gluteal muscles
    d. prevent edema

4. A tourniquet is kept at Joe's bedside, *in plain sight*, and is used _____.
    a. to reduce edema
    b. when the physician changes the dressing to prevent accidental bleeding
    c. if gross hemorrhage should occur

5. Joe could develop phantom limb sensation, which is a _____.
    a. mourning over the loss of his limb
    b. feeling that the limb is detached from the body
    c. sensation of the presence of an amputated limb

6. Patients who have had an amputation can develop flexion contractures of the stump. The nurse may assist in the prevention of these contractures by _____.
    1. assisting the patient in rolling from side to side
    2. checking the mattress to be sure it is soft and flexible
    3. having the patient lie in the prone position to create extension of the amputated stump
    4. placing a frame on the bed so the patient can extend his unoperated side
        a. 1, 2
        b. 1, 3
        c. 2, 3
        d. 2, 4

Mr. Warren had an amputation above his left knee because of long-standing vascular disease and the recent development of gangrene. The physician plans to fit a prosthesis to the stump at the time of surgery.

7. When Mr. Warren returns from surgery, there is a cast applied to the stump with a fitting for a pylon attachment. If the cast becomes dislodged from the stump but the dressing remains in place, you would immediately _____.
    a. wrap the stump with an elastic bandage and call the physician
    b. put the cast back on the stump, manually hold it in place, and call the physician
    c. cover the stump with a second dress-

ing and secure the gauze with adhesive tape
d. call the physician for orders as to the nursing action to be taken

8. A suspension harness, fitted around Mr. Warren's waist, is attached to the cast to keep it secure and in place. Unless ordered otherwise, Mr. Warren's harness is ____.
   a. kept tightened when he is both ambulatory and in bed
   b. slightly tightened when he is ambulatory and slightly loosened when he is in bed
   c. kept slightly loose at all times

9. Mr. Warren tells you that he has pain in his left foot, yet he has had an amputation of his left leg. As a nurse you know that ____.
   a. patients try to convince themselves that the amputation never took place by talking about an extremity that isn't there
   b. this is an example of phantom limb pain
   c. the physician must be called as Mr. Warren is not accepting his surgery

10. The rationale for a fitting of a temporary prosthesis in the operating room is that ____.
    a. it prevents postoperative hemorrhage and edema
    b. it aids in strengthening the unoperated extremity
    c. it provides a better stump to attach a permanent prosthesis
    d. it allows the patient out of bed as soon as possible

11. Before the stump can be fitted with a permanent prosthesis it must shrink and shape properly. To accomplish this, the physician usually orders ____.
    a. the patient to be ambulated frequently
    b. exercise of the extremity
    c. the stump dressing changed frequently
    d. an elastic bandage applied to the stump

12. Amputation of the arm can present difficulty with the posture, especially in those with an above-the-elbow amputation. These patients tend to ____.
    1. tilt the trunk of their body away from the side of the amputation
    2. tilt the trunk of their body toward the amputation
    3. develop a kyphosis
    4. develop a scoliosis
       a. 1, 3
       b. 1, 4
       c. 2, 3
       d. 2, 4

III. Fill-in and discussion questions.

Read each question carefully and place your answer in the space provided.

1. Two days ago Mr. Garner, age 49, had an amputation of his right leg below the knee. He had known that the surgery was going to be performed and had been provided with time to consider what was happening. He appeared to accept the fact that the surgery was necessary. However, he now appears depressed and has verbalized fears regarding what will happen to him. What might be some of the concerns that Mr. Garner, or any patient, may have before or after amputation of a limb? _____

_____
_____
_____
_____

2. List 3 diseases or events that might necessitate the amputation of a limb.

   1. _____   3. _____
   2. _____

3. Mr. Garner has told his physician that he is concerned about the phantom limb sensations of numbness and tingling. It is also very distressing, he says, to feel his leg and foot when he knows they have been amputated.

   a. Is this a usual sensation for an amputee? _____
   b. How long may this sensation last? _____
   c. Might he later ignore the sensation even though it is still present? _____

4. A patient is having a moderate amount of drainage from his stump. The physician examines the stump, changes the dressing and enters the following note in the chart: "a moderate amount of drainage is present and to be expected."
   a. If the drainage is near the top of the stump what could the nurse do to protect the bed clothes? _____
   _____
   _____
   _____

   b. What effect might the sight of drainage have on the patient and his visitors? _____
   _____
   _____
   _____

5. Good care of the stump is essential if ambulation and use of a prosthesis are to be successful. In teaching the patient about the care of his stump, the nurse must thoroughly explain the various aspects of stump care. What points would you cover if a patient is being shown stump care in preparation for discharge from the hospital?
   _____
   _____
   _____
   _____
   _____
   _____

UNIT FOUR
Disorders of cognitive, sensory, or psychomotor function

CHAPTER—15

The patient with neurological disturbance

Neurological nursing requires observational powers and bedside skills. The patient may be extremely ill and require detailed observation. Neurological lesions that change physical and/or mental functions are distressing to both the patient and his family, and the nurse must be alert for all opportunities to help the patient become self-sufficient. Intensive nursing care during the acute phase and a well-planned rehabilitation program can bring a return of function to many patients with a neurological deficit.

The following questions deal with the contents of Chapter 15.

I. True or false.

Read each statement carefully and place your answer in the space provided.

_____ 1. Normal cerebrospinal fluid is slightly opaque.
_____ 2. The normal cerebrospinal fluid pressure is 80 to 180 mm of H_2O.
_____ 3. A Queckenstedt test may be done during a lumbar puncture and is performed to determine changes in spinal fluid pressure when the jugular veins are compressed.
_____ 4. A cerebral angiogram is a relatively safe and painless procedure.
_____ 5. A pneumoencephalogram utilizes a radiopaque dye to visualize the structures of the brain.
_____ 6. A brain scan is an uncomfortable procedure.
_____ 7. Coughing is contraindicated in patients with increased intracranial pressure.
_____ 8. At times it is difficult to distinguish between some levels of consciousness as the patient could have characteristics of two or more levels.
_____ 9. The causative organism of meningitis is almost always a virus.
_____ 10. Encephalitis is an infectious disease of the central nervous system.
_____ 11. Another name for Parkinson's disease is paralysis agitans.
_____ 12. The symptoms of secondary parkinsonism are similar to those of idiopathic parkinsonism.
_____ 13. The symptoms of parkinsonism usually progress rapidly.
_____ 14. Patients with moderate physical disability due to parkinsonism should not be ambulated as this increases chances of early disability.
_____ 15. Once the cause of symptomatic epilepsy is removed, the disorder will presumably be corrected.
_____ 16. Psychomotor attacks, a form of

epilepsy, are characterized by periods of automatic activity.

_____ 17. Status epilepticus is a rapid progression of convulsive grand mal seizures; the patient does not regain consciousness between each seizure.

_____ 18. Migraine headaches appear to be due to a deficiency of neurohormones.

II. Multiple choice questions.

Select the most appropriate answer and place it in the space provided.

1. A myelogram is a contrast study performed to detect abnormalities of the _____.
   a. brain and spinal cord
   b. spinal canal
   c. vertebrae
   d. upper spinal column

2. Pain may be experienced *during* a myelogram because of the _____.
   a. manipulation of the spinal needle and contact of the needle with the nerve roots
   b. position assumed before and after the procedure
   c. removal of spinal fluid
   d. irritating property of the radiopaque dye

3. Herpes zoster or "shingles" is a(n) _____.
   a. bacterial infection
   b. skin infection that is highly contagious
   c. disease due to nerves
   d. acute viral infection

4. Typical grand mal seizures are characterized by a sequence of events. The seizure pattern may be described as a _____.
   a. clonic phase followed by a tonic phase
   b. tonic phase followed by a clonic phase
   c. rigid contraction of all body muscles followed by a deep sleep
   d. loss of consciousness followed by excessive salivation

5. A petit mal seizure is a convulsive disorder characterized by a(n) _____.
   a. loss of consciousness followed by rhythmical, jerking movements of the head, arms, and legs
   b. falling to the ground followed by a rigid contraction of muscles
   c. aura followed by rhythmical contraction of muscles
   d. brief loss of consciousness during which physical activity ceases

6. Jacksonian or focal seizures are characterized by _____.
   a. alternate and rhythmical, or jerking, movements beginning in the upper part of the body and "marching" to the lower extremities
   b. a loss of consciousness followed by a spread of the seizures from the lower to the upper extremities
   c. convulsive twitching or jerking movements beginning in one area and spreading to other areas
   d. convulsive movements of the entire body

7. The prevention of pressure on the lower part of the neck and axilla by proper positioning of the shoulder and arm will prevent _____.
   a. injury to the brachial plexus
   b. decubitus ulcers of the elbow and upper arm
   c. contractures of the forearm and wrist
   d. wristdrop

8. Hypostatic pneumonia may be prevented by _____.
   a. the administration of antibiotics
   b. frequent change of the patient's position
   c. keeping the patient in a supine position
   d. the administration of an expectorant

9. If a drug is given directly into the subarachnoid space of the spinal cord, this is called a(n) _____ injection.
   a. intrathoracic
   b. dural
   c. intrathecal
   d. epidermal

10. Contractures are always a serious problem in the patient immobile for long periods of time. Contractures may be prevented or at least minimized by _____.
    a. application of splints to prevent lengthening of muscles
    b. use of a firm mattress
    c. passive exercise to immobile limbs
    d. use of a bedboard

Clinical Situations

Mr. Ellis, age 29, is admitted to the hospital because of fever, lethargy, muscular weakness, headache, and diplopia. After examination by a neurologist a tentative diagnosis of encephalitis is made.

11. A lumbar puncture is performed on Mr. Ellis to obtain samples of cerebrospinal fluid. A lumbar puncture can also be performed to _____.
    1. administer an anesthetic
    2. test the patient's reflexes
    3. inject a drug
    4. inject air
    5. biopsy the spinal cord
       a. 1, 3, 4
       b. 1, 2, 5
       c. 2, 3, 5
       d. 3, 4, 5

12. Following the lumbar puncture, a patient's activity is usually restricted by keeping _____.
    a. him on bed rest with bathroom privileges
    b. him in a supine position for 8 hours
    c. the bed flat for 6 or more hours and the patient on complete bed rest
    d. the bed flat for 2 to 3 days but allowing the patient bathroom privileges

13. Mr. Ellis has the following signs and/or appearance: drowsy; can be aroused but then falls asleep; answers questions but answers are delayed; speech is chiefly incoherent; responds slowly to verbal commands. In assessing his level of consciousness he appears to be _____.
    a. stuporous
    b. somnolent
    c. comatose
    d. semicomatose

14. Mr. Ellis has a further change in his level of consciousness and is now unresponsive. Unresponsive patients may develop a drying of the cornea. This is usually caused by _____.
    a. paralysis of the upper eyelid
    b. low humidity
    c. warm air drafts around the patient's head
    d. absence of the blinking reflex and reduction in tear formation

15. Mr. Ellis is found to have a viral encephalitis; therefore, management of his disease is _____.
    a. symptomatic
    b. aimed at administering antiviral drugs
    c. directed toward preventing further infection by the same virus

Mr. Trenton is a 44-year-old insurance salesman who has been admitted to the hospital for evaluation of his headaches, dizziness, and the recent occurrence of a convulsive seizure.

16. Mr. Trenton is scheduled for a neurological examination. His physician performs a Romberg test during which the patient stands with his feet close together and his eyes closed. This is a test used to determine ____.
    a. difficulty with sensual perception
    b. a problem with the equilibrium
    c. the presence of a motor deficit
    d. inherited disorders of the brain and spinal cord

17. After a skull x-ray series and other neurological tests, Mr. Trenton is scheduled for a cerebral angiogram. This x-ray study is a(n) ____.
    a. visualization of the bony structures of the skull and cervical spine
    b. contrast study of the ventricles of the brain
    c. visualization of the cerebral artery
    d. study of the vascular system of the brain

18. For a few hours following the cerebral angiogram, Mr. Trenton may complain of difficulty in ____.
    a. swallowing and talking
    b. walking and climbing stairs
    c. seeing and hearing
    d. thinking clearly and speaking

19. Following a cerebral angiogram, a cold pack or ice collar is ordered to be applied to Mr. Trenton's neck to ____.
    a. decrease the possibility of an allergic reaction to the dye
    b. decrease the amount of blood going to the brain
    c. relieve the subcutaneous swelling and discomfort
    d. relieve the burning sensation felt during and after the procedure

20. Mr. Trenton had a grand mal seizure at 10:20 A.M. His physician was contacted and he examined Mr. Trenton approximately 35 minutes after his seizure. The physician states that the cerebral angiogram performed 2 days ago shows a brain tumor that has been causing his symptoms. Mr. Trenton's convulsive seizures would now be considered ____.
    a. idiopathic
    b. symptomatic

21. Epilepsy may be defined as a(n) ____.
    a. inability of certain neurons to transmit impulses
    b. abnormal electrical disturbance in a specific area(s) of the brain
    c. area of damage in the cerebellum
    d. abnormal electrical response in the neurons of the thalamus

22. The epileptic "cry" that immediately precedes a grand mal seizure is caused by ____.
    a. spasms of the respiratory muscles and the muscles of the throat and glottis
    b. fright—the patient knows what is coming as he has experienced it before
    c. a deep inhalation of air followed by mucus pooling in the lungs
    d. an alternating contraction and relaxation of the muscles of the diaphragm

Miss Burke, age 66, is a retired secretary who has had Parkinson's disease for approximately 7 years. Four years ago Miss Burke's symptoms became very pronounced, forcing her to retire earlier than anticipated. She lives alone and now finds it difficult to care for herself. Miss Burke has been admitted to the hospital for evaluation of her disease and possible change(s) in therapy.

23. The etiology of Miss Burke's parkinsonism is probably ____.
    a. symptomatic
    b. idiopathic
    c. secondary
    d. drug related

24. The area of the brain affected in Parkinson's disease is primarily the ____.
    a. basal ganglia
    b. thalamus
    c. cerebellum
    d. hypothalamus

25. When Miss Burke *first* began to have symptoms of Parkinson's disease she probably experienced ____.
    1. stumbling
    2. tremors of the hands
    3. severe weight loss
    4. stiffness
    5. difficulty in performing movements
        a. 1, 2, 4
        b. 1, 3, 5
        c. 2, 3, 4
        d. 2, 4, 5

26. As the disease progressed, Miss Burke most likely had which signs of the disease? ____.
    1. tremors of the head
    2. weight gain
    3. stooped posture
    4. masklike expression
    5. paralysis
        a. 1, 2, 5
        b. 1, 3, 4
        c. 2, 3, 4
        d. 2, 4, 5

27. Treatment of Miss Burke is aimed at ____.
    a. allowing her to rest as much as possible
    b. keeping her dependent on nursing personnel
    c. prolonging independence and delaying dependence
    d. showing her the importance of having certain tasks done for her

28. Miss Burke has been prescribed an anticholinergiclike drug—benztropin (Cogentin). Side effects that may be experienced while taking this drug include ____.
    a. dryness of the mouth and throat
    b. abdominal pain
    c. gastric distress and excessive nasal secretions
    d. edema of the extremities

29. The drug benztropin (Cogentin) does not control Miss Burke's symptoms, and the physician discontinues the drug and orders levodopa. After one week there is noticeable improvement and Miss Burke will be discharged and referred to the outpatient clinic. Discharge teaching must include the warning that she not take any vitamin preparations except those prescribed for her by her physician which will *not* contain ____.
    a. calcium
    b. vitamin B_1 (thiamine)
    c. phosphorus
    d. vitamin B_6 (pyridoxine)

Mrs. West, a 29-year-old mother of two, developed her first symptoms of multiple sclerosis at age 23. In the beginning her symptoms were vague and temporary. Now, symptoms are more pronounced and permanent. Mrs. West has been admitted because of a chronic urinary tract infection.

30. Multiple sclerosis is a progressive disease of the nervous system characterized by a ____.
    a. loss of myelin from some of the nerves in the central and peripheral nervous system
    b. degeneration of nerves in the peripheral nervous system resulting in paralysis
    c. buildup of phospholipids along the axons of nerves
    d. change in the axons of nerves in the central and peripheral nervous system

31. The symptoms of multiple sclerosis ____.
    1. are the same for all patients
    2. are worse at night than during the day
    3. usually appear gradually
    4. may be vague

5. may form a pattern of exacerbations and remissions
   a. 1, 2, 3
   b. 1, 4, 5
   c. 2, 3, 4
   d. 3, 4, 5

32. Mrs. West's urinary tract infection is controlled with medication and the physician decides to discharge her in several days. Even though she has had the disease for 6 years, she has not been told how to take care of herself or prevent further difficulties. One point that should be stressed in her discharge teaching is the importance of ____.
    a. staying in bed and only getting out of bed for meals and morning care
    b. avoiding milk, milk products, meat, and other protein foods
    c. avoiding infections and contact with those who have an infection
    d. not omitting the medications necessary to control her multiple sclerosis

Mr. Cooper is a 67-year-old retired auto worker who has had attacks of trigeminal neuralgia for the past 2 years. The attacks have become more severe and it was decided to admit him to the hospital for further evaluation of the disorder and possible surgery.

33. Attacks of trigeminal neuralgic pain may be caused by ____.
    a. seasonal allergies
    b. drugs
    c. degeneration of the seventh cranial nerve
    d. irritation of trigger spots

34. It is decided to perform surgery on Mr. Cooper and he is told he will have permanent numbness or a tingling sensation on the left side of his face. He is willing to accept this rather than endure the pain. Postoperatively Mr. Cooper will have difficulty eating; therefore, the nurse must ____.
    1. supervise his eating until he is used to the numb sensation as aspiration of food can occur
    2. explain how he must eat baby food for the rest of his life
    3. check the inside of his mouth for food particles after he has finished eating
    4. explain that he can no longer brush his teeth but must use mouthwash
       a. 1, 2
       b. 1, 3
       c. 2, 3
       d. 2, 4

III. Fill-in and discussion questions.

Read each question carefully and place your answer in the space provided.

1. VOCABULARY. Define the following terms.

   a. brachial plexus: _____

   b. cerebrospinal fluid: _____

   c. cisternal puncture: _____

   d. clonic: _____

   e. diplopia: _____

   f. edentulous: _____

g. encephalopathy: _____

h. gingivitis: _____

i. hypostatic pneumonia: _____

j. idiopathic: _____

k. intrathecal: _____

l. meningitis: _____

m. nuchal rigidity: _____

n. nystagmus: _____

o. sequelae: _____

p. tonic: _____

q. vesicles: _____

2. Label the 5 areas identified in the drawing below by filling in the blanks to the right of the drawing. The 5 areas are to be selected from the words given below the drawing.

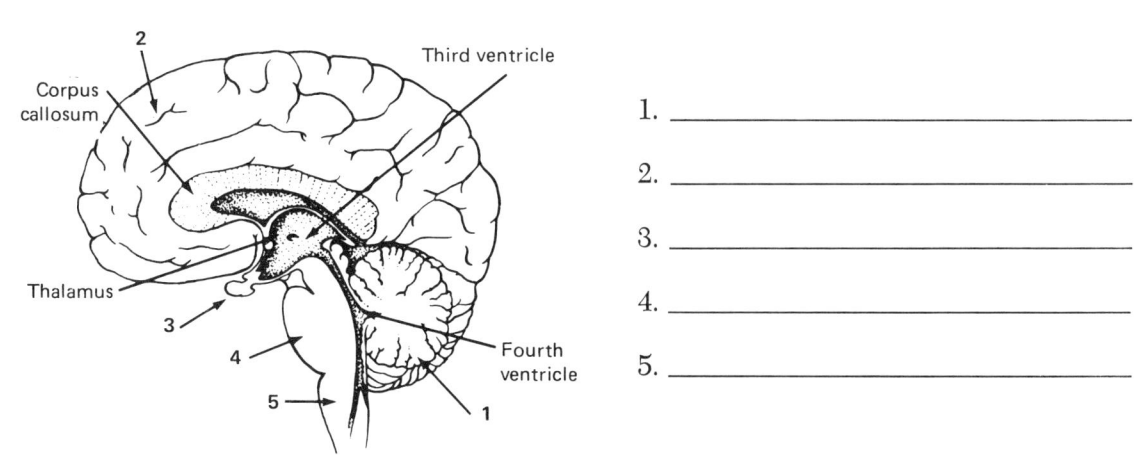

1. _____

2. _____

3. _____

4. _____

5. _____

pons   medulla   cerebrum   cerebellum   pituitary

75

3. Label the 5 areas identified in the drawing below by filling in the blanks to the right of the drawing. The 5 areas are to be selected from the words given below the drawing.

1. _____

2. _____

3. _____

4. _____

5. _____

visual area   speech area   cutaneous and muscular sensory area   hearing area   motor area

4. The neurological examination is an important diagnostic maneuver performed to identify and in some cases locate disorders of the nervous system. List 4 examining instruments or objects that may be used in the neurological examination.

   1. _____   3. _____

   2. _____   4. _____

5. Contrast studies are sometimes necessary to detect lesions or abnormalities of the brain and spinal cord. Name 3 such studies.

   1. _____   3. _____

   2. _____

6. Briefly describe 2 nursing measures that may be used to increase the amount of air a patient takes into his lungs with each breath.

   1. _____

   2. _____

7. Correct positioning of the patient with a long-term illness is important. Pillows are used to support the upper part of the body when the unconscious patient is on his side. The head is supported by a *small* pillow. Give 2 reasons why a standard-sized pillow is contraindicated in these patients.

   1. _____

   _____

   2. _____

   _____

8. Identify the location of the 3 meninges that lie between the bones of the skull and the brain tissue.

MENINGES	LOCATION

9. Nursing management of the patient with herpes zoster is aimed at keeping the patient as comfortable as possible. What suggestions might be given to the patient with this disorder with regard to his clothing? _____

10. Individuals with grand mal epilepsy usually experience a *prodromal* phase prior to a convulsive seizure. Briefly describe this phase and what may be experienced by the patient. _____

11. Individuals with grand mal epilepsy may also experience an *aura* immediately prior to the seizure. Explain what an aura is and what significance it may have in the diagnosis of epilepsy. _____

12. List—in order—the nursing actions taken if you entered a room and found a patient having a grand mal seizure.

1. _____
2. _____
3. _____
4. _____
5. _____

77

13. The *newly* diagnosed epileptic and/or his family must have a thorough explanation of his disease. Prepare a teaching plan for a patient by listing at least 3 points you could cover (some may need a physician's approval) in a teaching session.

   1. _____

   2. _____

   3. _____

14. Many epileptics suffer more acutely from the stigma attached to epilepsy than from the symptoms themselves. Briefly discuss the emotional difficulties that may be experienced with regard to employment, worry about attacks, social implications, and so on.

   _____

CHAPTER—16

The patient with cerebrovascular disease

Cerebrovascular disease, or disease of the blood vessels of the brain, is one of the major medical problems affecting adults in the United States. The frequency of cerebrovascular disease increases with age; thus, as the expected lifespan increases, it is expected that the incidence of cerebrovascular disease will increase.

Nursing management of the patient with cerebrovascular disease involves the formulation of short- and long-term goals. It is often necessary to utilize the entire medical team in an effort to attain these goals and plan for optimum patient care.

The following questions deal with the contents of Chapter 16.

I. True or false.

Read each statement carefully and place your answer in the space provided.

_____ 1. Cerebrovascular disease is one of the major health problems affecting adults in the United States.

_____ 2. A more common term for cerebrovascular accident is "stroke."

_____ 3. The patient with cerebrovascular disease is usually aware of the changes occurring in his physical and mental abilities.

_____ 4. The longer coma lasts, the poorer the prognosis.

_____ 5. Cerebrovascular accidents can occur with no previous warning.

_____ 6. The physician is able to predict the amount of permanent damage that will occur about 6 hours after a cerebrovascular accident.

_____ 7. The speech center of a right-handed person is located in the right side of the brain.

_____ 8. Aphasia is only caused by a cerebrovascular accident.

_____ 9. An endarterectomy may be performed for atherosclerosis of the carotid artery.

_____ 10. Transient ischemic attacks are indications of a bleeding disorder of the brain.

_____ 11. After the death of brain tissue has occurred, nothing can be done to repair the damaged tissue.

_____ 12. Most cerebral aneurysms occur in the circle of Willis.

_____ 13. The presence and location of a cerebral aneurysm can usually be seen on a plain x-ray of the skull.

_____ 14. Some cerebral aneurysms are inoperable because of their type (fusiform or saccular) and the length of time the patient has had the aneurysm.

_____ 15. The patient under medical treatment for a cerebral aneurysm is

usually placed on bed rest with bathroom privileges.
_____ 16. When a patient gets out of bed after a long period of immobilization, he should immediately progress from a lying to a standing position to prevent orthostatic hypotension.
_____ 17. An early start at rehabilitation is one of the best ways to prevent depression in the patient with a cerebrovascular accident.
_____ 18. Family attitudes are of utmost importance during the rehabilitation of the patient with a cerebrovascular accident.
_____ 19. Speech rehabilitation is most effective if it is started just before the patient is ready for discharge from the hospital.

II. Multiple choice questions.

Select the most appropriate answer and place it in the space provided.

1. The most common cause of death during prolonged coma is _____.
   a. infection of decubitus ulcers
   b. fever
   c. pneumonia
   d. paralysis

2. Transient ischemic attacks are _____.
   a. brief, fleeting attacks of neurological impairment
   b. moments of forgetfulness
   c. brief lapses of consciousness
   d. instances of memory loss similar to amnesia

3. The 4 major arteries of the brain are the 2 _____.
   1. external carotid arteries
   2. internal carotid arteries
   3. vertebral arteries
   4. thoracic arteries
      a. 1, 3
      b. 1, 4
      c. 2, 3
      d. 2, 4

CLINICAL SITUATIONS

Mr. Forman has had signs of cerebrovascular disease for the past 10 years. This was evidenced by signs of arteriosclerosis, impaired memory, personality changes, difficulty in concentration, and periods of confusion. He lives with his married daughter and son-in-law and has been able to care for himself and perform simple household tasks. Yesterday morning he complained of a headache. This morning he was found unconscious on the floor of his bedroom and was admitted by ambulance to the hospital.

4. The pathophysiology of cerebrovascular disease involves _____.
   a. an increase in oxygen-carrying ability of red cells
   b. an increase in arterial blood pressure thereby decreasing the amount of blood reaching the brain
   c. the increased ability of arteries to carry blood to brain cells
   d. the lessened ability of arteries to carry blood to brain cells

5. Mr. Forman has had a cerebrovascular accident. The most common causes of this disorder are _____.
   a. falling and head injuries
   b. cerebral thrombus and cerebral embolus
   c. cerebral anoxia and cerebral hypoxia
   d. hypotension and heart disease

6. Mr. Forman has paralysis of the right side of his body. This is called _____.
   a. hemiplegia
   b. paraplegia
   c. quadraplegia
   d. isoplegia

7. If Mr. Forman has paralysis of his right arm and leg, the hemorrhage or clot occurred _____.
   a. on the left side of his brain
   b. on the right side of his brain
   c. in the cerebellum
   d. in the occipital lobe
8. During the acute phase, nursing management of Mr. Forman will include _____.
   1. suctioning his mouth p.r.n. to clear secretions
   2. position changes every 4 to 6 hours
   3. intake and output
   4. placing the foot of the bed higher than the head
   5. use of an oropharyngeal airway if breathing is difficult
      a. 1, 3, 4
      b. 1, 2, 5
      c. 1, 3, 5
      d. 2, 3, 4
9. To prevent contractures and deformities of the legs and hips, the nurse can use _____.
   1. a soft mattress on the bed
   2. pillows between the knees
   3. trochanter rolls
   4. a pillow under the knees
   5. a footboard
      a. 1, 2, 3
      b. 1, 3, 4
      c. 2, 4, 5
      d. 2, 3, 5

Mark Evans is a senior in high school. Last evening while getting ready to go to work as a part-time dishwasher he collapsed in the living room of his home. He had complained of headaches—some mild and some severe—over the past several months. His father called the fire department rescue squad who immediately transported him to the hospital. Ten minutes after arrival in the emergency department he became comatose and slightly cyanotic. An oral airway was immediately inserted and oxygen given. He is tentatively diagnosed as having a ruptured cerebral aneurysm in the circle of Willis.

10. A lumbar puncture is performed. If Mark has a ruptured cerebral aneurysm the spinal fluid will be _____.
    a. clear
    b. cloudy
    c. grossly bloody
    d. absent
11. Mark is to be treated medically until surgery is possible. One of the nursing assistants asks if Mark is to have a back rub. Your answer will be _____.
    a. No. Passive exercises and back rubs are not given unless approved by the physician
    b. Yes, providing the back rub is given gently
    c. Yes. Press down on the mattress and insert your hand underneath the bony prominences and give a gentle massage
    d. No. Acutely ill patients are not given back rubs
12. The physician wishes to prevent any straining during bowel movements or instances of constipation and will most likely order a(n) _____.
    a. stool softener
    b. enema to be given daily
    c. soft diet
    d. cathartic
13. Mark's physician orders elastic stockings which are _____.
    a. used in place of passive exercises
    b. applied daily for 2 to 4 hours
    c. used to prevent thrombophlebitis
    d. of value in the prevention of varicose veins in immobilized patients
14. Mark is taken to surgery and a Selverstone clamp is applied to his left carotid artery. The purpose of the clamp is to _____.
    a. increase the pressure in the aneurysm
    b. improve circulation to the right side of the brain
    c. reduce blood flow to cerebral vessels on the left side of the brain
    d. totally stop blood flow to cerebral vessels

15. The clamp is slowly tightened over a period of 6 days. Now the clamp totally occludes the carotid artery. Mark will have to be observed for _____.
    a. signs of increased circulation to cerebral structures
    b. aphasia and hemiparesis
    c. signs of decreased circulation to his arms and legs
    d. paraplegia and muscular atrophy

III. Fill-in and discussion questions.
Read each question carefully and place your answer in the space provided.

1. VOCABULARY. Define the following terms.
    a. aphasia: _____

    b. arteriosclerosis: _____

    c. atherosclerosis: _____

    d. hemianopsia: _____

    e. infarction: _____

    f. intima: _____

    g. sequela: _____

2. Name 2 of the more common causes of cerebral (intracranial) hemorrhage.
    1. _____   2. _____

3. Give 8 signs and symptoms that may be present at the time of a cerebrovascular accident.
    1. _____   5. _____
    2. _____   6. _____
    3. _____   7. _____
    4. _____   8. _____

4. Mrs. Dent has a possible ruptured cerebral aneurysm. The nurse in charge of the special care unit instructs the nursing personnel to observe Mrs. Dent for signs of increased intracranial pressure. Give 5 signs of increased intracranial pressure that might be observed in Mrs. Dent should she develop this disorder.
    1. _____   4. _____
    2. _____   5. _____
    3. _____

5. Mrs. Adams has aphasia and some limited motion in her right leg following a cerebrovascular accident. At present she can speak, but often has difficulty naming objects or putting words together to ask or answer a question. What might the nurse do to help in the speech rehabilitation of Mrs. Adams?

CHAPTER—17

The patient with spinal cord impairment

A trauma to the spinal column may cause pressure on the spinal cord and spinal nerve roots. Symptoms of injury can vary from minor pain and discomfort to paralysis, which may be either temporary or permanent.

Nursing management of patients with a spinal column injury often requires a detailed and innovative approach. The patient who is immobilized for long periods, and in some cases permanently, will require an intensive program of skin care, nutrition, and the prevention of complications. In addition, a rehabilitation program with both immediate and long-range goals must become a part of the nursing care plan.

The following questions deal with the contents of Chapter 17.

I. True or false.

Read each statement carefully and place your answer in the space provided.

_____ 1. The posterior portion of the spinal cord contains motor nerve fibers.

_____ 2. The term hypoesthesia means increased sensation in an area.

_____ 3. The location and severity of an injury to the spinal cord determines how much function will be lost.

_____ 4. A lesion involving tissues surrounding or outside of the spinal cord is called an extramedullary lesion.

_____ 5. The function of an intervertebral disc is to protect the spinal cord.

_____ 6. The spinal cord ends at the level of the first or second lumbar vertebra.

_____ 7. Tumors of the spinal cord may be primary or metastatic.

_____ 8. Pott's disease is an arthritic condition of the spine.

_____ 9. The patient with a laminectomy and a spinal fusion is usually kept on bed rest longer than the patient who has had a simple laminectomy.

_____ 10. Following a lumbar laminectomy, the patient should begin exercising his spine and back muscles within 1 or 2 days.

_____ 11. A fracture bedpan should be used with postoperative laminectomy patients as they must avoid lifting their hips and straining their back.

_____ 12. Paraplegia and quadraplegia are caused by injury to the spinal cord.

_____ 13. Transection of the spinal cord at the lower thoracic level will result in quadraplegia.

_____ 14. Patients with a spinal cord injury

may lose control over bowel and bladder function.
_____ 15. Patients on prolonged bed rest should limit their fluid intake as they are prone to edema.
_____ 16. The quadraplegic patient should never be placed in an upright position because his paralysis will interfere with his ability to breathe.
_____ 17. Patients with a permanent spinal cord injury can achieve bladder control more easily than bowel control.

II. Multiple choice questions.

Select the most appropriate answer and place it in the space provided.

1. After an injury to the spinal cord, disturbance of motor and/or sensory function occurs _____.
   a. above and below the level of the injury
   b. above the level of the injury
   c. below the level of the injury

2. If a spinal cord injury occurs high in the cervical region _____.
   a. respiratory failure and death follows paralysis of the diaphragm
   b. there will be paralysis on one side of the body
   c. a sensory loss below the waist will follow
   d. the patient will be a paraplegic

3. Trauma may lead to bleeding within the spinal cord which will then result in _____.
   a. fracture of the vertebrae
   b. severing of nerve tracts
   c. compression of the spinal cord and nerve roots
   d. paralysis above the injury

4. The primary goal of rehabilitation of paraplegic and quadraplegic patients is to _____.
   a. prevent further deformities
   b. help the patients accept their physical liabilities
   c. show the patients that everyone can be rehabilitated if he tries
   d. help the patients use their remaining capacities to the fullest

CLINICAL SITUATIONS

Mrs. Finley is a 33-year-old housewife with two children. When lifting one of her children she felt a sudden pain in her back which radiated down her left leg to her heel. She has been on bed rest at home but has had little relief. She is now admitted for treatment of her back pain and her problem has been tentatively diagnosed as a herniated intervertebral disc.

5. X-ray contrast studies are ordered. The x-ray study performed for the diagnosis of spinal column abnormality or disease is a(n) _____.
   a. spinalgram
   b. aortogram
   c. myelogram
   d. vertebrogram

6. Herniated lumbar discs compress _____.
   a. cervical nerves
   b. spinal nerve roots
   c. peripheral nerves
   d. thoracic nerves

7. X-ray studies show Mrs. Finley has a ruptured intervertebral disc and conservative treatment will be tried first. The bed will require a _____.
   1. firm mattress
   2. bed board
   3. soft mattress
   4. double set of springs

   a. 1, 2
   b. 1, 4
   c. 2, 3
   d. 2, 4

8. Mrs. Finley is placed in pelvic traction which ____.
   a. increases the distance between the vertebrae
   b. pushes the herniated disc back into place
   c. decreases the distance between the vertebrae
   d. keeps the herniated disc in place
9. Mrs. Finley is allowed out of traction 3 times a day. When placing her back in traction the weights are ____.
   a. lowered gently before the pelvic harness is applied
   b. lowered gently after the harness is placed around the hips
   c. supported on a chair after the pelvic harness is applied
   d. kept off until she complains of pain
10. When Mrs. Finley is out of traction and moving in bed she should ____.
    a. only move her arms and not her legs
    b. pull herself up in bed by using a trapeze and raising her hips
    c. only roll on the side that does not have pain
    d. roll from side to side without twisting her spine
11. After one week in traction Mrs. Finley has had little relief from pain and a lumbar laminectomy with a spinal fusion is planned. In this surgery the ____.
    a. herniated disc will be repaired
    b. spinal cord will be fused
    c. herniated disc will be removed
    d. spinal nerve near the disc is clipped
12. Following surgery Mrs. Finley's position in bed will be changed by ____.
    a. log rolling from side to side
    b. use of a drawsheet under her shoulders
    c. having her use the trapeze
    d. placing a pillow in her lumbar region
13. Mrs. Finley is to wear a back brace when ambulating. The brace should be put on ____.
    a. while she is standing at the bedside
    b. while she is sitting in a straight-backed chair
    c. while she is still in bed
14. While using pillows to support the back when Mrs. Finley is on her side, the pillows are *not* placed or pressed ____.
    a. between the knees
    b. behind the shoulder blades
    c. behind the thoracic spine
    d. against the surgical dressing

Jack and his father were in an automobile accident. Jack suffered a severe spinal injury, whereas his father only sustained minor bruises and was released from the hospital after being examined by a physician. X-ray studies and a neurological examination show that Jack has an injury to his spinal cord at the thoracic-lumbar level.

15. At the scene of the accident movement and transportation of Jack—who is known to have an injury to his spine—is accomplished by ____.
    a. placing him on a rigid surface
    b. log rolling him onto the ambulance stretcher
    c. placing him facedown on an ambulance stretcher
    d. lifting him by his shoulders and knees
16. Jack is admitted to the neurology service and placed in a regular hospital bed with a firm mattress and bed board. He states he has no feeling and it is noted he has no movement below the waist. The paralysis may be temporary or permanent. If temporary it was most likely caused by ____.
    a. a temporary severance of the spinal cord
    b. the psychological trauma and fright of the accident
    c. edema present in the injured area which has compressed the cord
    d. temporary damage to spinal nerves

17. The physician says Jack can be turned from side to side. Therefore the nurse will ____.
    a. log roll him
    b. turn him with a drawsheet placed under his thoracic spine
    c. use pillows under his shoulders while rotating the lower part of his body
18. The physician decides to order a CircOlectric bed as Jack will be immobile for a long period of time. To prevent hypostatic pneumonia Jack should ____.
    a. have passive range-of-motion exercises to all 4 extremities
    b. engage in active range-of-motion exercises in all 4 extremities
    c. practice deep-breathing exercises hourly while awake
    d. be turned every 4 hours
19. If Jack receives any drugs by injection they are given ____.
    a. only by the intravenous route
    b. only in the gluteal muscles
    c. above the area of paralysis
    d. in the subcutaneous tissues of the thighs
20. Jack's father comes to see him and both notice an occasional jerking motion in Jack's legs. Jack and his father now believe that Jack is beginning to move his extremities. As a nurse you know that ____.
    a. this is a sign of a return of function to his legs
    b. both men are imagining the movement
    c. the movement is due to the contractures and skin breakdown Jack is developing
    d. the muscle movement is probably reflex spasms
21. Jack is eating poorly. When you ask him why, he doesn't seem to know. At this point you could ____.
    a. ignore the situation. Jack will eat when he is hungry
    b. have the dietician talk to Jack. He may prefer foods other than what have been offered on the menu
    c. ask Jack's father to talk to him about his poor eating habits
    d. ask the physician to order a different diet

III. Fill-in and discussion questions.

Read each question carefully and place your answer in the space provided.

1. VOCABULARY. Define the following terms.

    a. flaccid paralysis: _____

    b. hemiplegia: _____

    c. laminectomy: _____

    d. nucleus pulposa: _____

    e. paraplegia: _____

    f. quadraplegia: _____

g. spastic paralysis: _____

2. Describe the log-rolling technique used in turning a postoperative laminectomy patient. _____
_____
_____
_____
_____
_____

3. A patient who has had a spinal cord injury may become extremely depressed at some point during the recovery phase or during the rehabilitation program. Nurses must try to understand the patient and how this type of injury has affected his life. In the space below, list some activities that you have performed in the past 24 hours that you could not have performed if you were a paraplegic. _____
_____
_____
_____
_____

4. What steps can be used to help the paraplegic patient achieve bowel control? _____
_____
_____
_____
_____

CHAPTER—18

The patient with visual and hearing impairment

Patients with a handicap involving sight and/or hearing present specific problems in nursing management. Along with the medical or surgical problem there may also be a problem of communication with the hard of hearing or deaf patient. The visually handicapped patient may also have difficulty in the unfamiliar surroundings of the hospital.

Also to be considered are patients who suddenly acquire a visual or hearing loss. Not only must physical needs be met but the emotional impact of this sudden loss, and its effect upon the patient's future present special challenges in nursing management.

The following questions deal with the contents of Chapter 18.

I. True or false.

Read each statement carefully and place your answer in the space provided.

_____ 1. An ophthalmoscope is an instrument used to examine the interior of the eye.

_____ 2. A tonometer measures pressure behind the retina of the eye.

_____ 3. Deficiency of vitamin C can result in a form of night blindness.

_____ 4. Direct exposure of the eye to sunlamps can burn the eyelids and cornea.

_____ 5. Blind people develop extraordinary powers of hearing to compensate for the loss of vision.

_____ 6. Refractive errors are the most common type of eye disorder.

_____ 7. Bifocals are usually prescribed for astigmatism.

_____ 8. Cataracts are the most common cause of blindness.

_____ 9. The anterior chamber of the eye is filled with vitreous humor.

_____ 10. An iridectomy may be performed for acute glaucoma.

_____ 11. The sensory layer of the retina receives the visual stimuli that are transmitted to the brain.

_____ 12. Surgical treatment of a detached retina is usually attempted if conservative medical management and drug therapy fail to correct the problem.

_____ 13. Injury to one eye may result in the development of severe inflammation of the other eye.

_____ 14. The prognosis is more favorable for those with a sensorineural type of deafness than a conduction-type deafness.

_____ 15. Sensorineural deafness is usually irreversible and beyond surgical correction.

_____ 16. There is a partial vacuum in the middle ear which allows the transmission of sound.

_____ 17. Otosclerosis is a common cause

89

of hearing impairment among adults.
___ 18. Disorders of the inner ear are easier to treat than disorders of the middle and outer ear.
___ 19. Ménière's disease is due to a penetrating injury to the middle ear.
___ 20. Inner-ear deafness is a conduction-type deafness.

II. Multiple choice questions.

Select the most appropriate answer and place it in the space provided.

1. Which of the following methods may be of value in removing a foreign body from the eye? ___.
   1. irrigating the eye with water
   2. touching the object gently with a sterile swab
   3. using the corner of a clean handkerchief
   4. irrigating the eye with sterile normal saline
      a. 1, 2
      b. 1, 3
      c. 2, 3
      d. 2, 4

2. If an irritating chemical is splashed into the eye, the eye should immediately be ___.
   a. flushed copiously with water as soon as possible
   b. rinsed with a small amount of normal saline
   c. covered with a sterile patch until it is examined by a physician
   d. taped shut with the lid held in place with sterile tape

3. The term blindness is used for many legal purposes when central visual acuity is ___.
   a. one-half normal vision
   b. one-fifth normal vision without corrective lenses and one-half with corrective lenses
   c. 10/100 in the better eye with a corrective lens
   d. 20/200 or less in the better eye even when corrective lenses are worn

4. The refractive media of the eyes are the ___.
   1. lens
   2. retina
   3. vitreous body
   4. ciliary body
   5. aqueous humor
      a. 1, 2, 4
      b. 1, 3, 5
      c. 2, 3, 4
      d. 2, 3, 5

5. Symptoms of acute glaucoma include ___.
   1. severe pain in and around the eye
   2. blurred vision
   3. excess formation of tears
   4. fever
      a. 1, 2
      b. 1, 3
      c. 2, 3
      d. 2, 4

6. In a detached retina ___.
   a. all layers of the retina pull away from the choroid
   b. the sensory layer becomes separated from the pigmented layer
   c. the retina and choroid become detached from the muscle coat of the eye

7. Symptoms of detached retina include ___.
   1. feeling that a curtain is being drawn over the field of vision
   2. spots or moving particles before the eyes
   3. gaps in the vision
   4. flashes of light
      a. 1, 2
      b. 1, 3
      c. 2, 3
      d. all of these

90

8. After surgery on the eye, there may be an order for an enema or gentle laxative because ____.
   a. the patient has not been out of bed to the bathroom for several days
   b. drugs used prior to eye surgery often cause constipation
   c. straining at stool must be avoided
   d. the soft diet necessary after surgery leads to constipation

9. Conduction deafness is caused by any disease or injury ____.
   a. to the auditory nerve
   b. that interferes with the conduction of sound waves to the inner ear
   c. to the external ear and eardrum
   d. to the cochlea

10. The usual treatment for impacted cerumen is ____.
    a. warm water irrigations with a special syringe
    b. removal with a flexible cotton-tipped applicator
    c. application of warm packs to the side of the head
    d. removal with eardrops containing antibiotics

11. Select the correct progression describing the transmission of sound from the outer to the inner ear ____.
    a. tympanic membrane—malleus—incus—stapes—oval window
    b. tympanic membrane—incus—malleus—stapes—oval window
    c. tympanic membrane—incus—stapes—malleus—oval window

12. The middle ear connects with the nasopharynx by way of the ____.
    a. tympanic membrane
    b. external auditory canal
    c. eustachian tube
    d. auditory tube

13. In serous otitis media ____.
    a. infection occurs in the outer auditory canal and middle ear
    b. the inner ear becomes filled with fluid
    c. the bones of the middle ear fuse
    d. fluid forms in the middle ear

14. The Valsalva maneuver is a way of ____.
    a. releasing the pressure in the middle ear by creating a minute hole in the tympanic membrane
    b. equalizing pressure on both sides of the eardrum
    c. freeing the fused bones of the middle ear
    d. increasing pressure in the middle ear

15. Treatment of serous otitis media is surgical, by means of a ____.
    a. stapedectomy
    b. myringotomy
    c. tympanectomy
    d. myringoplasty

16. If facial paralysis occurs 12 to 24 hours after surgery on the ear, it is probably caused by ____.
    a. injury to the nerve
    b. edema at the site of surgery
    c. the external dressing being too loose
    d. the dressing in the ear canal being saturated with drainage

17. Ménière's disease is characterized by ____.
    1. facial paralysis
    2. tinnitus
    3. purulent drainage from the ear canal
    4. severe vertigo
    5. progressive hearing loss
       a. 1, 2, 4
       b. 1, 3, 5
       c. 2, 3, 4
       d. 2, 4, 5

CLINICAL SITUATIONS

Mrs. Collins, age 71, is admitted for cataract surgery. Both eyes are affected; however, the surgeon is going to operate on her right eye first and on her left eye in a few months.

18. A cataract is a condition in which the ____.
    a. lens of the eye becomes opaque thus reducing the amount of light reaching the retina
    b. ciliary muscles no longer expand and contract thereby reducing the amount of light transmitted through the lens
    c. retina degenerates, resulting in an increased loss of vision
    d. vitreous humor and lens are unable to transmit light because of the development of scar tissue

19. Cataract surgery involves ____.
    a. removal of the lens
    b. removal of the lens and ciliary body
    c. cutting a window into the lens and iris
    d. removal of the vitreous humor

20. Two major complications of cataract surgery are ____.
    a. hypotension and loss of the contents of the lens capsule
    b. loss of vision and increased intraocular pressure
    c. loss of vitreous humor and hemorrhage
    d. paralysis of the iris and hypertension

21. To prevent hemorrhage during the postoperative period, special care is taken to ____.
    a. keep the operative eye covered to prevent tearing of the sutures
    b. keep proper pressure applied to the eyeball by reinforcing the dressing as it becomes loose
    c. keeping the patient on his unoperative side
    d. prevent straining and any sudden movement of the head

Mr. Wilson was diagnosed as having early glaucoma at the time of his last eye examination. Eyedrops were prescribed for him and he was advised to have his eyes re-examined every 6 months.

22. Glaucoma is a(n) ____.
    a. disease of the eye resulting from an infection in the anterior chamber
    b. disorder involving the vitreous humor and retina
    c. absence of aqueous humor in the anterior chamber
    d. condition resulting from increased intraocular pressure

23. Mr. Wilson is diagnosed as having chronic glaucoma. In this case, the symptoms of glaucoma ____.
    a. will include pain which is usually severe
    b. may be absent
    c. do not appear until the glaucoma becomes acute
    d. cannot be controlled with medication

Mrs. Hunt, 32 years of age and the mother of 3 children, has had a progressive hearing loss for 2 years. After a thorough evaluation of her hearing loss she is diagnosed as having otosclerosis. Surgery has been recommended and she is admitted for a stapedectomy.

24. Otosclerosis results from ____.
    a. bony ankylosis of the stapes
    b. fixation of the stapes on the round window
    c. fixation of the malleus on the tympanic membrane
    d. bony deposits on the malleus and incus

25. Following surgery, Mrs. Hunt complains of nausea and dizziness. These complaints are ___.
    a. an indication that pressure in the ear is increasing and the patient will need to return to surgery
    b. not unusual and do occur after ear surgery
    c. an indication that the surgery is a failure

26. The surgeon orders Mrs. Hunt out of bed with assistance. The packing has been removed from the outer ear and a small cotton plug inserted. Mrs. Hunt states that she still cannot hear any better than before surgery. As a nurse you know that ___.
    a. this means the surgery will not help her hearing
    b. hearing improvement may take more time
    c. Mrs. Hunt can hear better, but is so used to a hearing loss it will take time for her to adjust to her improvement
    d. additional surgery will probably be necessary

27. The surgeon cautions Mrs. Hunt against blowing her nose suddenly or violently because this action could ___.
    a. rupture the tympanic membrane/malleus junction
    b. decrease pressure in the middle ear and thus interfere with the healing process
    c. increase drainage from the outer canal
    d. dislodge the prosthesis

III. Fill-in and discussion questions.

Read each question carefully and place your answer in the space provided.

1. VOCABULARY. Define the following terms.

    a. accommodation: _____

    b. astigmatism: _____

    c. cerumen: _____

    d. hyperopia: _____

    e. iridectomy: _____

    f. mastoiditis: _____

    g. miotic: _____

    h. myopia: _____

i. myringotomy: _____

j. oculist: _____

k. ophthalmologist: _____

l. optician: _____

m. optometrist: _____

n. otosclerosis: _____

o. photophobia: _____

p. presbyopia: _____

q. Valsalva maneuver: _____

2. MATCHING. In column B place the number identifying the eye disease named in column A.

COLUMN A

1. ptosis
2. keratitis
3. uveitis
4. ectropion
5. corneitis
6. hordeolum
7. conjunctivitis

COLUMN B

____ inflammation of the iris, ciliary body, choroid
____ inflammation of membrane lining the eyelids and front of eyeball
____ inflammation of the cornea
____ infection at the edge of the eyelid originating in a lash follicle
____ turning out of the eyelid
____ drooping of the upper eyelid

3. Label the 10 areas in the drawing below by filling in the blanks to the right of the drawing. The 10 areas are to be selected from the words given below the drawing.

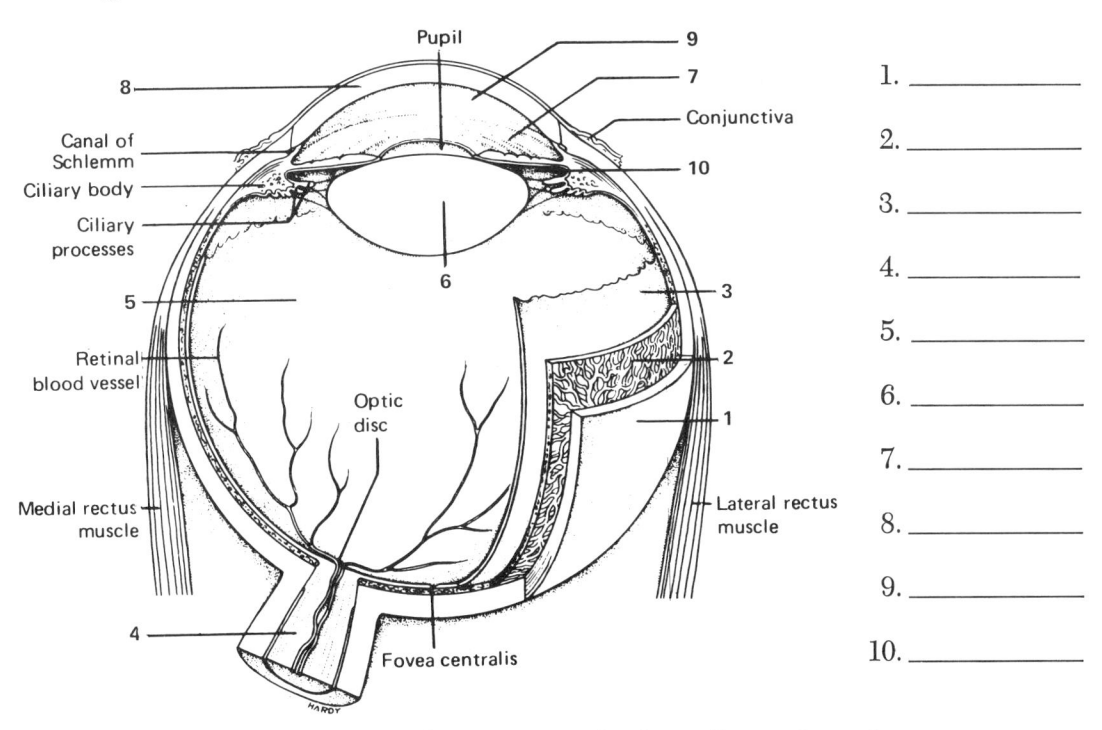

iris   posterior chamber   vitreous body   sclera   choroid

optic nerve   retina   lens   anterior chamber   cornea

1. _____
2. _____
3. _____
4. _____
5. _____
6. _____
7. _____
8. _____
9. _____
10. _____

4. Discuss how the nurse may help the newly blind patient begin to adjust to his immediate environment—that is, the hospital room—when first admitted to the hospital.

_____
_____
_____
_____
_____
_____
_____

5. To suddenly lose one's sight is a tremendous emotional shock. The newly blind person typically reacts with depression to the loss of vision. Name some of the things you have done in the past 24 hours that you could not have done if you had suddenly lost your sight. _____

_____
_____

6. Certain courtesies smooth the way for the blind person and make him feel more comfortable when with sighted individuals. Describe some of the courtesies which should be extended to the blind during social contact. _____

7. All patients with glaucoma, even after surgery, require continued supervision by an ophthalmologist. Give 5 general instructions that should be given to patients with this eye disease.

    1. _____

    2. _____

    3. _____

    4. _____

    5. _____

8. Postoperative care of patients who have had eye surgery must include nursing measures to prevent complications as well as help the patient through the postoperative period. Describe 2 nursing measures particular to the postoperative management of the patient with eye surgery.

    1. _____

    2. _____

9. Hearing loss, especially a total hearing loss, can seriously impair an individual's ability to protect himself. Name 2 common sounds that warn us of danger, yet would not be heard by the deaf.

   1. _____ 2. _____

10. Shouting may not be of value in trying to communicate with the hard of hearing patient. Describe the manner of speech that appears to work best when communicating with the hard of hearing. _____
_____
_____
_____

UNIT FIVE
Threats to adequate respiration

CHAPTER—19

The patient with a disease of the nose or the throat

Disorders of the nose and throat may be as minor as a mild case of laryngitis or a nosebleed, or as serious as cancer of the larynx which requires radical surgery. Nursing management of the patient with cancer of the larynx focuses not only on the physical demands of major surgery, but on the emotional trauma over the loss of one of man's greatest gifts—the gift of speech.

The following questions deal with the contents of Chapter 19.

I. True or false.

Read each statement carefully and place your answer in the space provided.

True 1. The sinuses drain through openings in the turbinate bones of the nose.

True 2. The entire nasal cavity is lined with a highly vascular mucous membrane.

False 3. The function of the sinuses is to provide an area of drainage for the cavities of the skull.

False 4. The olfactory area is contained in the paranasal sinuses.

True 5. The maxillary sinus is most often affected by sinusitis.

True 6. Surgery may be indicated in the treatment of chronic sinusitis with an opening made to provide drainage.

True 7. Nasal polyps are grapelike swellings that obstruct breathing and sinus drainage.

True 8. The supporting framework of the larynx consists of cartilage.

False 9. Those having hoarseness that persists beyond 6 to 8 weeks should seek medical advice as this can be a sign of cancer of the larynx. Seeking advice before this time is not necessary.

True 10. Cancer of the larynx metastasizes at a faster rate than most other cancers.

True 11. A laryngofissure may be performed if cancer of the larynx is detected early and the tumor has not metastasized.

False 12. Following a laryngectomy the patient may receive nasogastric feedings for about 2 weeks after surgery or until such time as he is able to swallow.

True 13. The patient with a permanent tracheal opening can never go swimming and must be careful to prevent water from entering his stoma when taking a shower.

__True__ 14. Patients who have had a tracheostomy without a laryngectomy can speak by covering the opening with their finger.

__True__ 15. A cuffed tracheostomy tube may be used when mechanical ventilation is necessary.

II. Multiple choice questions.

Select the most appropriate answer and place it in the space provided.

1. Sinusitis can lead to serious complications such as __c__.
   - a. headache
   - b. nausea
   - c. spread of infection to the middle ear
   - d. tonsillitis

2. Conditions that predispose to sinusitis are __a__.
   1. allergy
   2. nasal polyps
   3. antritis
   4. sneezing
   - a. 1, 2
   - b. 1, 3
   - c. 2, 3
   - d. 2, 4

3. Nosedrops used too frequently or over a long period of time can result in __a__.
   - a. "rebound" congestion
   - b. sinusitis
   - c. tonsillitis
   - d. bronchiectasis

4. The major complication of nasal surgery is __d__.
   - a. inability to breathe through the nose
   - b. fever
   - c. difficulty swallowing
   - d. hemorrhage

5. Following nasal surgery, the head of the bed is elevated to __B__.
   1. promote more comfortable breathing
   2. make it easier to swallow drainage
   3. decrease edema
   4. decrease nasal congestion
   - a. 1, 2
   - b. 1, 3
   - c. 2, 3
   - d. 2, 4

Clinical Situations

Mr. Carter, age 44, developed hoarseness about 8 months ago but as he was a heavy smoker he attributed this to smoking and did not seek medical advice. Several weeks ago he noted dysphagia in addition to his hoarseness. On advice of a friend he decided to see a physician. After an examination and thorough history, the physician had Mr. Carter admitted to the hospital. He was found to have cancer of the larynx and is scheduled for a laryngectomy and a radical neck dissection.

6. Following surgery Mr. Carter will breathe through __a__.
   - a. his nose or mouth but cannot talk
   - b. his mouth but not his nose
   - c. a tracheal stoma
   - d. a special electronic device

7. Compared to a tracheostomy tube, a laryngectomy tube is __a__.
   - a. shorter and wider
   - b. longer and tapered

8. Patients having had a radical neck dissection usually have less pain than patients with other major surgeries because __d__.
   - a. there are very few sensory nerves in the area of the neck
   - b. they are usually unresponsive the first few days after surgery and therefore feel no pain
   - c. of the edema around the operative site
   - d. sensory nerve endings are severed during surgery

9. To prevent extremes in movement of Mr. Carter's head, the nurse __b c__
   - a. places sandbags on both sides of his head as well as behind his neck
   - b. applies a cervical collar when moving or changing his position

    c. supports his head when moving or changing his position
    d. uses one pillow behind his neck and another behind his shoulders

10. The area around the stoma should be cleaned __B__.
    a. every 4 hours and whenever necessary using sterile water
    b. every 4 hours and whenever necessary using hydrogen peroxide
    c. once per shift
    d. with a normal saline and hydrogen peroxide mixture

11. If drainage catheters have been placed in the surgical incision they are __c__.
    a. covered with sterile dressings which are changed every 4 hours and p.r.n.
    b. connected to drainage bottles which are emptied every 8 hours
    c. connected to suction
    d. sealed with cotton and taped to the surgical dressing

12. Mr. Carter is to have nourishment by way of tube feedings. The temperature should be __B__.
    a. 40 to 50 degrees
    b. 90 to 100 degrees
    c. 100 to 120 degrees
    d. approximately 150 degrees

13. Tube feedings are __A__.
    a. allowed to flow in by gravity
    b. given through a large syringe and pushed through the tube by applying pressure on the barrel of the syringe

14. The tube feeding is followed by __B__.
    a. additional vitamins and minerals in liquid form
    b. approximately 50 ml. of water
    c. approximately 250 ml. of water
    d. 100 ml. of normal saline

15. Mr. Carter is given a pad and pen and has been using them to write notes. One day you notice he seems very depressed and he writes that he did not know his voice loss would be permanent. You know that the surgery *was* explained in detail, but it is most likely __d__.
    a. the sedatives given for his preoperative anxiety prevented him from understanding what was said
    b. the surgery was explained in technical terms
    c. the surgery was explained at the wrong time and should have been explained in the physician's office
    d. he had refused to accept the diagnosis when the physician was explaining the need for radical surgery

    Mrs. Martin, age 29, was admitted to the hospital for an open reduction of a compound fracture of her left ankle. She developed osteomyelitis and was given an antibiotic. After the fourth dose she had an allergic reaction (angioneurotic edema) and due to the severe edema of her face, throat, and tongue, and difficulty in breathing, a tracheostomy was performed.

16. The part of the tracheostomy tube that can be removed by the nurse is __A__.
    a. the inner tube
    b. the outer tube
    c. both of the above
    d. none of the above

17. If Mrs. Martin's outer tracheostomy tube should accidently come out, the nurse should first __b__.
    a. administer oxygen
    b. try to gently reinsert the tube
    c. call the physician
    d. insert the inner tube and if this will not go in, insert the outer tube

18. If the above action is not successful, the nurse would then __c__.
    a. call the physician and in the meantime give oxygen
    b. insert the inner tube
    c. insert a tracheal dilator until the physician arrives
    d. insert the outer tube

103

19. Mrs. Martin has an excessive amount of mucus secretion. This is considered a(n) __D__.
    a. abnormal reaction to the tracheostomy
    b. forewarning of impending tracheal edema
    c. indication of infection
    d. normal reaction to the irritation

20. Proper suctioning technique is absolutely necessary to ensure minimal trauma to the delicate mucous membrane lining of the trachea. When suctioning Mrs. Martin, suction is applied __a__.
    a. only when the catheter is withdrawn
    b. only when the catheter is inserted
    c. anytime the catheter is in the trachea
    d. only when there is mucus

III. Fill-in and discussion questions.

Read each question carefully and place your answer in the space provided.

1. Label the 10 areas identified in the drawing below by filling in the blanks to the right of the drawing. The 10 areas are to be selected from the words given below the drawing.

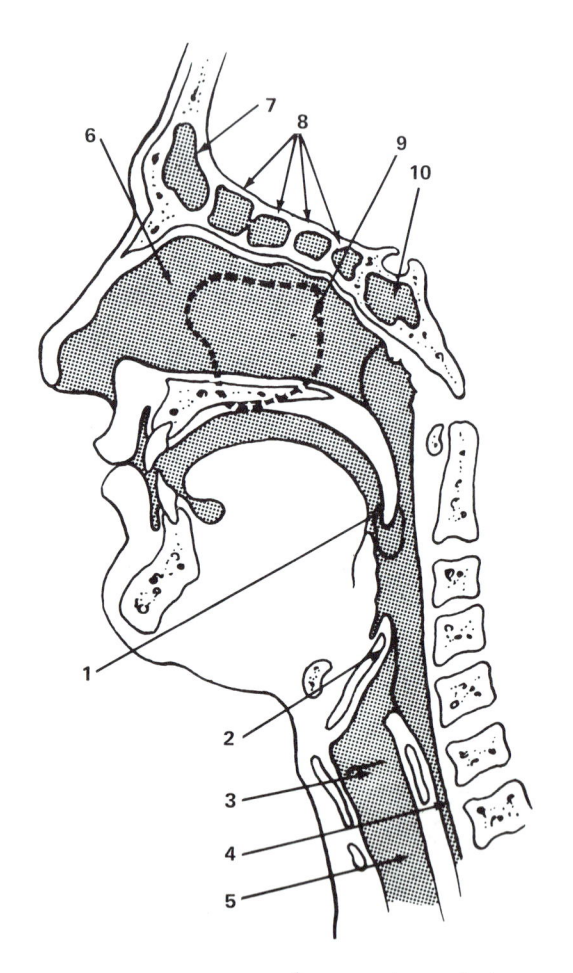

   1. Uvula
   2. Epiglottis
   3. Larynx
   4. Esophagus
   5. Trachea
   6. Nasal septum
   7. Frontal sinus
   8. Ethmoid sinus
   9. Maxillary sinus
   10. Sphenoid sinus

   esophagus   frontal sinus   ethmoid sinus   trachea   uvula

   epiglottis   larynx   maxillary sinus   nasal septum   sphenoid sinus

2. Fill in the blanks of the following questions with the correct word or words that will complete the statement.
   1. The surgery performed for a deviated nasal septum is called a _submucous resection_.
   2. An opening in the inferior meatus to provide sinus drainage is called a(n) _antrotomy_.
   3. The anatomical name for the voice box is _larynx_.
   4. Surgical removal of the larynx is called a _Laryngectomy_.
   5. The medical term for difficulty in swallowing is _____.
   6. An opening into the trachea is called a _tracheostomy_.
   7. The medical term for nosebleed is _Epistaxis_.
   8. Examination of the interior of the larynx with a lighted laryngoscope or with a mirror and external light source is a(n) _Indirect laryngoscopy_.
   9. The structure that closes off the trachea while food or fluid is swallowed is the _epiglottis_.
   10. The total laryngectomy patient may achieve speech by regurgitating swallowed air. This is called _Esophageal_ speech.

3. The exact etiology of cancer of the larynx is unknown, but it is believed that certain factors or conditions may be direct or indirect causes. Name 3 factors or conditions which may be related to the occurrence of this form of cancer.
   1. _Cigarette smoking_
   2. _alcohol_
   3. _industrial pollutants_

4. The permanent loss of one's voice is an extremely traumatic prospect. List any types or forms of communication you performed in the past 24 hours that could not be performed by a patient with a laryngectomy who has not yet learned esophageal speech or does not have an artificial electronic device to produce speech. _Talking, laughing,_

5. Name the 3 parts of a tracheostomy or laryngectomy tube.
   1. _____   3. _____
   2. _____

CHAPTER—20

The patient with acute respiratory disorder

Respiratory infections are the most common type of respiratory disorder. Usually, milder respiratory infections result in unpleasant symptoms and the inconvenience of loss of time from work, school, or social activities. On the other hand, the same illness causing minimal difficulty in most can become a serious illness in the debilitated or chronically ill patient.

One of the most vital needs is a continuous supply of oxygen. Severe disease in the network of the respiratory passages can interfere with the oxygen supply. Because many respiratory conditions can be prevented to a certain extent, the nurse needs to know what causes them to develop, how the severity can be reduced and how to care for the patient who becomes acutely ill.

The following questions deal with the contents of Chapter 20.

I. True or false.

Read each statement carefully and place your answer in the space provided.

True 1. The x-ray examination of the chest is an important test used for the diagnosis of respiratory disorders.

False 2. Bronchoscopy is similar to x-ray and shows the contents of the thoracic cavity.

False 3. There are no complications following a bronchoscopy and the patient can go home immediately after the procedure.

True 4. Arterial blood studies are of importance in the critical and acutely ill patient.

False 5. If the sputum is collected for culture of microorganisms, the container must be thoroughly washed with soap and water before it is given to the patient.

True 6. Gastric contents may be analyzed when tuberculosis is suspected.

True 7. The patient with pneumonia may have considerable difficulty breathing.

False 8. Patients with pneumonia should not be encouraged to cough as coughing causes pain.

True 9. Influenza is a respiratory infection caused by one of several viruses.

True 10. Automobile accidents are a frequent cause of rib fractures and other chest injuries.

II. Multiple choice questions.

Select the most appropriate answer and place it in the space provided.

1. Patients who have had a bronchoscopy are given nothing by mouth for several hours after the procedure because the __D__.
   a. dye used during the procedure usually causes nausea
   b. patient must remain in a head down position for 4 hours and, therefore, cannot eat or drink
   c. patient will be expectorating a copious amount of mucus after the procedure
   d. gag reflex was temporarily abolished with a local anesthetic

2. Bronchography is an x-ray visualization of the __c__.
   a. trachea by means of fluoroscopy
   b. bronchi by means of fluoroscopy
   c. bronchi by means of radiopaque dye
   d. larynx, trachea, and bronchi

3. Pleurisy with effusion is the __a__.
   a. collection of fluid between the pleural layers
   b. inflammation and swelling of the pleura
   c. presence of fluid in the alveoli and bronchioles
   d. collection of fluid in the lung

4. If a great deal of fluid accompanied by respiratory embarrassment would occur in the patient with pleurisy, the fluid may be removed by __c__.
   a. coughing
   b. suctioning
   c. thoracentesis
   d. turning the patient every 2 hours

5. Antibiotic therapy may be prescribed for individuals with a cold __D__.
   a. if they have had repeated colds within a short period of time
   b. if the cold occurs during the typical "cold and flu" season
   c. when the cold lasts more than a week
   d. as a prophylactic measure in those with a tendency to develop secondary infections

6. The usual treatment of rib fractures is __a__.
   a. support of the chest with an elastic bandage or adhesive strapping
   b. application of a cast
   c. administration of antibiotics
   d. application of a sling-type support to the chest and arms to limit motion in the chest and arms

7. Penetrating wounds of the chest are very serious and require immediate first aid because an open wound may __b__.
   a. result in bleeding
   b. permit air to enter the thoracic cavity
   c. cause infection
   d. result in severe pain

8. An important first aid measure in the treatment of penetrating wounds of the chest is __c__.
   a. covering the wound with sterile gauze
   b. giving the patient oxygen
   c. applying an airtight dressing over the wound
   d. relieving pain

9. Following a penetrating wound of the chest, surgery may be necessary to remove or repair injured tissues. This surgery is called a __c__.
   a. thoracentesis
   b. thorectomy
   c. thoracotomy
   d. pneumonectomy

CLINICAL SITUATION

Mrs. Baker, age 53, is brought to the emergency department at 2 A.M. by her husband. Mr. Baker tells the physician that his wife has been ill for several days but is now worse.

After examination, the physician decides to admit Mrs. Baker to a medical unit. An x-ray examination of the chest taken on admission shows bilateral pneumonia.

10. Symptoms of pneumonia usually include __c__.
    1. severe, sharp chest pain
    2. slowing of the pulse
    3. shaking chills
    4. decreased respiratory rate
    5. fever
        a. 1, 2, 4
        b. 1, 3, 4
        c. 1, 3, 5
        d. 2, 3, 4

11. The diagnosis of pneumonia is usually made by __D__.
    1. bronchogram
    2. respiratory function studies
    3. sputum cultures
    4. physical examination, patient history
    5. chest x-ray
        a. 1, 3, 4
        b. 2, 3, 5
        c. 3 only
        d. 3, 4, 5

12. The specific antibiotics for treatment of Mrs. Baker's pneumonia will depend upon the __a__.
    a. sensitivity of the causative organism to the drug
    b. seriousness of the illness
    c. symptoms Mrs. Baker exhibits
    d. cost of the antibiotic

13. To help liquify secretions, the air around Mrs. Baker should be __c__.
    a. cooled
    b. warmed
    c. humidified
    d. dried

14. Mrs. Baker's rectal temperature is 104°F. The physician decides to order hypothermia measures which could include the use of __B__.
    1. tepid sponges
    2. hyperthermia blanket
    3. humidification of the air
    4. aspirin
    5. hypothermia blanket
        a. 1, 2, 3
        b. 1, 4, 5
        c. 2, 3, 4
        d. 2, 4, 5

III. Fill-in and discussion questions.

Read each question carefully and place your answer in the space provided.

1. VOCABULARY. Define the following terms.
    a. bronchoscopy: _insertion of a bronchoscope for visual examination of the trachea & bronchi_
    b. empyema: _pus in the pleural space_
    c. hemothorax: _blood in the pleural space_
    d. pleurisy: _inflammation of the pleura_
    e. pneumothorax: _air in the thoracic cavity_

f. thoracentesis: _entry into the thoracic cavity to remove fluid_

2. Label the 11 areas identified in the drawing below by filling in the blanks to the right of the drawing. The 11 areas are to be selected from the words given below the drawing.

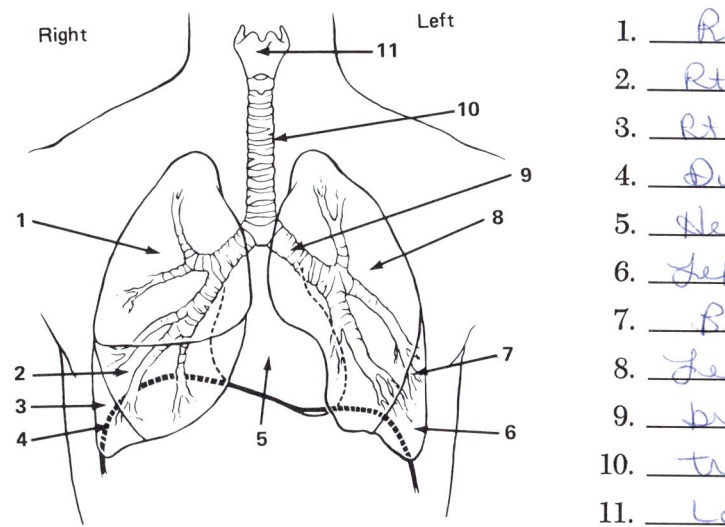

1. Right Upper Lobe
2. Rt. middle Lobe
3. Rt Lower Lobe
4. Diaphragm
5. Heart
6. Left Lower Lobe
7. Bronchiole
8. Left Upper Lobe
9. bronchus
10. trachea
11. Larynx

larynx   bronchiole   left upper lobe   left lower lobe   right upper lobe

bronchiole   middle lobe   heart   trachea   diaphragm   right lower lobe

3. Influenza (also called "flu") has occurred in outbreaks during the fall of the year. Many patients do not require hospitalization and may be treated at home. What is the usual treatment of the influenza symptoms listed below?

SYMPTOMS	TREATMENT
Headache, muscle aching	Aspirin or Acetoaminophen
Easing of dry cough	Steam or cool vapor inhalation
Control of coughing	Codeine or cough medicine
Type of diet	Extra fluids, frequent feedings
Recommended physical activity	Bed rest

4. Sputum samples may be collected on patients with respiratory disease. Briefly answer the following questions about sputum samples.
   1. For a single specimen, when is the sputum sample best taken? _In the Morning, on rising_
   2. Why is mouth care given before a single specimen is obtained? _To remove saliva & old food particles_
   3. What should be included in the notation made on the patient's chart after the sample is obtained? _Color, consistency, odor & amount of sputum_
   4. What type of container may be used to collect a sputum sample? _Waxed sputum cup or wide mouth bottle._

CHAPTER—21

The patient with chronic respiratory disorder

When the usual automatic function of breathing enters awareness and becomes a struggle, a vicious cycle ensues. The dyspneic patient is anxious because he has difficulty breathing and the more anxious he becomes, the more difficult it is for him to breathe. Patients with acute and chronic respiratory diseases experience varying degrees of anxiety. Acute anxiety often makes the patient uncooperative and nursing management difficult. Only through an understanding of the patient's constant struggle for air will the nurse develop the patience and empathy necessary in the care of individuals with acute and chronic respiratory disorders.

The following questions deal with the contents of Chapter 21.

I. True or false.

Read each statement carefully and place your answer in the space provided.

True 1. The more anxious the dyspneic patient becomes, the more difficult it is for him to breathe.

False 2. The most effective treatment of allergic rhinitis is the use of products containing a histamine and an antihistamine.

True 3. Allergic rhinitis is most severe when exposure to the allergen is at its height.

True 4. In a severe asthmatic attack, there may be cyanosis of the lips and nail beds.

False 5. Patients with asthma should limit their fluid intake as excess fluids tend to cause excess bronchial secretions.

True 6. The maintenance of good general health is important in reducing the frequency of asthma attacks.

False 7. Acute bronchitis is not uncommon and rarely spreads to other parts of the respiratory tract such as the trachea or lungs.

True 8. Nursing management of the patient with acute bronchitis is similar to the nursing management of any patient with an acute respiratory disorder.

True 9. The mucosal surface of the tracheobronchial tree is lined with cilia.

True 10. Repeated pulmonary infections can result in an alteration of lung structure.

False 11. In chronic obstructive pulmonary disease the lung surface appears smooth and shiny.

True 12. Chronic obstructive pulmonary disease can often be diagnosed by history alone.

True 13. Individuals with chronic obstructive pulmonary disease have a chronic lung infection.

False 14. Patients with chronic obstructive pulmonary disease can smoke and not damage their lungs as long as they smoke less than one pack of cigarettes per day.

True 15. Bronchopneumonia and chronic sinusitis may be precursors of bronchiectasis.

False 16. Surgery is indicated in all cases of bronchiectasis.

False 17. Except in more advanced cases, surgery is often indicated in the treatment of pneumoconiosis.

False 18. Early diagnosis of cancer of the lung is easily made by chest x-ray and the many early symptoms that clearly pinpoint the disease.

True 19. When the thoracic cavity is opened during surgery the lung collapses.

True 20. Tuberculosis is more common among persons of low social and economic status.

True 21. The tubercle bacilli—the microorganism causing tuberculosis—can be identified by microscopic examination of the sputum and other body fluids.

False 22. Tuberculosis is spread by contact with animals or insects that transmit the disease from person to person.

False 23. The onset of tuberculosis is rapid with a definitive set of signs and symptoms of the disease.

False 24. Every individual with a positive tuberculin test has active tuberculosis.

True 25. Education of the public has helped reduce the incidence of tuberculosis.

II. Multiple choice questions.

Select the most appropriate answer and place it in the space provided.

1. Allergic rhinitis is caused by _a_.
    a. allergy to a specific antigen
    b. any irritating substance found in the air
    c. sneezing
    d. viruses

2. In allergic rhinitis the tissues of the nose swell and there is itching and a watery discharge. These symptoms are caused by _c_.
    a. the irritant directly affecting the nasal mucosa
    b. the localized effect of antihistamines
    c. the immediate release of histamine
    d. mucous cells reacting to an antibody

3. Acute bronchitis is usually viral in origin but still may be treated with antibiotics _a_.
    a. as a prophylaxis against a secondary bacterial infection
    b. to keep the number of viruses to a minimum
    c. as a prevention against the spread of a viral infection to other parts of the body
    d. to increase the body's resistance to infection

4. Cilia play an important role in clearing air passages of mucus and secretions by _d_.
    a. preventing irritants from entering the bronchi and bronchioles
    b. keeping excess tracheal secretions from gravitating into the bronchi and bronchioles
    c. propelling secretions from the trachea to the bronchi and bronchioles where a cough will clear the secretions
    d. propelling excess secretions to the trachea where a cough will raise the secretions

5. Chronic bronchitis is common among those __d__.
   1. who smoke
   2. with recent respiratory infections
   3. with a history of allergy
   4. who live in heavily polluted areas
      a. 1, 2
      b. 1, 3
      c. 2, 4
      d. all of these
6. Medical treatment of chronic bronchitis is generally directed toward the __b__.
   a. prevention of recurrent irritation of the bronchial mucosa
   b. adjustment to a different way of life
   c. clearing the trachea and bronchi of mucus and secretions
   d. keeping the patient symptom-free by eliminating all pollutants and irritants from the environment
7. Postural drainage helps remove secretions by __c__.
   a. increasing the blood supply to the bronchi
   b. increasing pressure in the thoracic cage
   c. gravity
8. The medical management of bronchiectasis may include __d__.
   1. antitussives
   2. antibiotics
   3. humidification of the air
   4. postural drainage
   5. special breathing exercises
      a. 1, 2, 3
      b. 1, 4, 5
      c. 2, 4, 5
      d. 2, 3, 4
9. Treatment of a lung abscess may include __c__.
   1. bronchodilators
   2. surgical drainage of the abscess
   3. expectorants
   4. postural drainage
   5. antibiotics
      a. 1, 2, 5
      b. 1, 3, 4
      c. 2, 4, 5
      d. all of these
10. Unless the physician specifically states otherwise, patients who have had a pneumonectomy are not __b__.
    a. turned on the operative side
    b. turned on the unoperative side
    c. allowed to lie on their backs
    d. allowed in a semi-Fowler's position

Clinical Situations

Mrs. Sinclair, age 34, is brought by ambulance to the emergency department. She began having an asthmatic attack at home and her husband called the rescue squad which gave initial first aid (oxygen) and brought her to the hospital. Mrs. Sinclair has a history of asthma with attacks that are more severe in the spring and summer months.

11. Bronchial asthma is typified by __c__.
    1. fever
    2. wheezing
    3. production of thick, tenacious sputum
    4. cough
    5. dilatation of the bronchi
       a. 1, 2, 5
       b. 1, 3, 4
       c. 2, 3, 4
       d. all of these
12. Treatment of Mrs. Sinclair may include the administration of oxygen. As a nurse you know that __c__.
    a. oxygen is used on all patients with asthma as it relieves bronchospasms and lowers the respiratory rate
    b. oxygen is never used on the asthma patient as it decreases the respiratory rate and raises the CO_2 level in arterial blood
    c. the physician should specify how the oxygen is to be administered and the liter flow to be used

113

13. Mrs. Sinclair is given aminophylline by the intravenous route. While the drug is administered she should be observed for side effects which may include __a__.
    a. hypotension, cardiovascular collapse
    b. hypertension, anxiety
    c. tremors, bradycardia
    d. restlessness, bronchodilatation

14. Mrs. Sinclair is also given epinephrine 1:1000, 0.3 ml. subcutaneously. Some of the side effects she may experience are __a__.
    a. anxiety, tachycardia
    b. hypotension, cardiovascular collapse
    c. bradycardia, dizziness
    d. drowsiness, bronchospasm

15. Mrs. Sinclair has experienced relief with medications and her physician orders isoproterenol (Isuprel) by nebulizer. Instructions regarding the use of a hand-held nebulizer should include, __b__.
    a. "you squeeze the bulb as you exhale"
    b. "while breathing in, the bulb is squeezed"
    c. "the lips must be closed around the nebulizer spout"
    d. "you must be lying down to use the nebulizer"

16. Asthmatic attacks that are prolonged or recur in rapid succession are called __c__.
    a. progressive asthma
    b. successive asthma
    c. status asthmaticus

17. At night, Mrs. Sinclair frequently presses her call light for insignificant reasons such as a sip of water or an adjustment of her covers or pillow. As a nurse you know that she is probably __c__.
    a. afraid of the dark
    b. worried about her family but is afraid to talk
    c. anxious and wants someone to be with her
    d. a demanding patient

Mr. Johnson, an unemployed 56-year-old construction worker, has chronic obstructive pulmonary disease (COPD). He is admitted to the hospital for evaluation of his disease because his general physical condition has deteriorated in the past several months.

18. Mr. Johnson has pulmonary emphysema, a chronic obstructive respiratory disorder. In this disease there are specific morphologic changes in and of the __c__.
    a. bronchi
    b. bronchioles
    c. alveoli
    d. pleura

19. While the exact cause of chronic obstructive pulmonary disease is unknown, many patients have a history of __a__.
    a. chronic bronchitis
    b. pneumonia
    c. tuberculosis
    d. sore throat

20. The first sign of chronic obstructive pulmonary disease is usually __d__.
    a. headache
    b. dry cough
    c. mental confusion
    d. exertional dyspnea

21. Mr. Johnson is given aminophylline in an effort to __d__.
    a. liquify bronchial secretions
    b. reduce coughing episodes
    c. dilate the alveoli
    d. reduce bronchospasm

22. Mr. Johnson coughs frequently and raises thick, tenacious sputum. Drugs or treatments that may be used to enhance the removal of excess secretions include __b__.
    1. expectorants
    2. antitussives
    3. humidity control
    4. postural drainage
    5. air conditioning of the environment
        a. 1, 2, 3
        b. 1, 3, 4
        c. 2, 3, 4
        d. 2, 4, 5

23. Mr. Johnson appears to have some difficulty breathing but his physician states that oxygen should not be given to patients with COPD unless absolutely necessary. The rationale for this statement is that oxygen will __b__.
    a. increase the respiratory rate leading to a decrease in carbon dioxide in the blood
    b. decrease the respiratory rate leading to further retention of carbon dioxide

24. If it becomes necessary to give Mr. Johnson oxygen, it is best given by __b__.
    a. mask at 4 to 6 liters per minute
    b. nasal cannula at 2 to 3 liters per minute
    c. nasal cannula at 6 to 8 liters per minute
    d. mask at 1 to 2 liters per minute

25. In giving encouragement to Mr. Johnson, the nurse should emphasize __b__.
    a. long-range improvement
    b. day-to-day progress

26. Mr. Johnson is to be taught abdominal breathing. When breathing in this manner __a__.
    a. the chest remains still and the abdomen rises and falls with each breath
    b. both the chest and the abdomen move simultaneously
    c. the patient alternates his breathing pattern: first using chest muscles, then abdominal muscles
    d. the abdominal muscles are pulled in while the chest expands

Mr. Davis is a 49-year-old automobile sales manager. As part of a routine physical examination a chest x-ray was taken. The x-ray showed a suspicious area and Mr. Davis is admitted for further examination and diagnostic studies.

27. Mr. Davis' second chest x-ray indicates a possible tumor in the right bronchus. Other diagnostic studies or tests that may be performed include __d__.
    1. biopsy
    2. sputum examination
    3. bronchoscopy
    4. surgical exploration
       a. 1, 2
       b. 1, 3
       c. 2, 4
       d. all of these

28. A diagnosis of bronchiogenic carcinoma has been confirmed and Mr. Davis is scheduled for exploratory surgery. The tumor is small and a right middle lobectomy is performed. One of the *most important* nursing tasks in the postoperative period is __a__.
    a. the maintenance of a patent airway
    b. the administration of oxygen
    c. support of the incision when the patient coughs
    d. turning the patient every 4 hours

29. Dilaudid, a narcotic analgesic, is ordered for Mr. Davis. Before and after administration of this drug it is important to __b__.
    a. check Mr. Davis' surgical dressing
    b. check for respiratory depression
    c. check the narcotic book and take a narcotic count

30. Mr. Davis has two chest catheters—one anterior and one posterior. Each catheter is connected to a separate underwater seal drainage. Each underwater seal consists of two bottles which are positioned as follows: __c__
    a. on a platform 2 to 4 inches below the level of the bed
    b. higher than the level of the bed
    c. never raised from floor level

31. If a break in the drainage system should occur, the nurse should __b__.
    a. place one clamp on the tubing near the bottle
    b. lower the drainage bottles below the level of the bed
    c. raise the drainage bottles above the level of the bed
    d. place a clamp on the tubing as close to the chest wall as possible

32. Failure of the fluid in the glass tubing in the drainage bottle to rise and fall with each inspiration and expiration could mean the chest catheter is plugged or the __a__.
    a. lung has completely re-expanded
    b. drainage system is full
    c. chest catheter is in the pleural space
    d. drainage system is functioning correctly

33. On checking Mr. Davis' chest catheters and surgical dressing you note a small amount of swelling around the catheter where it enters the chest. On palpation you note some crepitation. This is usually considered __a__.
    a. normal
    b. abnormal

Betty Cole, age 24, is being treated for active tuberculosis as an outpatient in the county health department clinic. The diagnosis was confirmed one month ago. The tuberculosis was originally diagnosed during a pre-employment physical which included a chest x-ray.

34. In addition to sputum examination, laboratory diagnosis of tuberculosis may be confirmed by __d__.
    a. blood drawn early in the morning
    b. salivary samples taken after coughing
    c. smears of nasal secretions
    d. gastric fluid obtained by gastric lavage

35. The usefulness of drug therapy in treating Betty Cole lies in a drug's ability to __d__.
    a. halt the growth of tubercle bacilli and destroy all bacilli entering the body
    b. destroy all tubercle bacilli present in the body
    c. stop the tubercle bacillus from being drug resistant
    d. decrease the growth and multiplication of the tubercle bacillus

36. An important aspect of teaching that should be stressed when giving Betty instructions about her drugs is __c__.
    a. what signs the patient looks for to show the drug is effective
    b. an explanation of how the drug works
    c. that the drug must be taken regularly and over a long period of time to be effective
    d. that the drug's effectiveness will depend on her attitude toward treatment

III. Fill-in and discussion questions.

Read each question carefully and place your answer in the space provided.

1. VOCABULARY. Define the following terms.
    a. allergen: *a substance that produces an allergy may be food, inhalant, animal*
    b. allergic rhinitis: *reaction of nasal mucosa to various allergens commonly found in the environment*
    c. attenuated: *to weaken, reduce the virulence of a pathogenic organism.*
    d. bronchitis: *inflammation of the mucous membrane lining of the bronchi*
    e. bronchodilator: *drug producing broncho dilatation or dilatation of the bronchi*

f. bronchospasm: _spasm of the bronchus, thus reducing the lumen & cutting down on the amount of air that can pass thru_

g. bulla (plural, bullae): _a blister or bleb_

h. crepitation: _crackling or grating sound_

i. dyspnea: _labored or difficult breathing_

j. extrinsic: _coming from without_

k. humidification: _supplying moisture to the air_

l. malaise: _a general feeling of discomfort_

m. mucopurulent: _consisting of mucous & pus_

n. suppuration: _the formation of pus_

o. thorax: _the chest cavity_

2. Name 4 possible causes of chronic obstructive pulmonary disease.
   1. _Chronic bronchitis_
   2. _smoking_
   3. _repeated pulmonary infections_
   4. _aging process_

3. The 3 questions below apply to the drawing on the right.

   1. Which tube is connected to the patient, 1 or 2? _2_

   2. As the patient inhales or exhales, the water rises and falls in which tube? _2_

   3. Which tube is open to the atmosphere? _1_

4. The 3 questions below apply to the drawing to the right.

   1. Which tube goes to the patient, 1 or 2? __1__

   2. Which tube is open to the atmosphere, 1 or 2? __2__

   3. Which bottle will contain drainage from the patient, A or B? __A__

5. Name 3 early symptoms of tuberculosis.
   1. _fatigue_
   2. _night sweats_
   3. _anorexia_

6. Why are the symptoms in question 5 misleading and not indicative of tuberculosis?
   Those symptoms can be associated with other causes such as poor nutrition

UNIT SIX
Insults to cardiovascular integrity

CHAPTER—22

The patient with a blood or lymph disorder

Many individuals with disorders of the blood or related disorders are chronically ill; others such as those with leukemia may be acutely ill. Nursing management of patients with blood disorders will frequently require intensive nursing care skills. Many patients with leukemia or Hodgkin's disease are young, which may create a difficult emotional situation for both parents and nursing personnel.

The following questions deal with the contents of Chapter 22.

I. True or false.

Circle either the word true or false given to the right of the statement. If the word false has been circled, make the statement true by changing the underlined word(s) and place your answer in the space provided.

1. A red blood cell that is <u>hypochromic</u> contains less than the normal amount of hemoglobin. — (True) / False

2. When referring to the size of a blood cell, a <u>microcytic</u> cell is larger than a normal cell. — True / (False) — macrocytic

3. Women usually have <u>fewer</u> red blood cells than men. — (True) / False

4. <u>Chronic</u> leukemia has an insidious onset. — (True) / False

5. Patients with idiopathic thrombocytopenic purpura have an <u>increased</u> number of platelets. decreased — (True) / (False)

6. Hemophilia is transmitted from <u>mother</u> to son as a recessive sex-linked characteristic. — True / (False)

7. Polycythemia vera is a disease characterized by a <u>decrease</u> in the production of red blood <u>cells and hemoglobin</u>. — True / (False)

8. Agranulocytosis is a condition characterized by an <u>increased</u> production of white blood cells. — (True) / (False)

121

9. Multiple myeloma is a <u>malignant</u> disease of plasma cells. **True** False

10. Lymphosarcoma is characterized by overgrowth of <u>monocytes</u> in the lymph nodes, spleen, and <u>lymphoid</u> tissues. True **False** — lymphocytes

II. True or false.

Read each statement carefully and place your answer in the space provided.

__T__ 1. Many patients with a blood disorder are prone to bleeding.
__F__ 2. The red color of blood is caused by iron contained in the plasma.
__F__ 3. The body is unable to conserve iron and once red blood cells are broken down the iron is excreted in the feces.
__T__ 4. The treatment of iron-deficiency anemia includes the administration of iron.
__F__ 5. The body requires large amounts of vitamin B_{12}.
__T__ 6. If pernicious anemia is not treated properly, degenerative changes in the nervous system can develop.
__T__ 7. Blood loss, either acute or chronic, can cause anemia.
__T__ 8. Aplastic anemia can occur with the use of certain drugs.
__F__ 9. Leukemia is probably due to a bacterial invasion of the bone marrow.
__T__ 10. With proper therapy, patients with chronic leukemia may live 5 or more years.
__T__ 11. The administration of injections may cause oozing of blood and ecchymosis if the patient is prone to bleeding.
__F__ 12. Even patients with a mild form of hemophilia die before reaching puberty.
__T__ 13. Patients with polycythemia vera should be observed for symptoms of thrombosis.
__F__ 14. Hodgkin's disease is thought to be caused by the inhalation of air pollutants.
__T__ 15. Infectious mononucleosis is a condition that primarily affects lymphoid tissues.

III. Multiple choice questions.

Select the most appropriate answer and place it in the space provided.

1. When studying the formation of blood cells, a specimen is taken of __c__.
    a. arterial blood
    b. venous blood
    c. bone marrow
    d. none of the above

2. Anemia may be defined as a(n) __a__.
    a. decrease in the number of red blood cells and a deficiency of hemoglobin
    b. iron deficiency
    c. decrease in blood cells
    d. loss of blood

3. Individuals living at very high altitudes have a(n) __c__.
    a. increased amount of plasma
    b. decreased number of white cells
    c. increased number of red blood cells
    d. decreased number of red blood cells

4. According to the laboratory results, which patient would not be considered anemic? __d__
    a. patient A: hemoglobin 10.8 Gm.
    b. patient B: hemoglobin 11 Gm.
    c. patient C: hemoglobin 12.3 Gm.
    d. patient D: hemoglobin 14.6 Gm.

5. Old red blood cells are destroyed by the __b__.
    a. platelets
    b. spleen
    c. gastrointestinal tract
    d. white blood cells

6. Each red blood cell survives approximately __d__.
   a. 21 days
   b. 4 weeks
   c. 8 weeks
   d. 120 days

7. Patients with pernicious anemia lack __b__.
   a. vitamin B_{12} in their bone marrow
   b. the intrinsic factor which is found in gastric juices
   c. the extrinsic factor manufactured by cells of the stomach
   d. vitamin B_6 and B_{12} in their diet

8. Pernicious anemia can be controlled by __b__.
   a. diet alone
   b. diet and the administration of vitamin B_{12}
   c. the daily administration of iron
   d. taking iron and a diet containing above average amounts of meat and eggs

9. Treatment of anemia due to blood loss usually includes __c__.
   1. a diet high in iron
   2. replacement of blood by transfusion
   3. correction of the underlying cause
   4. administration of vitamin B_{12}
      a. 1, 2
      b. 1, 3
      c. 2, 3
      d. 2, 4

10. Sickle cell anemia, an example of a hemolytic anemia, occurs chiefly in __b__.
    a. Caucasians
    b. Blacks
    c. Mediterranean inhabitants
    d. American Indians

11. Aplastic anemia is the term used to describe a condition in which __a__.
    a. the activity of the bone marrow is depressed
    b. the bone marrow fails to produce lymphocytes
    c. the bone marrow fails to produce normocytic, hypochromic red blood cells
    d. anemia is present due to a chronic blood loss

12. The objectives of the treatment of aplastic anemia include __a__.
    1. supplying the missing elements of the blood
    2. removal of the causative agent, if known
    3. giving drugs to reverse the anemia process
    4. restoring lost iron by giving oral iron tablets
    5. prevention of infection
       a. 1, 2, 5
       b. 1, 3, 4
       c. 2, 3, 4
       d. 2, 4, 5

13. Normally there are between __c__ and ____ leukocytes per cubic ml. of blood. ____
    a. 2000   4000
    b. 3000   5000
    c. 5000   7000
    d. 8000   12,000

14. Chronic leukemia often begins with __d__.
    a. hemorrhage from the gastrointestinal tract
    b. liver enlargement
    c. neurological symptoms
    d. painless enlargement of one or more lymph nodes

15. If the gums of the leukemic patient bruise easily, oral care can be given with a __c__.
    a. toothbrush
    b. toothpick
    c. moistened cotton applicator
    d. dental floss

16. Purpura results from a(n) __b__.
    1. lack of platelets
    2. lack of red blood cells
    3. abnormality of bone marrow
    4. abnormality of blood vessels
       a. 1, 3
       b. 1, 4
       c. 2, 3
       d. 2, 4

17. Treatment of polycythemia vera includes __a__.
    a. measures to reduce the volume of circulating whole blood
    b. whole blood transfusions
    c. transfusions of platelets
    d. measures to encourage the bone marrow to manufacture more red blood cells

18. Treatment of agranulocytosis includes __a__.
    a. removing the causative factor
    b. administering platelets by transfusion
    c. administering drugs capable of depressing the bone marrow
    d. keeping the patient with other patients to maintain his morale

19. Usually the first symptom(s) of multiple myeloma is __c__.
    a. sores that do not heal
    b. fatigue, weakness, and afternoon temperature elevation
    c. vague bone pain in the pelvis, spine, or ribs
    d. personality change, tendency to bleed

20. Diagnosis of multiple myeloma is made by __d__.
    1. sputum samples
    2. skeletal x-ray examinations
    3. lymph node biopsy
    4. urine samples
        a. 1, 2
        b. 1, 3
        c. 2, 3
        d. 2, 4

21. During discharge teaching, the patient with multiple myeloma must have 2 points emphasized, __a__.
    1. adequate hydration by increasing fluid intake
    2. frequent ambulation
    3. limiting fluids
    4. out of bed only to the bathroom and for meals
        a. 1, 2
        b. 1, 4
        c. 2, 3
        d. 2, 4

22. Treatment of Hodgkin's disease includes __d__.
    1. x-ray therapy
    2. antineoplastic drugs
    3. antibiotics
    4. transfusions
        a. 1, 2
        b. 2, 3
        c. 3, 4
        d. all of these

CLINICAL SITUATION

Tom, age 16, began to complain of fatigue and weakness. One day while at school he told one of his teachers that he was too tired to even walk home. The teacher sent him to the school infirmary. He was seen by the school nurse who called Tom's parents and recommend he visit his physician as soon as possible. Tom's parents took him to their family physician who sent Tom to a laboratory for routine blood work. The following day the physician called Tom's parents and said that the initial studies showed that Tom is acutely ill. Further studies confirmed the physician's suspicions; Tom has acute leukemia.

23. In acute leukemia, symptoms begin abruptly and often coincide with __c__.
    a. taking drugs toxic to the bone marrow
    b. contact with another person who has acute leukemia or some other form of cancer
    c. an acute upper respiratory infection
    d. a urinary tract infection

24. Although the leukemia patient has more leukocytes, he is less able to fight infection because the leukocytes are __a__.
    a. immature and not effective in fighting infection
    b. older and cannot be triggered to fight infection

25. Besides peripheral blood studies, another test performed to establish the diagnosis of leukemia is a __b__.
    a. chest x-ray
    b. bone marrow specimen
    c. urinalysis
    d. bone survey
26. In acute leukemia, anemia is __c__.
    a. rarely present
    b. usually mild
    c. usually severe
27. Treatment for Tom will most likely include __d__.
    1. antibiotics
    2. antineoplastic drugs
    3. blood transfusions
    4. vitamin B$_{12}$ for secondary anemia
    a. 1, 3, 4
    b. 2 only
    c. 2, 3, 4
    d. 1, 2, 3
28. Antineoplastic drugs are used in the treatment of leukemia because they __a__.
    a. interfere with the multiplication of rapidly dividing cells
    b. kill cancer cells
    c. prevent cancer cells from multiplying

IV. Fill-in and discussion questions.

Read each question carefully and place your answer in the space provided.

1. VOCABULARY. Define the following terms.

    a. anemia: *decrease in number of red blood cells & lower than normal hemoglobin*

    b. erythrocytes: *red blood cells*

    c. hemolysis: *destruction of red blood cells*

    d. hyperchromic: *more hemoglobin than normal*

    e. hypochromic: *less hemoglobin than normal*

    f. macrocytic: *larger than normal size red blood cell*

    g. microcytic: *smaller than normal size red blood cell*

    h. normocytic: *normal size of red blood cell*

    i. petechiae: *small hemorrhage spots*

    j. phlebotomy: *removal of blood from a vein*

k. purpura: _small hemorrhage areas in skin, mucous membrane & subcutaneous tissue_

l. splenomegaly: _enlargement of spleen_

m. viscous: _thick_

2. List 3 ways in which red blood cells can be *lost* or *destroyed*.
   1. _Chronic blood loss_
   2. _Rapid blood loss_
   3. _hemolysis_

3. Give 3 typical signs of anemia.
   1. _fatigue_
   2. _pallor_
   3. _weakness_

4. Name the 3 types of white blood cells.
   1. _lymphocytes_
   2. _monocytes_
   3. _granulocytes_

5. Patients with leukemia may or may not know their diagnosis or prognosis. Many physicians prefer to inform their patients of the diagnosis and often—as treatment progresses—the prognosis. Discuss how a patient might feel if he is told he has acute leukemia. Use either an actual nurse-patient experience you may have had or try to relate how you may feel if this were to happen to you.

6. If it is believed a patient is having a transfusion reaction, he should be observed for what signs or complaints?
   1. _hives_
   2. _chills_
   3. _fever_
   4. _dyspnea_
   5. _restlessness_

CHAPTER—23

The patient with heart disease: anatomy; diagnostic tests

People often have intense reactions to the diagnosis of heart disease. They may be frightened because of past experience with a family member, friend, or neighbor. Often, their past experience with heart disease will be compared to what is happening to them at the present. Their fears may be out of proportion to the seriousness of their illness. Frequently, all that is necessary will be for them to follow the physician's advice about slowing down the hectic pace of their lives. Other individuals may choose to ignore a physician's advice believing that nothing can be done for them.

Through proper education, patients can be taught to view their disease correctly and to recognize the importance of following the physician's suggestions and prescribed changes in their life styles. For many of these patients, the results of faithful adherence to a medical regimen will be encouraging.

The following questions deal with the contents of Chapter 23.

I. True or false.

Read each statement carefully and place your answer in the space provided.

__T__ 1. The term "heart attack" has no precise meaning but is often used to refer to a myocardial infarction.

__T__ 2. In the United States, cardiovascular disease is the leading cause of death.

__F__ 3. Blood is pumped out of the heart during diastole.

__T__ 4. Insufficient blood supply to the heart and its arteries is an important factor in some forms of heart disease.

__T__ 5. When filling out a request slip for an ECG, the nurse should enter all drugs taken by the patient on the request slip.

__F__ 6. The preparation for an ECG includes fasting for a minimum of 2 hours.

__T__ 7. The preparation for a vectorcardiogram is the same as for an electrocardiogram.

__F__ 8. There is no special preparation of the patient having an angiocardiogram

__F__ 9. Arteriograms rarely cause discomfort to the patient, and he can ambulate as soon as he returns to his room.

__T__ 10. A cardiac catheterization procedure is not without danger.

II. Multiple choice questions.

Select the most appropriate answer and place it in the space provided.

1. The mitral valve is located between the __b__.
   a. right atrium and right ventricle
   b. left atrium and left ventricle

2. Rectal temperatures may be contraindicated in patients with heart disease as insertion of a rectal thermometer can produce vagal stimulation with consequent __d__.
   a. diarrhea
   b. constipation
   c. tachycardia
   d. bradycardia

3. Fluctuation and especially increase in the daily weight of a cardiac patient is usually indicative of __a__.
   a. edema
   b. an overdose of cardiac drugs
   c. a development of an infection
   d. constipation

4. A vectorcardiogram is usually performed when __d__.
   a. the patient has a cardiac arrest
   b. the patient has been placed on a cardiac monitor
   c. an ECG technician is not available
   d. an ECG shows questionable heart damage

5. The angiocardiogram is used in diagnosing __c__.
   a. presence of edema
   b. abnormalities of the blood vessels in the extremities
   c. abnormalities of the heart and great vessels
   d. variations in heart sounds

6. Dye is injected during an arteriogram. For several minutes after the dye is injected the patient will usually feel __c__.
   a. chilly
   b. very cold
   c. extremely warm
   d. intense pain throughout his entire body

7. Patients having an arteriogram may also develop a headache which is due to __b__.
   a. the dye irritating the sinus membranes
   b. dilatation of cerebral blood vessels
   c. constriction of cerebral blood vessels
   d. a drop in blood pressure

8. A cardiac catheterization is performed to __a__.
   1. measure the pressure in the chambers of the heart
   2. obtain cardiac blood samples for analysis of oxygen and carbon dioxide
   3. determine the location of the mitral valve
   4. measure the amount of blood in all chambers of the heart
      a. 1, 2
      b. 1, 3
      c. 2, 3
      d. 2, 4

III. Fill-in and discussion questions.

Read each question carefully and place your answer in the space provided.

1. VOCABULARY. Define the following terms.

   a. atria (singular, atrium): _upper chambers of the heart_

   b. bradycardia: _slow pulse rate, usually below 60_

   c. Cheyne-Stokes respirations: _irregular resp - shallow that increased in rate & depth then decreased followed by a period of apnea_

d. chordae tendineae: cords which connect edges of atrioventricular valves, to papillary muscles

e. diastole: period of relaxation — atria & ventricals fill

f. electrocardiogram (ECG): graphic recording of the electrical activity going on in the heart.

g. endocardium: Inside lining of the heart that comes in contact c̄ the blood

h. hypoxia: lack of adequate oxygen in inspired air

i. myocardium: Muscle layer of the heart

j. orthopnea: difficulty breathing in any but a sitting or standing position

k. pericardium: outer layer of heart sac

l. systole: Contraction phase of the cardiac cycle

m. tachycardia: rapid pulse rate, usually over 100

n. tachypnea: rapid respiratory rate

o. ventricles: lower chambers of the heart

2. The pulse is an important measurement in the evaluation of a cardiac patient. When the pulse rate is being counted what 2 characteristics should also be noted?
   1. Pulse rhythm
   2. Pulse quality

3. What is a pulse deficit? Numerical difference between apical & radial pulse

CHAPTER—24

The patient with heart disease

Patients with heart failure may be chronically or critically ill. The chronically ill patient has probably been ill for many years, is seen by a physician frequently, has taken many different types of medications and has probably been told to follow a specific diet. The patient with pulmonary edema is an example of a critically ill patient and an acute emergency, for he is literally drowning in his own body fluids. Both critically and chronically ill patients require skilled nursing management—one needing the skills required in an emergency, the other needing the patience and understanding required for the nursing management of the chronically ill.

The following questions deal with the contents of Chapter 24.

I. True or false.

Read each statement carefully and place your answer in the space provided.

_F_ 1. When the patient shows symptoms of heart failure, his condition is described as compensated heart failure.

_T_ 2. The treatment of congestive heart failure involves locating and, if possible, correcting the cause.

_T_ 3. In time, changes in the blood vessels can lead to congestive heart failure by interfering with the blood supply to the heart muscle.

_T_ 4. Excess sodium contributes to the problem of edema by holding water in the tissues.

_F_ 5. Congestive heart failure is only seen in those with arteriosclerotic heart disease.

_T_ 6. Diuretics are drugs that help rid the body of excess fluid.

_F_ 7. The patient with congestive heart failure should be weighed weekly.

_F_ 8. Patients with congestive heart failure do not have their position changed every 2 hours because they are usually too ill for this maneuver.

_F_ 9. When giving fluids to the patient with congestive heart failure, the fluid should be chilled but ice should not be added.

_T_ 10. Diuretics administered intravenously may initiate diuresis in 5 to 10 minutes.

_T_ 11. Salt substitutes may contain potassium which, if taken in excess, could cause cardiac arrhythmias.

_T_ 12. Digitalization is a term used to describe the achievement of a therapeutic effect of digitalis.

_F_ 13. Digitalis preparations are relatively safe drugs with few side effects.

_T_ 14. The relief of the symptoms of pulmonary edema is urgent because the patient can literally drown in his own secretions.

II. Multiple choice questions.

Select the most appropriate answer and place it in the space provided.

CLINICAL SITUATIONS

Mr. Harrison, age 67, is a retired insurance salesman. For the past several years he has been seen by his physician for symptoms of congestive heart failure. Because his symptoms have become more serious, his physician has decided to admit him to the hospital for evaluation of his cardiac status.

1. Heart failure develops when the __c__.
   a. patient reaches middle age
   b. heart meets the demands of the body but the blood pressure is low
   c. heart is unable to meet the demands of the body
   d. patient has had two or more heart attacks

2. Patients with congestive heart failure retain excessive amounts of __c__.
   a. bicarbonate
   b. acid
   c. sodium
   d. urine

3. The *first* symptoms of congestive heart failure that Mr. Harrison noticed were probably __a__.
   a. fatigue, dyspnea
   b. fever, tachycardia
   c. bradycardia, double vision
   d. cyanosis, rash

4. It is noted that Mr. Harrison has pitting edema. Pitting edema __d__.
   a. is found only in the legs
   b. is painful and uncomfortable
   c. occurs when the patient has difficulty breathing
   d. occurs when pressure is exerted and the part pressed becomes indented

5. Dependent edema is edema that __a__.
   a. appears in the ankles and feet after long periods of sitting or standing
   b. occurs when the patient has compensated heart failure
   c. is seen only in left-sided heart failure
   d. cannot be helped with drugs

6. It has been decided to measure Mr. Harrison's central venous pressure. To do this, a catheter is inserted into his __b__.
   a. left ventricle
   b. right atrium
   c. inferior vena cava

7. Normal central venous pressure is __b__.
   a. 0 to 20 cm. of water
   b. 5 to 12 cm. of water
   c. 10 to 50 cm. of water
   d. 10 to 100 cm. of water

8. Treatment for Mr. Harrison will involve __c__.
   a. surgery
   b. measures to reverse the damage to his heart muscle
   c. measures to help his heart function as effectively as possible
   d. the administration of drugs that will completely correct all symptoms of the disease

9. Mr. Harrison's diet will probably be restricted in __d__.
   a. fluids
   b. calcium
   c. potassium
   d. sodium

10. Mr. Harrison has an order for a digitalis preparation—digoxin. Digitalis and related drugs are given to __a__.
    a. slow and strengthen the heart rate
    b. rid the body of edema
    c. decrease the cardiac output
    d. rid the body of excess sodium
11. Oxygen is ordered to be given to Mr. Harrison as needed. Administration of oxygen improves ventilation when oxygenation is impaired by __D__.
    a. refusal of the patient to cough and deep breath
    b. peripheral edema
    c. poor ventilation in the room
    d. congestion and sluggish circulation through the lungs
12. When Mr. Harrison asks if something can be done to stop him from sliding down in bed when the head of the bed is raised, you could __B__.
    a. raise the knee gatch
    b. put a footboard on his bed
    c. put his bed in a flat position
    d. turn him on his side
13. A diuretic is ordered for Mr. Harrison. When patients receive this type of drug they should be observed for __C__.
    a. signs of renal failure and pitting edema
    b. difficulty in breathing and cyanosis
    c. signs of hypokalemia and hyponatremia
    d. signs of hyperkalemia and hypernatremia

Mrs. Graves, age 61, is admitted to the hospital with acute pulmonary edema. She has had heart disease for the past 10 years but has not always followed her physician's advice, taken the medications prescribed for her, or adhered to a low sodium diet.

14. Acute pulmonary edema occurs when there is a weakening of the __b__.
    a. right ventricle
    b. left ventricle
    c. pulmonary artery
    d. pulmonary vein
15. Mrs. Graves has severe dyspnea and orthopnea. She is also raising sputum typical of a patient with pulmonary edema—sputum that is __c__.
    a. mucopurulent
    b. thick and tenacious
    c. frothy and pink-tinged
    d. thin and watery
16. Mrs. Graves' physician orders morphine to be given stat. Morphine is used to __a__.
    a. relieve anxiety and slow the respiratory rate
    b. relieve the pain associated with pulmonary edema
    c. dilate the bronchi
    d. increase the blood flow to the heart
17. Mrs. Graves will be more comfortable __a__.
    a. in a semi-Fowler position
    b. lying on her side
    c. lying prone
18. To relieve Mrs. Graves' hypoxia the physician will order __d__.
    a. Demerol or another non-narcotic analgesic
    b. carbon dioxide inhalations
    c. morphine
    d. oxygen
19. The physician orders rotating tourniquets to be started immediately. The purpose of this procedure is to __d__.
    a. increase arterial pressure
    b. decrease venous pressure
    c. increase venous return to the heart
    d. retard venous return to the heart
20. Rotating tourniquets are applied __c__.
    a. at the ankles and wrists
    b. tightly enough to interfere with arterial blood flow
    c. tightly enough to interfere with venous return
    d. only when the patient appears deeply cyanotic

21. Rotating tourniquets are applied __b__.
    a. to all 4 extremities
    b. to 3 extremities
    c. to 2 extremities
22. Rotating tourniquets are rotated every __b__.
    a. 5 minutes
    b. 15 minutes
    c. 30 minutes
    d. hourly
23. After 8 hours, the physician orders the rotating tourniquet procedure terminated. The procedure that is followed is to remove __c__.
    a. all tourniquets immediately
    b. 2 tourniquets immediately, and the remaining tourniquets in ½ an hour
    c. one tourniquet every 15 minutes
    d. one tourniquet every 45 minutes

III. Fill-in and discussion questions.

Read each question carefully and place your answer in the space provided.

1. Give 2 causes of congestive heart failure.
    1. Rheumatic fever, MI
    2. Inflammation of pericardium, Hypothyroidism

2. Give 3 signs of *Hypo*kalemia.
    1. Muscle cramps, muscle weakness, cardiac arrythmias
    2. postural hypotension, malaise, anorexia,
    3. vomiting, abd distention, thirst, shallow respirations

3. Give 2 signs of *Hypo*natremia.
    1. Oliguria, anuria, decreased skin turgor, hypotension
    2. dry mucous membrane, tachycardia, apprehension.

4. The patient with congestive heart failure should have a thorough explanation of his limitations, restrictions, and physician's orders before he is discharged from the hospital. Give at least 4 general points the nurse should cover during discharge teaching.
    1. Limit salt intake, avoid foods high in sodium
    2. avoid all drugs not prescribed or ordered by doctor
    3. Limit activities as doctor orders
    4. Take daily weights

CHAPTER—25

The patient with inflammatory or valvular disease of the heart

Patients with cardiac disease such as rheumatic fever or rheumatic valvular disease, bacterial endocarditis, or pericarditis share certain commonalities. These disorders are inflammatory and often follow infection elsewhere in the body. The treatment of these diseases is often slow and tedious with the patient requiring long-term medical management.

These diseases are often found in young adults who must forgo their usual job, family, and social responsibilities and often face a loss of income. The young patient may have difficulty handling a prolonged period of inactivity and following the rigid framework of medical treatment.

The following questions deal with the contents of Chapter 25.

I. True or false.

Read each statement carefully and place your answer in the space provided.

__T__ 1. Pericarditis is an inflammatory cardiac disease.

__F__ 2. Rheumatic fever rarely causes permanent damage to the heart or its valves.

__T__ 3. Sometimes the symptoms of rheumatic fever are so mild the disease may escape detection.

__T__ 4. Rest is very important during the active stage of rheumatic fever.

__F__ 5. The mitral valve lies between the right atrium and the right ventricle.

__F__ 6. All patients with mitral stenosis are suitable candidates for mitral valve surgery.

__T__ 7. In mitral insufficiency the wall of the left ventricle usually becomes distended.

__T__ 8. In older patients, aortic stenosis may be caused by arteriosclerosis

__T__ 9. Prevention of streptococcal infections in rheumatic fever patients is very important because every new infection carries the risk of a recurrence of the disease.

__F__ 10. Almost every patient with rheumatic fever develops permanent heart damage.

__T__ 11. Patients whose heart valves have been damaged are susceptible to bacterial endocarditis.

__T__ 12. Any patient with damaged heart valves should have antibiotics before and after any event that might cause bacteremia.

134

II. Multiple choice questions.

Select the most appropriate answer and place it in the space provided.

1. Rheumatic fever is an inflammatory cardiac disease usually found in those between the ages of __a__.
   a. 5 and 15
   b. 15 and 30
   c. 30 and 45
   d. 40 and 70

2. Rheumatic heart disease refers to the __d__.
   a. symptoms that persist for 5 or more years after the disease
   b. heart murmur that may be found when the patient reaches adulthood
   c. cardiac symptoms of rheumatism
   d. cardiac manifestations of rheumatic fever

3. Although the precise cause of rheumatic fever is unknown, it is believed to be related to __c__.
   a. any bacterial infection
   b. a staphylococcus infection
   c. a streptococcus infection
   d. upper respiratory infections that are viral in origin

4. Laboratory tests that may be used to diagnose rheumatic fever include __a__.
   1. sedimentation rate
   2. antistreptolysin O titer
   3. prothrombin time
   4. Lee-White clotting time
   a. 1, 2
   b. 2, 3
   c. 3, 4
   d. all of these

5. Drugs that may be used to relieve the symptoms of rheumatic fever include __d__.
   1. narcotics
   2. salicylates
   3. antineoplastic drugs
   4. corticosteroids
   a. 1, 2
   b. 1, 4
   c. 2 only
   d. 2, 4

6. The valves between the atria and the ventricles prevent the __a__.
   a. blood from flowing back into the atria each time the ventricle contracts
   b. blood from flowing into the ventricle each time the atria contracts

7. The aortic valve __a__.
   a. prevents blood pumped into the aorta from flowing back toward the heart
   b. prevents blood pumped from the ventricle from flowing into the aorta

8. Endocarditis usually leads to __b__.
   a. inflammation of the chordae tendineae without permanent damage to the heart
   b. permanent scarring and deformity of the heart valves, particularly the mitral and aortic valves
   c. scarring of the pulmonary valve
   d. inflammation of the middle layer of the heart

9. The most common aftermath of rheumatic fever is __c__.
   a. aortic stenosis
   b. endocarditis
   c. mitral stenosis
   d. stenosis of the pulmonary valve

10. Insufficiency of a valve means it does not __d__.
    a. open properly
    b. push blood into heart chambers
    c. propel blood out of heart chambers
    d. close properly

11. In which person might bacterial endocarditis become a strong possibility? __b__
    a. a patient with infectious hepatitis
    b. a heroin addict
    c. those with severe upper respiratory infections
    d. people with a history of thrombosis

135

12. The treatment of bacterial endocarditis will include __a__.
    a. large doses of the antibiotic to which the organism is sensitive
    b. the administration of the only effective drug—penicillin
    c. having the patient drink excess fluids to mechanically remove bacteria
    d. a low sodium, low carbohydrate diet
13. Acute pericarditis can result in a collection of fluid in the __c__.
    a. myocardium
    b. endocardium
    c. pericardial space
    d. ventricle
14. If there is fluid in the pericardial sac the physician may __d__.
    a. order postural drainage
    b. order IPPB treatments
    c. place the patient on anticoagulants
    d. perform a pericardial paracentesis

III. Fill-in and discussion questions.

Read each question carefully and place your answer in the space provided.

1. VOCABULARY. Define the following terms.
    a. bacteremia: _bacteria in the blood_
    b. chorea: _uncontrollable, uncoordinated purposeless movement_
    c. familial: _occurring or affecting members of a family_
    d. myocarditis: _Inflammation of the myocardium_
    e. pericarditis: _Inflammation of the pericardium_
    f. polyarteritis: _arthritis in several joints_
    g. stenosis: _narrowing_
    h. tamponade: _pressure or compression of a part of an organ_

2. Give 3 important points of nursing management to be considered when a patient is receiving antibiotics by intramuscular injection for a long period of time, for example, the patient with bacterial endocarditis.
    1. _Give on time, as ordered_
    2. _rotate sites_
    3. _observe for allergic reaction_

CHAPTER—26

The patient with cardiovascular disease: coronary artery disease; functional heart disease; hypertension

The myocardium has its own blood supply through a system of coronary arteries. Blood flows through these vessels and through branches over the surface of the heart, then into smaller arteries and capillaries in the cardiac muscle and finally to the systemic circulation through the coronary veins. Disease of these coronary arteries produces a variety of symptoms, the first of which is usually angina pectoris. Angina pectoris serves as a warning that the myocardium is not receiving enough blood.

Hypertension is a cardiovascular disease in that generalized arteriosclerosis usually results in hypertension, and hypertension can result in damage to the heart and hasten atherosclerotic heart disease.

The following questions deal with the contents of Chapter 26.

I. True or false.

Read each statement carefully and place your answer in the space provided.

_T_ 1. The myocardium receives its blood supply from the coronary arteries.

_T_ 2. Usually there are 2 main coronary arteries, a right and a left.

_T_ 3. In patients with coronary artery disease, the development of collateral circulation in the coronary arteries is of critical importance in the survival of myocardial tissue.

_F_ 4. Unlike other arteries of the body the coronary arteries do not undergo degenerative changes.

_T_ 5. Coronary artery disease is due to multiple causative factors rather than a single cause.

_T_ 6. Attacks of angina are usually over in 5 minutes or less.

_F_ 7. A coronary occlusion results from a clot in a coronary vessel breaking loose.

_T_ 8. Nitroglycerin may be used to relieve attacks of angina that do not disappear quickly with rest.

_F_ 9. Vasodilating drugs cannot be used to prevent anginal attacks.

_T_ 10. There may be an association between smoking and heart disease. Therefore, patients with

137

heart disease should stop smoking.
- _T_ 11. Some patients with angina may find that their symptoms remain the same for years.
- _T_ 12. Symptoms associated with heart disease can also be caused by anxiety.
- _F_ 13. Normally the walls of the aorta are inelastic, to prevent pressure on the contents of the thorax by the forceful flow of blood through this large vessel.
- _T_ 14. Blood pressure can normally fluctuate with a change in position or posture.
- _T_ 15. Death from malignant hypertension usually results from damage to the heart, brain, and kidneys.
- _F_ 16. Heredity does not play a role in the development of primary hypertension.
- _T_ 17. Obese people have a higher incidence of hypertension than those of normal weight.
- _F_ 18. Patients with hypertension should never be taught to take their own blood pressure since this will usually increase their anxiety and concern about their disease.
- _F_ 19. When the nurse is taking the blood pressure of a patient with known hypertension, she should not tell him his blood pressure, because patients should not be aware of their condition.
- _T_ 20. Treatment of secondary hypertension includes the removal of the cause, if possible.

II. Multiple choice questions.

Select the most appropriate answer and place it in the space provided.

1. The coronary arteries originate from the _c_.
   a. aortic arch near the subclavian artery
   b. carotid arteries
   c. aorta, immediately above the aortic valve
   d. myocardium

2. The young individual who has not had the opportunity to develop collateral circulation of his myocardial blood supply has a greater chance of _c_.
   a. becoming acutely ill from a coronary occlusion
   b. developing atherosclerosis
   c. dying instantly following a coronary occlusion
   d. developing angina

3. The pathologic change which is usually responsible for coronary disease is _a_.
   a. atherosclerosis
   b. angina pectoris
   c. development of collateral circulation
   d. a coronary thrombosis

4. The symptoms of coronary artery disease result from _a_.
   a. an insufficient supply of blood to the myocardium
   b. exercise, stress
   c. emotional instability
   d. dilatation of the coronary arteries

5. When myocardial ischemia and the resulting pain are fleeting, the condition is called _d_.
   a. coronary thrombosis
   b. myocardial thrombosis
   c. cardiac arrest
   d. angina pectoris

6. A sudden loss of blood supply to a portion of the myocardium from an occluded coronary artery may lead to necrosis of that part of the myocardium. This area of necrotic tissue is called _d_.
   a. coronary sclerosis
   b. coronary insufficiency
   c. a myocardial occlusion
   d. a myocardial infarction

7. The chief symptom of myocardial ischemia is _d_.
    a. dyspnea
    b. cyanosis
    c. diaphoresis
    d. pain

8. Anginal pain is a warning that the _b_.
    a. coronary artery is dilated
    b. myocardium is not receiving enough blood
    c. coronary artery is sclerotic
    d. myocardium is infarcted

9. The pain of angina usually subsides _b_.
    a. in 20 to 30 minutes
    b. as soon as the patient rests
    c. in 30 to 45 minutes
    d. as soon as the patient learns to forget about his pain

10. A drug often used to relieve attacks of angina is _c_.
    a. meperidine (Demerol)
    b. aspirin
    c. nitroglycerin
    d. morphine

11. To prevent an attack when he is about to undertake an activity that usually causes angina, the patient may _d_.
    a. sit down and rest before the activity
    b. rest after the activity
    c. take an analgesic
    d. take nitroglycerin

12. Surgery may be attempted to correct the pathology caused by diseases of the blood vessels that serve the heart muscle. Basically, the techniques usually used involve a _a_.
    a. bypass of the diseased portion of the artery
    b. removal of the diseased conorary artery
    c. anastomosis of the diseased coronary artery to a healthy coronary artery

13. The treatment of functional heart disease may involve _b_.
    a. talking to the patient and telling him his disease is due to a mental rather than a physical problem
    b. gradually helping the patient understand that his symptoms may be due to anxiety
    c. not providing symptomatic relief until the patient accepts his problem

14. Systolic blood pressure is determined by the _c_.
    a. size of the left ventricle and its ability to eject blood into the pulmonary circulation
    b. pressure exerted by the blood against the wall of the aorta
    c. rate and volume of ventricular ejection and the ability of the aorta to distend
    d. ability of the heart to pump blood

15. Diastolic blood pressure is the pressure recorded _b_.
    a. after the mean arterial pressure
    b. during the period of ventricular relaxation
    c. during the period of ventricular contraction
    d. after atrial contraction

16. Pulse pressure is the _a_.
    a. numerical difference between the systolic and diastolic pressures
    b. pressure of blood against the wall of an artery
    c. numerical difference between the arterial and venous pressure
    d. pressure of blood against the wall of the aorta

17. Arterial pressure is regulated by the __b__.
    1. cerebral cortex
    2. kidneys
    3. endocrine glands
    4. cerebellum
    5. autonomic nervous system
        a. 1, 2, 3
        b. 2, 3, 4
        c. 2, 3, 5
        d. 5 only

18. A person having a sustained systolic pressure of __a__ mm. Hg or above and a sustained diastolic pressure of __a__ mm. Hg or above is usually considered hypertensive.
    a. 150   90
    b. 180   110
    c. 200   100
    d. 250   100

19. The term malignant hypertension is used to describe hypertension __c__.
    a. due to a malignancy
    b. due to a tumor of the adrenal glands (pheochromocytoma)
    c. that has an abrupt onset, followed by severe symptoms and complications
    d. associated with pregnancy

20. Many of the drugs used in the treatment of hypertension __b__.
    a. dilate the larger arteries such as the aorta
    b. relax constricted arterioles so that peripheral resistance is reduced
    c. work directly on the peripheral nervous system
    d. depress higher brain centers

21. Patients taking antihypertensive drugs may note side effects early in therapy. One side effect associated with a change in position is __d__.
    a. a sudden hypertensive episode
    b. blanching of the extremities
    c. flushing and a feeling of warmth
    d. postural hypotension

22. The treatment of secondary hypertension is aimed at __c__.
    a. a plan of lifelong control of the problem including diet, weight reduction, and drug therapy
    b. finding the drug(s) which will control the hypertension
    c. removing the cause, if possible
    d. changing the patient's lifestyle

23. For the cardiac patient, rehabilitation means __b__.
    1. evaluating how much and what kind of activity the patient's heart will allow him to do
    2. learning what he cannot do before learning what he can do
    3. learning to take the good with the bad
    4. helping him live as fully and contentedly as possible within his limitations
        a. 1, 2
        b. 1, 4
        c. 2, 3
        d. 2, 4

III. Fill-in and discussion questions.

Read each question and place your answer in the space provided.

1. Coronary artery disease is thought to be caused by many factors. List 6 factors which may increase the risk of coronary artery disease.
    1. Sex
    2. Heredity
    3. Obesity
    4. Diet
    5. Hypertension
    6. Smoking

2. Attacks of angina may demonstrate a variety of characteristics. Briefly describe the typical as well as the varieties of anginal pain. _Heavyness in chest, pain in chest that radiates to arms, or jaw, elbows. Indigestion_

3. Hypertension is divided into 2 main categories. Name these 2 categories and give the etiology of each.

TYPE OF HYPERTENSION	ETIOLOGY
1. Essential (Primary)	150/90 unknown
2. Malignant	

4. Although some patients will have no symptoms, others may experience a variety of symptoms of hypertension. List 4 symptoms that may be experienced by the patient with hypertension.
   1. Morning headache
   2. Dizzyness
   3. Fatigue
   4. Malaise

CHAPTER—27

The patient with peripheral vascular disease: thrombosis and embolism

The term *peripheral vascular disease* refers to diseases of the blood vessels supplying the extremities. Whether the disease involves the veins, arteries, or lymphatics or all three, patients with peripheral vascular disease experience similar problems. Pain is common, but the type of pain may vary.

The long-term nature of peripheral vascular disease is discouraging. Treatment is tedious, sometimes painful, and not always successful. The patient may require long hospitalization and/or an extended period of convalescence and limitation of activities at home.

The following questions deal with the contents of Chapter 27.

I. True or false.

Read each statement carefully and place your answer in the space provided.

__T__ 1. Pain is a symptom commonly seen in patients with a peripheral vascular disease.

__F__ 2. Leg pain caused by peripheral vascular disease is severe pain and, therefore, these patients are given narcotics.

__F__ 3. Excessive vasodilatation can result in ischemia.

__T__ 4. Atherosclerosis is the gradual occlusion of the lumen of an artery by fatty deposits.

__F__ 5. Trophic changes are changes in the blood vessels.

__T__ 6. Warm gloves and socks provide extra warmth to an extremity and, therefore, may increase the blood supply to an area.

__F__ 7. Exercise is not allowed for persons with peripheral vascular disease.

__T__ 8. Patients with peripheral vascular disease are vulnerable to infection.

__F__ 9. Raynaud's disease is more common among men than women.

__T__ 10. If Raynaud's disease becomes severe and of long duration, trophic changes may occur.

__F__ 11. Smoking is contraindicated in patients with Raynaud's disease because it causes vasodilatation.

__F__ 12. Buerger's disease is more common among women.

__T__ 13. Patients with Buerger's disease may develop gangrene which may necessitate the amputation of an extremity.

_F_ 14. Arteries in the extremities have valves that keep blood flowing in one direction only.
_T_ 15. There may be a familial tendency toward varicose veins.
_T_ 16. Varicose veins are made worse by anything that causes constriction or pressure on the legs.
_T_ 17. The treatment of varicose veins is usually surgical.
_F_ 18. Varicose ulcers, while unsightly, are not painful.
_T_ 19. Venous stasis can lead to the development of thrombophlebitis.
_T_ 20. Anticoagulant drugs may be ordered for the patient with thrombophlebitis.
_T_ 21. A lung scan may be performed to diagnose and locate the site of a pulmonary embolism.
_T_ 22. The middle layer of an artery is called the media.
_T_ 23. Aneurysms are treated surgically whenever possible since there is no other cure for this problem.
_F_ 24. Presence of back pain following repair of an abdominal aortic aneurysm is not serious and is usually referred pain from the incision.

II. Multiple choice questions.

Select the most appropriate answer and place it in the space provided.

1. Changes that may occur in an ischemic part if the diminished blood supply is severe and persistent will include __d__.
   1. coldness
   2. pallor
   3. redness
   4. cyanosis
   5. pain
      a. 1, 2, 4
      b. 1, 4, 5
      c. 2, 3, 5
      d. all of these

2. The flow of blood to an extremity that is affected by peripheral vascular disease can be increased by __a__.
   a. placing the extremity in a dependent position
   b. elevating the extremity
   c. wearing elastic stockings
   d. keeping the extremity quiet

3. Blood supply to an extremity affected by peripheral vascular disease can be increased by an interruption of sympathetic stimuli, which is accomplished by __a__.
   a. the administration of drugs
   b. keeping the extremity elevated
   c. applying warm soaks
   d. keeping the patient on bed rest

4. Vasoconstriction, which must be avoided in peripheral vascular disease, can be caused by __a__.
   a. smoking
   b. exposure to heat
   c. walking
   d. drinking alcohol

5. Atherosclerotic plaques __a, d__
   a. erode the inner wall of the artery, ultimately causing rupture
   b. are deposited in the middle or muscular layer of the artery
   c. pose no danger to the young individual
   d. gradually reduce the size of the lumen of arteries

6. Buerger-Allen exercises involve __a, c__
   a. walking slowly and increasing speed until pain is noted
   b. brisk walking and jogging
   c. a raising and lowering of the legs to promote circulation
   d. sit-up exercises combined with 15 minute walks

7. A complication of peripheral vascular disease is __d__.
   a. fatigue
   b. anemia
   c. cool extremities
   d. leg ulcers

8. To lessen the pain of peripheral vascular disease the nurse should __d__.
   1. place the legs in a dependent position
   2. cool the extremities with ice packs to relieve burning
   3. place a blanket roll under the knees
   4. elevate the legs 45°
      a. 1, 2
      b. 2, 3
      c. 3, 4
      d. 1 only

9. Varicose ulcers usually appear __b__.
   a. anywhere on the leg
   b. on the lower leg over a vein
   c. in the heel area
   d. on or near the toes and instep

10. The treatment of varicose ulcers may include __d__.
    1. administration of vasodilating drugs
    2. application of a gelatin paste boot
    3. treatment of the varicose veins that led to the ulcer
    4. a low sodium diet
    5. removal of the cause
       a. 1, 2, 5
       b. 1, 3, 4
       c. 2, 3, 4
       d. 2, 3, 5

11. All patients who are unable to walk about should have leg exercises while in bed to prevent __a__.
    a. thrombophlebitis and phlebothrombosis
    b. varicose veins
    c. peripheral ischemia
    d. thromboangiitis obliterans

12. Patients susceptible to thrombophlebitis are __d__.
    1. the elderly
    2. patients with infections
    3. those with heart disease
    4. patients who are dehydrated
       a. 1, 2
       b. 1, 3
       c. 2, 3
       d. all of these

13. Thrombophlebitis and phlebothrombosis can be prevented by __a__.
    a. changing position frequently and exercising the legs
    b. taking vasodilating drugs and wearing support hose
    c. stopping smoking and adhering to a low sodium diet

14. A patient with thrombophlebitis complains of a cramp in her leg and asks if someone could massage her leg to relieve the spasm. You would __b__.
    a. massage the leg
    b. not massage the leg

15. The reason you took the nursing action in question 14 is __b__.
    a. the pain of a leg cramp leads to anxiety which has a profound effect on the cardiovascular system; therefore, the leg cramp should be relieved by massage
    b. massage might dislodge a clot and result in an embolism; therefore, the leg should not be massaged

16. When an embolus suddenly occludes a large artery in an extremity, the extremity will __c__.
    1. be a deep red color
    2. appear white and be devoid of color
    3. be extremely painful
    4. feel cold
    5. feel warm
       a. 1, 2, 4
       b. 1, 3, 5
       c. 2, 3, 4
       d. 3 only

17. Initial care of the patient with an embolus in an extremity may include __b__.
    1. keeping the extremity warm
    2. keeping the extremity cool
    3. elevating the extremity
    4. placing the extremity in a dependent position
       a. 1, 3
       b. 1, 4
       c. 2, 3
       d. 2, 4

18. Predisposing conditions to pulmonary embolism are __d__.
    1. prolonged bed rest
    2. fracture or trauma to the lower extremities
    3. recent surgery
    4. thrombophlebitis and phlebothrombosis
    5. the postpartum state
       a. 1, 2, 5
       b. 1, 3, 4
       c. 2, 3, 4
       d. all of these

19. Symptoms of a pulmonary embolism include __b__.
    1. hemoptysis
    2. bradycardia
    3. Cheyne-Stokes respirations
    4. chest pain
    5. dyspnea
       a. 1, 2, 3
       b. 1, 4, 5
       c. 2, 3, 4
       d. all of these

20. The patient with a pulmonary embolism may receive drug therapy which may include __a__.
    a. heparin
    b. antitussives
    c. vasodilators
    d. narcotics to depress the cough reflex

21. An aneurysm of a blood vessel occurs when the __a & c__.
    a. wall of the blood vessel is repeatedly traumatized resulting in a tearing of the intima
    b. intima and media become rigid
    c. elasticity of the vessel is weakened by disease or trauma

22. Patients should deep breathe and cough after surgery; however, patients having a revascularization procedure __c__.
    a. should be encouraged to support their incision with a pillow
    b. must not cough or deep breathe after surgery
    c. should not have support of their incision unless this measure is approved by the physician

CLINICAL SITUATIONS

Mr. Gavin, age 67, has had Buerger's disease for the past 20 years. Because of the severity of the disease he had to retire early, at age 60.

23. Buerger's disease is a(n) __a__.
    a. inflammation of blood vessels and formation of clots and fibrosis of arteries
    b. disease primarily of veins with the formation of atherosclerotic plaques
    c. narrowing of arteries or veins secondary to an infection around or near the blood vessels

24. Symptoms of Buerger's disease include __b__.
    1. intermittent claudication
    2. pale extremities
    3. cold extremities
    4. trophic skin changes
    5. pain that disappears with exercise
       a. 1, 2, 3
       b. 1, 3, 4
       c. 2, 3, 5
       d. 2, 4, 5

25. Mr. Gavin had been a heavy smoker for years. He finally gave up smoking 5 years ago. He asks you what would happen if he began smoking again. As a nurse you know that the resumption of smoking leads to __c__.
    a. the chance of developing a malignancy in the affected areas
    b. further damage to the arteries and arterial dilatation
    c. an exacerbation of the disease

26. Treatment for Mr. Gavin will include __b__.
    1. keeping his extremities warm
    2. special exercises
    3. long walks
    4. a low sodium diet
    5. avoiding prolonged periods of standing
        a. 1, 2, 3
        b. 1, 2, 5
        c. 1, 4, 5
        d. 1, 3, 4

27. Drugs that may be used to treat the narrowing of the patient's arteries are __b__.
    a. adrenergic drugs
    b. adrenergic-blocking drugs
    c. cholinergic drugs
    d. muscle relaxants

28. If Mr. Gavin's legs are elevated, this would __b__.
    a. decrease his pain
    b. increase his pain

29. Surgery may ultimately be considered if drugs do not relieve the vasospasm. The surgery performed would be a(n) __a__.
    a. sympathectomy
    b. parasympathectomy
    c. arterectomy
    d. venous resection

Diane Parsons, age 22, has been having increasing pain in her fingertips for the past several months. She finally seeks the advice of her physician who diagnoses the problem as Raynaud's disease.

30. The patient with Raynaud's disease may experience an attack of arterial constriction when __a__.
    a. exercising
    b. exposed to warm temperatures
    c. resting
    d. exposed to cold temperatures

31. When Diane has an attack, her hands become __a__.
    a. cold, blanched, wet with perspiration
    b. warm, red, numb
    c. swollen, cool, dry

32. As Diane's disease progresses, she may have trophic changes of the fingers, which may include __b__.
    a. thickening of the nails
    b. ulcers and superficial gangrene
    c. discoloration of the palms
    d. brown spots on the palms and fingernails

33. Diane asks her physician if surgery is performed for Raynaud's disease. He tells her that surgery may be performed in some cases and it is called a __c__.
    a. release of a vascular occlusion
    b. parasympathectomy
    c. sympathectomy
    d. arterial bypass

Mrs. Wagner, a 36-year-old housewife and mother of two has had varicose veins for several years. The varicose veins first appeared during her second pregnancy. She has not sought treatment for her problem.

34. Varicose veins occur because of __c__.
    a. inflammation of the veins due to irritation
    b. heavy smoking, lifting heavy objects
    c. incompetency of the valves in the veins
    d. blood clots in the venous system

35. Symptoms of varicose veins include __d__.
    1. red streaking along the pathway of the vein
    2. tired, heavy feeling in the legs
    3. swollen, tortuous veins
    4. edema of the legs
    5. fever
        a. 1, 2, 3
        b. 1, 4, 5
        c. 2, 3, 5
        d. 2, 3, 4

36. Mrs. Wagner decides to have surgery for her varicose veins and is admitted to the hospital. She is scheduled for surgery tomorrow morning. An important aspect of the postoperative treatment of patients with varicose veins is __b__.
    a. complete bed rest for 72 hours
    b. early ambulation
    c. raising the head of the bed higher than the foot to prevent bleeding
    d. keeping the patient prone the first 12 hours after surgery

37. The name of the surgery performed on Mrs. Wagner is a(n) __c__.
    a. veinectomy
    b. arterectomy
    c. vein ligation and stripping
    d. arterial ligation and plication

38. Discharge teaching for Mrs. Wagner should include which of the following facts? __b__
    1. it is best to avoid prolonged periods of standing in one area
    2. varicose veins tend to recur in the same vein if the physician's advice is not followed
    3. if possible, the legs should be elevated when sitting
    4. vasodilating drugs and anticoagulants will need to be taken the rest of her life
        a. 1, 2
        b. 1, 3
        c. 2, 4
        d. all of these

III. Fill-in and discussion questions.

Read each question and place your answer in the space provided.

1. VOCABULARY. Define the following terms.
    a. embolism: *a clot carried in the blood stream from one area to another*
    b. intermittent claudication: *pain caused by ischemia, usually in calves, relieved by resting*
    c. lymph: *colorless fluid circulating in the lymphatic system*
    d. lymphedema: *accumulation of tissue fluid due to obstruction of lymph vessels*
    e. phlebothrombosis: *presence of clots in vein with little or no inflammation*
    f. stasis: *stagnation, stoppage of flow*
    g. thrombophlebitis: *inflammation of a vein*

h. thrombosis: _blood clot inside blood vessel_

2. Explain why the long-term nature of peripheral vascular disease is discouraging for many patients. _____

3. It is important for the patient with peripheral vascular disease to understand how to care for himself and thoroughly understand the importance of certain health measures. In the column on the left are areas that should be covered when teaching the patient. In the space at the right describe the points to be covered.

Feet	
Toenails	
Corns, calluses	
Shoes	
Socks, stockings	
Garters	
Standing	

4. List 5 symptoms of thrombophlebitis
    1. Swelling
    2. Redness
    3. Warmth
    4. Pain
    5. Fever

5. Give 3 causes of lymphedema
    1. Burns
    2. Excessive Radiation
    3. _____

6. A patient has surgery for the removal of an embolus occluding a major artery in his leg. What observations or tasks are performed to check circulation in the operated extremity? Color, temp, peripheral pulses

UNIT SEVEN

Disturbances of ingestion, digestion, absorption, and elimination

CHAPTER—28

Introduction, diagnostic tests, functional disorders

Patients with disorders of the gastrointestinal functions have a wide variety of health problems. The similarities among these patients involve disturbances in ingesting, digesting, and absorbing nutrients and eliminating waste products from the gastrointestinal tract. The following questions deal with the contents of Chapter 28.

I. True or false.

Read each statement carefully and place your answer in the space provided.

__T__ 1. A tarry stool indicates bleeding in the upper gastrointestinal tract.

__F__ 2. Histamine depresses gastric secretions.

__F__ 3. An enema is never given to obtain a stool specimen because the fluid used will dilute the specimen and render it worthless for examination.

__T__ 4. It is important to save any fecal material that is unusual in appearance.

__F__ 5. Normally, the barium a patient swallows leaves the stomach in 20 to 30 minutes and the stomach will be entirely free of barium in less than 1 hour.

__T__ 6. A laxative and an enema are usually given prior to x-ray examination of the bowel.

__T__ 7. Endoscopy refers to examination of certain organs through a hollow instrument passed through one of the body openings.

__F__ 8. Visualization of the small intestine is called a sigmoidoscopy.

__F__ 9. Passing an endoscope into a body cavity is uncomfortable but never painful.

__F__ 10. For an esophagoscopy and gastroscopy, nothing is taken by mouth for 1 hour before the procedure.

__T__ 11. Gastrointestinal decompression is the emptying or draining of the contents of the stomach or intestines.

__T__ 12. Another name for a nasogastric tube is a Levin tube.

__F__ 13. Immediately after insertion, the intestinal decompression tube must be anchored in place by taping the tube to the patient's nose and pinning the end to the bedding.

__T__ 14. Gastrointestinal decompression usually causes the loss of large amounts of fluids and electrolytes.

__T__ 15. Regurgitation of gastric contents into the esophagus causes burning which at times can be severe.

153

__T__ 16. Some people who are nervous may find that eating helps them to relax.

__F__ 17. Anyone not having a bowel movement at least once every 2 days would be considered to have a problem with constipation.

II. Multiple choice questions.

Select the most appropriate answer and place it in the space provided.

1. Bright red blood, mixed with stool is an indication of __B__.
   a. bleeding in or near the esophagus or stomach
   b. bleeding near the rectum
   c. cancer
   d. ulcerative colitis

2. A gastric analysis is useful in __A__.
   a. determining the ability of the stomach to secrete hydrochloric acid
   b. analyzing the contents of the last meal eaten before the procedure
   c. analyzing the ability of the stomach to mechanically digest food
   d. determining the ability of the stomach to absorb nutrients

3. Preparation for a gastric analysis includes __D__.
   a. fasting for 24 hours
   b. administration of an enema
   c. fasting from solid food for 8 hours and from liquids for 1 hour
   d. withholding food and fluids for 8 hours

4. Two methods used for gastric analysis are the __A__.
   1. basal secretion method: specimens collected for four-15 minute periods
   2. total collection method: specimens collected hourly for 12 hours
   3. stimulated secretion: injection of histamine
   4. water tolerance: use of water to produce histamine secretion
      a. 1, 3
      b. 1, 4
      c. 2, 3
      d. 2, 4

5. When histamine is given as part of a gastric analysis, what drug should be immediately available in case the patient has a reaction to the histamine? __A__
   a. epinephrine
   b. atropine
   c. an antihistamine

6. Occult blood is blood __B__.
   a. found only in the stool
   b. not visible to the naked eye
   c. visible in the stool
   d. found in the lower intestinal tract

7. Prior to x-ray examination or fluoroscopy of the gastrointestinal tract, the area to be examined should be as empty as possible so the __C__.
   a. contrast media can enter the bowel
   b. patient has minimal cramps during and after the procedure
   c. contrast media can clearly outline the area
   d. procedure takes less time

8. Feces present in the bowel during a sigmoidoscopy __B__.
   a. prevent insertion of the endoscope
   b. prevent adequate visualization during the examination
   c. make the procedure more painful

9. A tube using a balloon filled with air at its tip to facilitate passage along the gastrointestinal tract is a __C__.
   a. Cantor tube
   b. Levin tube
   c. Miller-Abbott tube
   d. Blakemore-Sengstaken tube

10. The tube using a balloon filled with mercury to facilitate passage along the gastrointestinal tract is a __A__.
    a. Cantor tube
    b. Levin tube
    c. Miller-Abbott tube
    d. Blakemore-Sengstaken tube
11. Tubes used for *intestinal* decompression are the __B__.
    1. Cantor tubes
    2. Levin tubes
    3. Miller-Abbott tubes
    4. Blakemore-Sengstaken tubes
    a. 1, 2
    b. 1, 3
    c. 2, 4
    d. all except 4
12. When a tube is inserted for intestinal decompression, the patient may be __D__.
    a. given fluids orally
    b. ambulated after the tube is clamped
    c. placed in a prone position to hurry the passage of the tube
    d. placed in various positions to facilitate passage of the tube
13. When a gastrointestinal tube is passed, the patient __A__.
    a. may have a few sips of water to facilitate passage of the tube
    b. cannot be given water while the tube is being passed
14. Nasogastric tubes are __d__.
    a. routinely irrigated with normal saline
    b. routinely irrigated with water
    c. both a and b
    d. none of these
15. When a patient has gastrointestinal decompression for several days, an accurate record of intake and output is necessary so that __C__.
    a. electrolyte losses are documented
    b. renal function can be evaluated
    c. the patient's needs for parenteral fluids can be accurately determined
16. The function of the gastrointestinal tract is affected by the __C__.
    a. autonomic nervous system
    b. the patient's emotions
    c. both a and b
    d. none of these
17. Anorexia nervosa is a severe disorder in which the patient __D__.
    a. cannot eat without vomiting
    b. is consistently nauseated and, therefore, cannot eat
    c. becomes nauseated at the sight and smell of food
    d. has an aversion to food
18. When used correctly, the term diarrhea means __B__.
    a. more than 4 bowel movements per day
    b. frequent, loose, watery stools
    c. frequent stools accompanied by abdominal cramps
19. When used correctly, the term constipation means __a__.
    a. hard, dry, infrequent stools
    b. no bowel movement for 2 or more days
    c. infrequent bowel movements accompanied by abdominal distention
20. Water is normally absorbed from the stool while it is in the __D__.
    a. duodenum
    b. jejunum
    c. ileum
    d. colon
21. In differentiating between normal and abnormal function of the gastrointestinal tract, the most reliable criterion is the __C__.
    a. frequency of the bowel movements
    b. color of the stools
    c. consistency of the stools
22. Hypermotility of the large intestine leads to __C__.
    a. diarrhea
    b. cramps
    c. both a and b
    d. none of these

23. Treatment of an irritable colon may include __a__.
    1. tranquilizers
    2. antispasmodics
    3. antidiarrheals
    4. laxatives
    5. enemas
       a. 1, 2, 3
       b. 1, 3, 4
       c. 2, 3, 4
       d. 2, 4, 5

III. Fill-in and discussion questions.
Read each question carefully and place your answer in the space provided.

1. Label the 17 areas identified in the drawing below by filling in the blanks to the right of the drawing. The 17 areas are to be selected from the words given below the drawing.

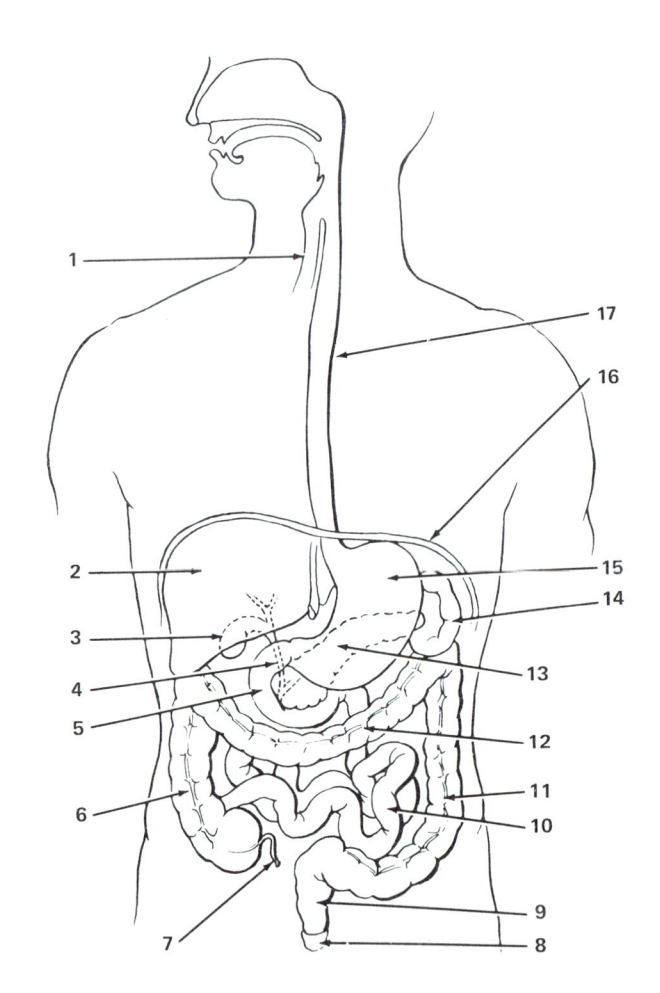

1. Trachea
2. Liver
3. gallbladder
4. common duct
5. duodenum
6. ascending colon
7. appendix
8. Anus
9. Rectum
10. small bowel
11. descending colon
12. transverse colon
13. pancreas
14. spleen
15. Stomach
16. diaphragm
17. esophagus

anus   diaphragm   pancreas   small bowel   common duct   trachea   rectum

transverse colon   appendix   spleen   ascending colon   liver   stomach

esophagus   duodenum   gallbladder   descending colon

2. Why is clean rather than aseptic technique used in a gastrointestinal procedure such as an enema? _gastrointestinal tract is laden c̄ bacteria + food injested is not sterile_

3. After a patient has had a barium enema, it is important to note if the contrast media (barium) has been expelled from the colon. How might the nurse check to see if the barium has been passed? _✓ check if patient is having regular bowel movements   ✓ for barium in stool_

4. The nurse's role in the preparation of a patient having a sigmoidoscopy includes the following:
   1. _Enemas, explaining procedure & knee chest position_
   2. _Positioning patient_
   3. _Draping patient_

5. List 3 uses of gastrointestinal suction.
   1. _Withdrawing specimens from stomach for diagnostic purposes_
   2. _Prevention + treatment of post op distention_
   3. _Removal of accumulated contents of gastro intestinal tract._

CHAPTER—29

The patient with ulcerative colitis, peptic ulcer

The patient with ulcerative colitis or peptic ulcer may require intensive medical and sometimes surgical management of his disease. Those with severe ulcerative colitis often experience a great deal of anxiety due to the symptoms of their disease. Frequent stools, often accompanied by cramps, leave the patient weak and debilitated. Many cannot keep employment, and the embarrassment of having to use the bathroom frequently often forces them to curtail social activities.

Peptic ulcer is a common disease among adults and is often related to the stress and strain of living in a highly competitive society. Actually, peptic ulcer occurs widely throughout the world in primitive as well as highly technical societies.

The following questions deal with the contents of Chapter 29.

I. True or false.

Read each statement carefully and place your answer in the space provided.

_F_ 1. Ulcerative colitis is caused by a bacterial infection of the bowel.

_T_ 2. Although it can occur at any age, ulcerative colitis is most common during young adulthood and middle life.

_T_ 3. When ulcerative colitis is in an acute stage, cathartics are contraindicated as part of the patient preparation for a barium enema.

_T_ 4. Corticosteroid preparations may be used in the treatment of ulcerative colitis if the patient does not respond to other measures.

_F_ 5. Corticosteroid drugs are only given by the oral route.

_F_ 6. Corticosteroid drugs can cure ulcerative colitis if given when symptoms first begin.

_T_ 7. The cardiac orifice of the stomach is located between the stomach and the esophagus.

_F_ 8. When the sphincters located at the cardiac and pyloric orifices of the stomach relax, the orifice closes.

_T_ 9. Gastric ulcers may be malignant or benign.

_T_ 10. The dietary management of a patient with a peptic ulcer may range from a milk and cream diet to a liberal diet of the patient's choice.

_T_ 11. Rest and relaxation are of prime importance in the treatment of a peptic ulcer.

_F_ 12. A vagotomy is the removal of the vagus nerve.

_F_ 13. A Cantor tube is usually inserted prior to surgery for a peptic ulcer to drain the contents of the stomach.

___T___ 14. Hemorrhage is the most frequent complication of a peptic ulcer.

II. Multiple choice questions.

Select the most appropriate answer and place it in the space provided.

CLINICAL SITUATIONS

Martha, age 20, has had gastrointestinal problems since she was 12 years old. Presently, she has marked symptoms of ulcerative colitis, for example, severe diarrhea, weight loss, and anemia. Her condition has been followed by her family physician.

1. The term *ulcerative colitis* refers to __C__.
   a. an inflammatory process in the sigmoid colon
   b. an ulcerative disorder of the terminal ileum
   c. inflammation and ulceration of the colon
   d. a condition with alternating bouts of diarrhea and constipation

2. The cause of ulcerative colitis is __B__.
   a. thought to be an auto-immunity factor
   b. most likely due to multiple causes
   c. bacterial
   d. inability to cope with everyday problems of living

3. Martha's symptoms __B__.
   a. definitely indicate ulcerative colitis
   b. could also be seen in other intestinal disorders

4. An examination used to diagnose ulcerative colitis is __D__.
   a. barium swallow
   b. biopsy
   c. insertion of a Miller-Abbott tube and gastric analysis
   d. sigmoidoscopy

5. It is decided to initially provide supportive treatment for Martha. This mode of treatment is designed to __A__.
   a. give the bowel a chance to rest and correct anemia and nutrition
   b. heal the bowel by the administration of antidiarrheal drugs and special diet
   c. help Martha emotionally accept her disease
   d. cure the disease

6. The diet usually ordered for a patient with ulcerative colitis is a __B__.
   a. soft diet
   b. bland diet
   c. liquid diet
   d. high residue diet

7. Martha's physician suggests bed rest and also plans to try drug therapy. Drugs that might be ordered are __D__.
   1. tranquilizers
   2. atropine or other cholinergic blocking agents
   3. sedatives
   4. corticosteroids
   5. kaolin, pectin
   a. 1, 2, 4
   b. 2, 3, 5
   c. 3, 4, 5
   d. all of these

8. Antispasmotic drugs are given with caution to the patient with ulcerative colitis because these drugs could cause __C__.
   a. constipation
   b. spasms of the colon
   c. marked dilatation of the colon

Martha's symptoms become more severe and her physician decides to admit her to the hospital for further evaluation. After a lengthy history, evaluation of past treatment and x-rays, it is decided that surgery is necessary.

9. The surgical treatment of severe, intractable ulcerative colitis includes a(n) __A__.
   a. total colectomy and permanent ileostomy
   b. exploratory laparotomy and removal of the diseased portion of the ileum
   c. hemicolectomy
   d. temporary ileostomy or colostomy

10. An antibiotic may be ordered prior to surgery to __B__.
    a. control the infection that caused the disease
    b. reduce the number of bacteria in the bowel and lessen the possibility of infection as a complication of surgery
    c. prevent infection prior to surgery

11. While awaiting surgery it is important that Martha maintain adequate dietary and fluid intake. This can be accomplished by __C__.
    a. letting her select a diet with no food restrictions or limitations
    b. ordering a low carbohydrate diet along with extra protein supplements
    and extra portions of fruit and vegetables
    c. serving small portions of food the patient enjoys in an environment that is odor free

Mr. Hill, age 29, is an accountant for a large chemical firm. He often works long hours and takes work home on weekends. Two months ago he noticed a burning sensation in his epigastrium.

12. Tests that may confirm the diagnosis of a peptic ulcer include __C__.
    1. barium enema
    2. G.I. series
    3. sigmoidoscopy
    4. endoscopic examination
       a. 1, 2
       b. 2, 4
       c. 1, 4
       d. all of these

13. Mr. Hill is found to have a peptic ulcer and his physician decides to try conservative therapy first. This approach is designed to __A__.
    a. provide optimum conditions for healing of the lesion
    b. heal the lesion in 2 to 3 weeks
    c. stop bleeding and pain
    d. differentiate between a malignant or benign lesion

14. The prime focus in the medical management of a peptic ulcer is on __D__.
    1. reduction of pepsin
    2. neutralization of stomach acid
    3. reduction of hypermotility
    4. reduction in gastric secretions
       a. 1, 2, 3
       b. 1, 2, 4
       c. 1, 3, 4
       d. 2, 3, 4

15. Dietary management is instituted to __B__.
    a. reduce gastric motility
    b. neutralize hydrochloric acid
    c. absorb pepsin
    d. reduce gastric secretions

16. Sodium bicarbonate is an antacid but is not recommended for use in the treatment of gastric disorders because __C__.
    a. the drug is not absorbed as rapidly as preparations such as Maalox or Gelusil
    b. large amounts encourage excess secretion of hydrochloric acid
    c. large amounts produce alkalosis

17. Mr. Hill is given a cholinergic blocking agent to reduce gastric hypermotility and secretion. Side effects of these drugs include __B__.
    1. dry mouth
    2. double vision
    3. difficulty voiding
    4. urinary retention
       a. all but 1
       b. all but 2
       c. all but 3
       d. all but 4

18. Mr. Hill does not respond to treatment and is readmitted to the hospital for surgery. The types of surgery usually performed for a peptic ulcer not responding to medical treatment are __D__.
    1. vagotomy
    2. gastroenterostomy
    3. subtotal gastrectomy
    4. total gastrectomy
       a. 1, 2
       b. 1, 3
       c. 2, 3
       d. all except 4

19. A vagotomy may be performed to __D__.
    a. reduce blood supply to the area
    b. promote healing in the surgical area
    c. prevent food from irritating the stomach
    d. reduce gastric motility and secretion

20. When Mr. Hill returns from surgery there is an order to connect his nasogastric tube to suction. The nasogastric tube is __C__.
    a. irrigated hourly
    b. irrigated every 2 hours and when needed
    c. not irrigated unless there is an order for this procedure

21. During the first 24 hours, the color and amount of drainage coming from the nasogastric tube should be checked every __A__.
    a. hour
    b. 2 to 4 hours
    c. 4 hours
    d. 8 hours

22. Once Mr. Hill is allowed small amounts of oral food and fluids, he is observed for fullness, distention, and vomiting. Should such symptoms occur it may mean __B__.
    a. there is still hypermotility and excess secretions
    b. the foods are not progressing normally through the gastrointestinal tract
    c. the surgery was probably unsuccessful

23. The dumping syndrome is a complication of gastric surgery and symptoms appear to be due to __D__.
    a. hypermotility of the stomach
    b. excessive gastric secretions
    c. an obstruction near the pylorus
    d. a rapid emptying of large amounts of food and fluid into the jejunum

III. Fill-in and discussion questions.

Read each question carefully and place your answer in the space provided.

1. List 8 symptoms of ulcerative colitis.
    1. Diarrhea
    2. fever
    3. wt loss
    4. anemia
    5. dehydration
    6. nausea - vomiting
    7. May be incontinent
    8. Blood & mucus in feces

2. A patient asks you what foods can or cannot be eaten on a bland diet. Place a √ in front of the foods allowed on a bland diet.

- ___ apple
- ✓ milk
- ___ cola beverage (carbonated)
- ___ french fries
- ✓ mashed potatoes
- ___ grapefruit juice
- ✓ chicken
- ✓ cream of asparagus soup
- ✓ beets (cooked)
- ✓ creamed spinach
- ___ bacon and eggs (fried)
- ✓ butter
- ✓ cottage cheese
- ___ pizza
- ✓ eggs (poached)
- ___ coffee
- ✓ banana
- ___ beer
- ___ pork chops
- ✓ gelatin dessert
- ✓ buttermilk
- ___ vegetable soup

3. A complication of peptic ulcer is hemorrhage. Give 4 signs that might be seen in a patient with a severe blood loss.

   1. pallor
   2. weak rapid pulse
   3. thirst — collapse
   4. sweating

4. Another complication of peptic ulcer is obstruction due to edema, spasm, inflammation, and the formation of scar tissue. Give 3 symptoms that may be seen in the patient with a severe pyloric obstruction.

   1. nausea - vomiting
   2. pain
   3. abd - distention

5. A peptic ulcer may penetrate tissue so deeply that perforation occurs. List 4 of the immediate symptoms of peptic ulcer perforation.

   1. Excruciating pain
   2. Abd - boardlike
   3. profuse perspiration
   4. rapid shallow breathing

6. An hour or 2 after perforation other symptoms occur. Give 4 symptoms that now may be seen in the patient with a perforated peptic ulcer.

   1. fever
   2. abd distended
   3. pulse weak & rapid
   4. face flushed

CHAPTER—30

The patient with cancer of the gastrointestinal tract

Cancer of the digestive tract is a major cause of illness and death. It occurs commonly in every area of the gastrointestinal tract although cancer is rare in the small intestine. Cancer of the mouth, esophagus, stomach, or rectum is more common in men, whereas cancer of the colon is slightly more common in women.

The following questions deal with the contents of Chapter 30.

I. True or false.

Read each statement carefully and place your answer in the space provided.

__F__ 1. One of the earliest symptoms of cancer of the gastrointestinal tract is pain.

__T__ 2. The appearance of blood in the stool is an early sign of rectal cancer.

__T__ 3. Compared to the normal population, individuals with ulcerative colitis have a higher incidence of cancer of the colon.

__F__ 4. Leukoplakia, a patch of white thickened tissue, is an oral cancer found exclusively in smokers.

__F__ 5. Cancer of the mouth is rarely cured even when detected early.

__T__ 6. One complication of oral surgery for cancer is hemorrhage from large arteries.

__T__ 7. Obstructing cancer of the esophagus may necessitate a temporary or permanent gastrostomy.

__T__ 8. A gastrostomy can be performed under local anesthesia if the patient cannot tolerate a general anesthesia.

__T__ 9. Some gastrostomy patients can eat a regular diet that is first converted to liquid form by use of a food blender.

__T__ 10. Treatment of cancer of the colon is primarily surgical.

__F__ 11. Patients who have had an abdominoperineal resection will have a temporary colostomy.

__F__ 12. Patients who have had an abdominoperineal resection usually have less pain after surgery than the average patient because many pelvic nerves were severed during surgery.

__T__ 13. Following an abdominoperineal resection, sitz baths may be ordered to promote healing of the perineal wound.

163

II. Multiple choice questions.

Select the most appropriate answer and place it in the space provided.

1. One of the earliest signs of cancer of the esophagus is __c__.
   a. dyspepsia
   b. weight loss
   c. dysphagia
   d. anemia

2. Symptoms of cancer of the stomach are __d__.
   a. indigestion, bright red blood in the stool
   b. flatulence, weight gain
   c. weight loss, signs of a bowel obstruction
   d. usually vague during the early stages of the disease

3. The earliest warning sign of cancer of the large intestine is/are __a__.
   a. change in bowel habits
   b. weight loss
   c. clay-colored stools
   d. flatulence when eating certain foods

4. A prominent and common symptom of rectal cancer is __a__.
   a. bright red blood in the stool
   b. tarry stools
   c. weight loss
   d. abdominal distention

5. Cancer of the digestive tract is diagnosed by a careful history. Additional tests may include __d__.
   1. physical examination
   2. biopsy
   3. endoscopic examination
   4. x-ray examination
   5. cytologic examination of exfoliated cells
      a. 1, 2, 3
      b. 1, 2, 4
      c. 3, 4, 5
      d. all of these

6. The final diagnosis of a malignant tumor is established by __c__.
   a. x-ray evidence of a tumor
   b. x-ray evidence collaborated by endoscopic evidence of a new growth
   c. microscopic examination of a section of the tumor

7. Probable causative factors of cancer of the stomach appear to be __b__.
   a. age, past history of gastric surgery
   b. heredity, chronic inflammation
   c. smoking, eating of fish and other foods high in iodine
   d. repeated bouts of gastroenteritis, drug abuse

8. Gastric carcinoma may be diagnosed by __d__.
   1. gastric analysis
   2. fluoroscopy
   3. barium swallow
   4. gastroscopy
      a. 1, 2, 3
      b. 1, 3, 4
      c. 2, 3, 4
      d. all of these

9. If a patient has a total gastrectomy he will most likely require lifetime injections of __a__.
   a. vitamin B_{12}
   b. B complex
   c. iron
   d. vitamin B and C

CLINICAL SITUATIONS

Mr. Quinn, age 47, noticed a small swelling under his tongue about 3 months ago. His dentist found the lesion during a routine dental examination and called it to Mr. Quinn's attention. The dentist suggested that Mr. Quinn see his physician immediately, especially since he admitted to having the swelling for several months. Now concerned over this growth, Mr. Quinn makes an appointment to see his family physician who refers him to a specialist in oral tumors.

10. Mr. Quinn will require surgery for the oral lesion which has been diagnosed as malignant. The surgery may be mutilating and interfere with normal breathing. What procedure *might* be performed to reduce the possibility of respiratory obstruction in the postoperative period? _B_
    a. IPPB
    b. tracheostomy
    c. oxygen by nasal catheter
    d. laryngectomy

11. Surgery for oral cancer will prevent Mr. Quinn from taking oral fluids and food until healing is complete; therefore, the calorie and fluid intake is usually maintained by _C_.
    a. intravenous therapy
    b. gastrostomy feedings
    c. nasogastric feedings

12. When Mr. Quinn returns from the operating room, care must be taken to facilitate oral drainage. Until the patient awakens from anesthesia he is kept _B_.
    a. on his back with the head of the bed elevated
    b. on his side or abdomen
    c. in Trendelenburg's position

13. To lessen pain while coughing the nurse can _a_.
    a. supply firm support to Mr. Quinn's head and neck
    b. support Mr. Quinn's incision
    c. place Mr. Quinn on his side before beginning coughing and deep-breathing exercises
    d. keep the head of the bed elevated

14. Mr. Quinn expectorates small amounts of dark red blood when coughing or clearing his mouth of saliva. This is _a_.
    a. to be expected
    b. not to be expected and a physician should be notified

15. During the postoperative period Mr. Quinn's temperature should be taken _b_.
    a. orally
    b. rectally

16. Oral irrigations are ordered for Mr. Quinn _c_.
    a. because he cannot use a toothbrush for several weeks
    b. because use of toothpaste might cause an infection
    c. to clean the mouth and wash away old blood and debris

Mrs. Travis is 46 years old and has had a weight problem for many years. To lose weight she frequently goes on a fad or crash diet but often regains the weight several months later. She recently gained 30 pounds, went on a severe diet, lost 40 pounds and now notices she has difficulty eating and swallowing. She attributes this problem to her recent crash diet and weight loss. She mentioned her problem to a friend who is a nurse. Her friend strongly recommended that she seek medical advice.

17. Mrs. Travis is admitted to the hospital because her physician suspects a tumor of the esophagus. Diagnosis of cancer of the esophagus is made by _B_.
    1. barium swallow
    2. gastric analysis
    3. esophagoscopy
    4. duodenal washings
        a. 1, 2
        b. 1, 3
        c. 2, 3
        d. 2, 4

18. If a special diet is ordered for Mrs. Travis before surgery, it will probably be a _d_.
    a. low residue, high vitamin house diet
    b. soft, bland, low calorie diet
    c. house diet
    d. high calorie, high protein, soft-to-liquid diet as tolerated

19. Treatment of cancer of the esophagus usually depends on the __B__.
    a. age of the patient and the evidence of lung involvement
    b. extent of the lesion and evidence of metastasis
    c. the size of the tumor

20. Mrs. Travis' tumor is operable and in the lower third of her esophagus. The surgical procedure that will probably be performed is __d__.
    a. use of a section of duodenum to bypass the tumor
    b. resection of two-thirds of the esophagus and replacement with a section of the duodenum
    c. anastomosis of the esophagus to the duodenum
    d. resection of the esophagus and anastomosis of the remaining two-thirds to the stomach

21. If a patient is too ill to withstand surgery now or in the future for this type of cancer, the patient may be fed __B__.
    a. intravenously
    b. by means of a gastrostomy
    c. orally, but only given liquids

22. Several days after surgery, Mrs. Travis will be allowed to take oral fluids and must be observed for __a__.
    a. regurgitation of fluid, dyspnea
    b. nausea, vomiting, constipation
    c. abdominal cramps, diarrhea
    d. abdominal distention, pulsating mass in her abdomen

Mr. Allen, a 77-year-old retired bookkeeper, has inoperable cancer of the esophagus. He is admitted in a malnourished and debilitated state due to his inability to swallow anything but liquids for the past several months.

23. A temporary gastrostomy is to be performed on Mr. Allen to provide a means of meeting his nutritional requirements. A tube will be inserted into his stomach __C__.
    a. by way of the esophagus but bypassing the tumor
    b. by way of the duodenum
    c. through the abdominal wall

24. The skin around the gastrostomy tube may become irritated due to leakage of gastric contents and may be protected with __B__.
    a. antibiotic creams
    b. ointments such as zinc oxide
    c. water-soluble ointments

25. After the gastrostomy Mr. Allen will first be given __a__.
    a. small amounts of tap water
    b. clear liquids such as water, juice, liquid gelatin
    c. liquids and blended foods diluted with water

26. Once healing around the tube has taken place the catheter may be __B__.
    a. clamped and opened only for feedings
    b. removed and inserted for feedings

27. Mr. Allen is now able to tolerate a regular gastrostomy feeding, the volume of which is usually __C__.
    a. 50 to 100 ml.
    b. 100 to 200 ml.
    c. 300 to 500 ml.
    d. 350 to 1000 ml.

Miss Stuart, age 43, is admitted to the hospital with the diagnosis of rectal cancer and is to have an abdominoperineal resection in an attempt to cure or least control the spread of the cancer.

28. What structures are removed in an abdominoperineal resection? __a__
    1. rectum
    2. anus
    3. sigmoid colon
    4. transverse colon
    5. ascending colon
        a. 1, 2, 3
        b. 1, 3, 4
        c. 2, 4, 5
        d. all of these

29. In an abdominoperineal resection what part of the colon is used to form a permanent colostomy? __a__
    a. sigmoid colon
    b. transverse colon
    c. ascending colon

30. Miss Stuart returns from the operating room with 2 dressings—an abdominal and a perineal. The perineal wound dressing __c__.
    a. should remain dry and have very little drainage on the dressing
    b. may have a small amount of serous drainage requiring reinforcement of the dressing
    c. may have profuse serosanguinous drainage

31. Miss Stuart's temperature should be taken every 4 hours during the first several days after surgery. Her temperature is taken __a__.
    a. orally
    b. rectally

32. Miss Stuart had an indwelling catheter inserted in her bladder before surgery. During the immediate postoperative period the urinary output is measured hourly and the physician called if the output falls below __a__.
    a. 30 ml. per hour
    b. 100 ml. per hour
    c. 600 to 700 ml. per 8 hour period
    d. 1000 ml. per 8 hour period

33. Because of her surgical incision Miss Stuart finds it difficult to find a position of comfort, but she will probably be comfortable lying __c__.
    a. prone
    b. supine
    c. on her side

34. The indwelling catheter also __b__.
    a. encourages healing by keeping the colostomy wound dry
    b. prevents soiling of the perineal wound with urine
    c. prevents a bladder infection

35. Once Miss Stuart is allowed out of bed she is made more comfortable sitting in a chair by __b__.
    a. using blankets to soften the seat of the chair
    b. placing a rubber ring or foam rubber pad on the seat
    c. elevating her legs on a footstool
    d. placing a pillow behind her head

36. Dressings will be worn over the perineal area __d__.
    a. for 1 to 2 weeks
    b. permanently as a means of supporting the area
    c. until diarrhea stops and the stool is formed
    d. until healing occurs and drainage ceases

III. Fill-in and discussion question.
Read the following question carefully and place your answer in the space provided.
1. Discuss how the nurse may be helpful in minimizing the patient's distress over his appearance after radical surgery for oral cancer. _provide privacy when pt first attempts to eat & swallow, provide plenty of tissues to prevent drooling, show him how to tilt head to aid in swallowing, help him pay special care to grooming._

CHAPTER—31

The patient with an ileostomy or a colostomy

An ostomy is a surgical opening of the bowel through the skin. There are two main types: *ileostomy* and *colostomy*. Fecal material drains from both openings (*stomas*).

Patients with an ostomy often have to make great adjustments to the changes in their body image. While no adjustment is easy, the nurse can play an important role in the manner in which these patients adjust to their condition. The nurse is the first person who cares for the ostomate's stoma. When the nurse understands the patient's problems and accepts the changes in his body image, the patient may begin to express his feelings and accept the changes in his body function.

The following questions deal with the contents of Chapter 31.

I. True or false.

Read each statement carefully and place your answer in the space provided.

__T__ 1. An ostomate is an individual with a colostomy or ileostomy.

__F__ 2. The patient with a stoma still has sphincter control; therefore, he will only be incontinent of feces a short time after surgery.

__F__ 3. Patients usually accept an ileostomy stoma after they have cared for their stoma for a few days.

__T__ 4. It is often beneficial to have a member of the local ostomy group visit a new ostomate.

__F__ 5. An ileostomy appliance can be removed at night.

__T__ 6. Changes in color and size of a colostomy stoma may vary with activity and emotional status.

__F__ 7. The bowel is very sensitive to pain and a stoma must be handled with particularly great care.

__T__ 8. A transverse double-barreled colostomy is usually temporary.

__T__ 9. A colostomy of the ascending colon will have fecal drainage similar in consistency to an ileostomy.

__F__ 10. When irrigating a colostomy, sterile technique is necessary since the stoma is prone to infection.

__T__ 11. It is essential that the colostomy patient be assisted with the irrigation procedure because the effectiveness of the irrigation is the basis for establishing control.

__T__ 12. A special diet may be prescribed for colostomy patients with excessive gas or frequent bowel movements.

__F__ 13. Colostomy patients will have to purchase special clothing to hide

169

the bulge created by their colostomy appliances.

__F__ 14. Gas-forming foods should be avoided by the patient with an ileostomy but need not be avoided by the patient with a colostomy.

II. Multiple choice questions.

Select the most appropriate answer and place it in the space provided.

1. The care of a patient with an ostomy should be __a__.
   1. patient-centered
   2. nurse-centered
   3. living-oriented
   4. hospital-oriented
   - a. 1, 3
   - b. 1, 4
   - c. 2, 3
   - d. 2, 4

2. The *overall* plan for care of the patient with an ostomy is adapted to the __d__.
   - a. family of the patient
   - b. type of stoma
   - c. nurse's ability to teach the patient about his stoma
   - d. individual patient

3. One of the first steps in explaining stoma care to the new ostomate is __d__.
   - a. giving the patient illustrated books to read about stoma care
   - b. having the patient watch another ostomate give himself care
   - c. showing the patient the various types of ostomy appliances
   - d. encouraging the patient to help with his stoma care

4. Ostomates should receive the equipment and instruction in its use and care __c__.
   - a. after discharge from the hospital in the outpatient clinic or physician's office
   - b. when the patient is able to accept the stoma
   - c. while hospitalized and prior to discharge

5. Fecal drainage from an ileostomy is __a__.
   - a. liquid
   - b. semi-formed
   - c. solid

6. After surgery an ileostomy requires __b__.
   - a. a temporary covering over the stoma until regularity is established
   - b. immediate and lifetime application of a collecting appliance

7. A particular problem for the patient with an ileostomy is __d__.
   - a. constipation
   - b. fluid retention
   - c. kidney failure
   - d. electrolyte imbalance

8. The size of an ileostomy stoma __b__.
   - a. remains unchanged
   - b. is larger immediately after surgery than it will be later
   - c. is smaller immediately after surgery than it will be later

9. A permanent ileostomy appliance is usually kept in place by __a__.
   - a. a gum or adhesive plus a belt
   - b. adhesive tape, preferably the hypoallergenic type
   - c. Montgomery straps

10. The best time to change an ileostomy appliance is __a__.
    - a. when the bowel is quiet
    - b. early in the morning, right after breakfast
    - c. immediately after the largest meal of the day
    - d. at the time the individual usually had a bowel movement

11. A relatively inexpensive yet effective deodorant for an ileostomy pouch is __c__.
    a. carbon tetrachloride
    b. paragoric
    c. two crushed aspirin tablets
    d. washing the pouch daily in benzine

12. Absence of an ileal flow may indicate __b__.
    a. an improper diet
    b. an intestinal obstruction
    c. that the patient is not applying the proper adhesive
    d. that the patient will need a laxative or stool softener

13. Functions of the large bowel include __a__.
    1. storage of feces
    2. reabsorption of water
    3. absorption of nutrients
    4. digestion of food
       a. 1, 2
       b. 1, 3
       c. 2, 3
       d. 2, 4

14. Fecal material in the transverse colon is normally __b__.
    a. liquid
    b. semiliquid to pasty
    c. semisolid
    d. solid

15. A cecostomy is usually performed __a__.
    a. to relieve intestinal obstruction
    b. after a colostomy or ileostomy
    c. before a colostomy
    d. to treat diverticulitis

16. The drainage from a cecostomy will be __d__.
    a. solid
    b. soft
    c. semisolid
    d. liquid

Clinical Situation

Mrs. Loring, age 63, has diverticulitis and her physician decides to perform a temporary ascending double-barreled colostomy. The surgical procedure has been explained and Mrs. Loring has been told that she will probably have the colostomy for 8 to 12 months.

17. A double-barreled colostomy consists of 2 stomas, one of which connects with __a__.
    a. either the distal or proximal portion of the colon
    b. the ileum and the other with the colon
    c. the ascending colon
    d. the descending colon

18. In a double-barreled colostomy, fecal drainage will come from the __b__.
    a. distal opening or loop
    b. proximal opening or loop

19. A single-barreled colostomy has only a proximal loop or opening, as the distal portion __c__.
    a. has been sutured to the internal abdominal wall
    b. has been anastomosed to the terminal ileum
    c. usually has been surgically removed

20. To determine which is the distal and which is the proximal loop, the nurse __a__.
    a. should ask the physician to diagram and identify the stomas
    b. must remember that the distal loop is on the left and the proximal on the right side of the umbilicus
    c. should mark "D" (for distal) and "P" (for proximal) on the dressing to identify each loop

21. *Control* of fecal evacuation in Mrs. Loring is based on __b__.
    1. the location of the stoma
    2. whether the colostomy is single- or double-barreled
    3. the function of that portion of the bowel
    4. the type of appliance worn over the stoma

    a. 1, 2
    b. 1, 3
    c. 2, 3
    d. 2, 4

22. Mrs. Loring is to be taught how to irrigate her colostomy. A colostomy is usually irrigated with __c__.
    a. normal saline
    b. distilled water (sterile)
    c. tepid tap water
    d. water and 60 ml. of mineral oil

23. Cramping may be a problem during the irrigation procedure. Causes of cramping are __a__.
    1. irrigating fluid that is introduced too rapidly
    2. irrigating fluid that is too cold
    3. air in the tubing of the irrigating set
    4. improper diet
    5. too little irrigating fluid

    a. 1, 2, 3
    b. 1, 3, 4
    c. 2, 3, 4
    d. 2, 4, 5

24. The maximum amount of irrigating fluid recommended for an entire irrigation is __b__.
    a. 500 to 1000 ml.
    b. 2 quarts
    c. 3 quarts
    d. 1 gallon

25. Mrs. Loring asks how long it usually takes for the *entire* colostomy irrigation procedure so she can plan her housework around the irrigation. Your answer is approximately __c__.
    a. 10 minutes
    b. ½ hour
    c. 1 hour
    d. 3 hours

26. The physician orders a distal as well as a proximal loop irrigation. When the distal loop is irrigated the irrigating fluid will leave the body by way of the __a__.
    a. anus
    b. proximal loop
    c. distal loop

27. The irrigation of the distal loop should be conducted with the patient __c__.
    a. sitting in a chair so the returns can be collected in an emesis basin
    b. remaining in bed
    c. sitting on a bedpan or on the toilet seat

III. Fill-in and discussion questions.

Read each question carefully and place your answer in the space provided.

1. Give 3 diseases and disorders which may require an ileostomy or colostomy.
    1. _ulcerative colitis_
    2. _Intestinal Obstruction_
    3. _Diverticulitis_
    Multiple polyposis

2. Almost every patient finds it difficult to accept a stoma but *how* the patient will react will depend on many factors. If a patient will not look at his stoma soon after surgery it is best not to force him to do so. What might the nurse do to make the patient more at ease during this time? _Carry out dressing changes quickly + promptly - controlling odors. Allow pt to express feelings_

172

3. Patients with a colostomy or an ileostomy may have difficulty adjusting to their stomas and some of the changes necessary in their life. Describe how you might feel at this point in your life if (a) you had a colostomy or abdominoperineal resection for cancer, or (b) you had an ileostomy for ulcerative colitis.

CHAPTER—32

The patient with an intestinal or rectal disorder

The patient with an intestinal or rectal disorder may have symptoms ranging from mild discomfort to the alarming experience of bleeding from the rectum. Regardless of the symptomatology, many patients with intestinal problems fear cancer, and rightly so, since gastrointestinal cancer is a major cause of illness and death.

Appendicitis, a common intestinal disorder of the adolescent and young adult, is one of the most common surgical emergencies. Other intestinal pathologies such as inguinal hernia or hemorrhoids are more common in the middle-aged adult.

The following questions deal with the contents of Chapter 32.

I. True or false.

Read each statement carefully and place your answer in the space provided.

__T__ 1. The appendix is located at the tip of the cecum.
__F__ 2. Appendicitis is more common in the elderly patient.
__T__ 3. The peritoneum is a serous sac lining the abdominal cavity.
__T__ 4. The two most common causes of peritonitis are perforation of the appendix and perforation of a duodenal ulcer.
__F__ 5. The most common type of hernia is an incisional hernia.
__T__ 6. Congenital defects account for a large portion of hernias.
__F__ 7. Women develop more inguinal hernias than men, whereas men are more likely to develop femoral hernias.
__F__ 8. A reducible hernia is a surgical emergency.
__T__ 9. Postoperative recovery for patients with hernia repairs is usually rapid.
__T__ 10. The majority of patients with an esophageal hiatus hernia can be treated medically.
__T__ 11. In the elderly, cancer is the most common cause of intestinal obstruction.
__T__ 12. Symptoms of a severe bowel obstruction can arise suddenly.
__F__ 13. Diverticula are more common in the small intestine than the large intestine.
__T__ 14. The cause of diverticulosis is unknown.
__T__ 15. Diverticulosis is often asymptomatic.
__F__ 16. Regional enteritis occurs most commonly in the elderly patient.
__F__ 17. Use of mineral oil or any stool softener is contraindicated in patients with hemorrhoids.
__T__ 18. Many patients have difficulty voiding after rectal surgery.
__T__ 19. Usually an individual is unaware that he has a pilonidal sinus until it becomes infected.

II. Multiple choice questions.

Select the most appropriate answer and place it in the space provided.

1. The pain of appendicitis usually occurs in the __B__.
   a. left lower quadrant
   b. right lower quadrant
   c. left upper quadrant
   d. right upper quadrant

2. The abdominal area typically tender in those with appendicitis is called __C__.
   a. the para-umbilical area
   b. the right upper quadrant
   c. McBurney's point

3. Management of the patient with peritonitis usually includes __a__.
   1. gastric decompression
   2. antibiotics
   3. anticoagulants
   4. replacement of fluids and electrolytes
   5. nasogastric feedings
      a. 1, 2, 4
      b. 1, 2, 5
      c. 2, 3, 4
      d. 3, 4, 5

4. The patient with acute peritonitis __d__.
   1. will have severe abdominal pain
   2. will have a subnormal temperature
   3. may be given sips of water and other clear liquids but no food
   4. will have a tender but soft abdomen
      a. 1, 2
      b. 1, 4
      c. 2, 3
      d. 1 only

5. Individuals prone to the development of incisional hernias are __a__.
   a. obese or elderly patients
   b. young, overly active postoperative patients
   c. individuals refusing to ambulate after surgery
   d. patients with large surgical incisions

6. If the protruding structures of a hernia can be replaced in the abdominal cavity, the hernia is said to be __d__.
   a. incarcerated
   b. strangulated
   c. unstrangulated
   d. reducible

7. A hernia that cannot be returned to the abdomen because of the edema of the protruding structures and constriction of the opening through which they emerged is called a(n) __a__.
   a. incarcerated hernia
   b. strangulated hernia
   c. unstrangulated hernia
   d. reducible hernia

8. If the blood supply to the viscera of an incarcerated hernia is cut off, it is called a(n) __c__.
   a. reducible hernia
   b. irreducible hernia
   c. strangulated hernia
   d. unstrangulated hernia

9. Postoperatively, the patient with a herniorrhaphy is encouraged to __d__.
   1. move and exercise his extremities
   2. change his position frequently
   3. deep breathe
   4. cough
      a. all but 1
      b. all but 2
      c. all but 3
      d. all but 4

10. Male patients may develop scrotal pain and swelling after a(n) __B__.
    a. incisional herniorrhaphy
    b. inguinal herniorrhaphy
    c. umbilical herniorrhaphy
    d. femoral herniorrhaphy

11. Symptoms of an esophageal hiatus hernia—heartburn, belching, and substernal pressure after eating—are more severe when the __a__.
    a. patient lies flat
    b. patient has an empty stomach

    c. hernia has returned to a normal position
    d. patient is thin and malnourished

12. Medical treatment of an esophageal hiatus hernia usually includes __a__.
    1. antacids
    2. antibiotics
    3. an ulcer-type diet
    4. a 6-inch elevation of the head of the bed
    5. the wearing of an abdominal support
       a. 1, 2, 3
       b. 1, 3, 4
       c. 2, 4, 5
       d. 3, 4, 5

13. Patients with an esophageal hiatus hernia may bleed, have melena or hematemesis if they __c__.
    a. have an infection of the esophagus
    b. are obese
    c. have secondary reflex esophagitis
    d. are elderly and malnourished

14. Patients who do not respond to medical treatment for an esophageal hiatus hernia may be treated surgically. Surgery involves __a__.
    a. replacing the stomach or other protruding organs into the abdomen and repairing the defect
    b. putting the esophagus in proper position and suturing it to the diaphragm

15. The symptoms of regional enteritis include __c__.
    1. abdominal distention
    2. pain in the right lower quadrant
    3. fever
    4. a palpable mass in the left lower quadrant
    5. diarrhea
       a. 1, 2, 5
       b. 1, 2, 3
       c. 2, 3, 5
       d. 3, 4, 5

16. Intestinal malabsorption results in __a__.
    1. weakness
    2. passage of abnormal stools
    3. weight loss
    4. constipation
    5. weight gain due to edema
       a. 1, 2, 3
       b. 1, 3, 4
       c. 1, 4, 5
       d. 2, 4, 5

17. Intestinal malabsorption may be due to __a__.
    1. a deficiency of digestive enzymes
    2. colitis
    3. celiac disease
    4. regional ileitis
       a. 1, 3
       b. 2 only
       c. 2, 4
       d. all of these

18. Factors predisposing to the development of hemorrhoids include __d__.
    1. pregnancy
    2. chronic constipation
    3. intra-abdominal tumors
    4. heredity factors
       a. 1, 2
       b. 2, 3
       c. 3, 4
       d. all of these

19. Two factors that make hemorrhoids worse are __d__.
    1. cold weather
    2. straining at stool
    3. bland foods
    4. constipation
       a. 1, 2
       b. 1, 3
       c. 2, 3
       d. 2, 4

20. The symptoms of internal hemorrhoids can also resemble __c__.
    a. ulcerative colitis
    b. regional enteritis
    c. cancer of the rectum
    d. diverticulitis

21. Sitz baths are important in the postoperative management of patients having rectal surgery as the baths __B__.
    a. clean the rectal area and prevent infection by keeping the area free of bacteria

b. increase circulation to the rectal area, reducing congestion, swelling and relieving pain
   c. make it easier to remove rectal packing by soothing the irritated areas and softening the external dressing
22. Following surgery the patient having surgery for a pilonidal sinus will be placed in a __b__ position.
   a. supine
   b. prone
   c. lateral Sims's

CLINICAL SITUATIONS

Mrs. Flynn is admitted to the hospital with severe abdominal pain. An x-ray examination of her abdomen is done immediately and the examining physician feels she has a bowel obstruction.

23. When the bowel is obstructed, the portion proximal to the obstruction __c__.
   a. becomes quickly emptied of intestinal contents
   b. contracts
   c. becomes distended with intestinal contents
   d. ceases peristaltic activity
24. If Mrs. Flynn's bowel obstruction had been high in the gastrointestinal tract she would have experienced __d__.
   a. upper abdominal pain
   b. lower abdominal pain and urinary retention
   c. severe diarrhea
   d. vomiting of the contents of the stomach and small bowel
25. Patients with a mechanical bowel obstruction rapidly become dehydrated because __a__.
   a. of vomiting and the inability to take oral fluids
   b. water is absorbed through the intestinal wall at a rapid rate
   c. the kidneys begin to excrete the excess water
26. A bowel obstruction usually must be corrected surgically. Two surgeries that could be performed immediately to relieve Mrs. Flynn's obstruction are __c__.
   1. abdominoperineal resection
   2. cecostomy
   3. colostomy
   4. colectomy
      a. 1, 2
      b. 1, 3
      c. 2, 3
      d. 2, 4
27. Mrs. Flynn is to have intestinal decompression prior to surgery. This will be accomplished by __c__.
   a. a nasogastric tube in the stomach
   b. keeping Mrs. Flynn without food or fluids and administering intravenous fluids
   c. passing a long tube such as a Miller-Abbott tube

Mr. Jarvis, a 51-year-old mechanic, has had vague abdominal complaints for several years and finally sees a physician when his discomfort becomes worse. After a series of x-ray examinations, his physician tells him he has diverticulitis. Two weeks later, Mr. Jarvis develops severe abdominal cramps and is admitted to the hospital.

28. Medical treatment of acute diverticulitis usually starts with __b__.
   1. intravenous therapy
   2. nothing by mouth
   3. soft diet
   4. enemas
   5. antibiotics
      a. 1, 2, 4
      b. 1, 2, 5
      c. 1, 4, 5
      d. 3, 4, 5
29. As inflammation subsides, Mr. Jarvis will be given a __a__.
   a. low residue diet
   b. bland diet
   c. soft diet
   d. house diet

30. Medical management of Mr. Jarvis will also include avoiding constipation by __a__.
    1. increasing his fluid intake
    2. use of stool softeners
    3. administering daily laxatives of the bulk-forming type
    4. a diet high in residue foods
        a. 1, 2
        b. 1, 3
        c. 2, 3
        d. 2, 4

31. If Mr. Jarvis does not respond to medical management, surgery will be necessary. The surgery performed will most likely be a(n) __B__.
    1. removal of the diseased portion of the colon
    2. abdominoperineal resection
    3. temporary colostomy
    4. ileostomy
        a. 1, 2
        b. 1, 3
        c. 1 only
        d. 2 only

III. Fill-in and discussion questions.
Read each question carefully and place your answer in the space provided.

1. VOCABULARY. Define the following terms.
    a. diverticula: _sacs or pouches caused by herniation of the intestinal mucosa thru weakened intestinal wall_
    b. diverticulitis: _inflammation or infection of diverticula_
    c. diverticulosis: _prescence of diverticula_
    d. fecalith: _hard mass of feces_
    e. hernia: _protrusion of intestines thru defect in abd. wall_
    f. herniorrhaphy: _operation to repair hernia_
    g. hirsute: _hairy_
    h. paralytic ileus: _paralysis of the intestines_
    i. peritonitis: _inflammation of the peritoneum_
    j. regional enteritis: _inflammation of the terminal ileum of the sm. intestine_
    k. steatorrhea: _high content of fat in the stool_

1. volvulus: _Twisting or kinking of the intestine_

2. Why are laxatives or enemas contraindicated when an individual has abdominal pain that could be indicative of appendicitis? _Both increase peristalsis & may cause appendix to rupture_

3. Name 5 signs of peritonitis.
   1. _Severe abd pain_
   2. _nausea & vomiting_
   3. _fever_
   4. _pulse rapid & weak_
   5. _leukocytosis_

CHAPTER—33

The patient with disorder of the liver, gallbladder, or pancreas

Disorders of the liver, gallbladder, and pancreas are common problems of the gastrointestinal tract. Disorders of the liver and pancreas, especially cirrhosis and pancreatitis, tend to be chronic illnesses requiring long-term treatment, sometimes with only minimal results. On the other hand, treatment of gallbladder disease is usually surgical, producing an immediate cure of the problem.

The following questions deal with the contents of Chapter 33.

I. Correct the false statements.

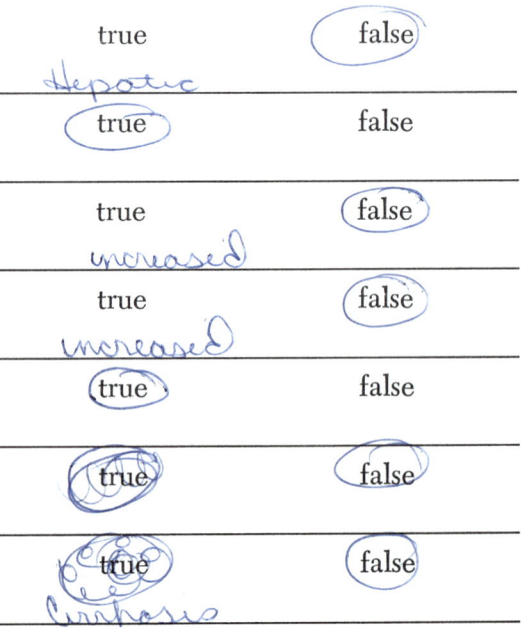

Circle the word true or false given to the right of the statement. If the word false has been circled, change the underlined word(s) to make the statement true. Place your answer in the space provided.

1. The liver receives arterial blood from the <u>mesenteric</u> artery. — true / **(false)** — *Hepatic*

2. The portal vein transports blood from the <u>intestines</u> to the liver. — **(true)** / false

3. The total serum bilirubin level is <u>decreased</u> in liver disease. — true / **(false)** — *increased*

4. The serum ammonia level is <u>decreased</u> in liver failure. — true / **(false)** — *increased*

5. Red blood cells are broken down by <u>reticuloendothelial</u> cells. — **(true)** / false

6. Another term for itching of the skin is <u>pruritus</u>. — **(true)** / false

7. <u>Hepatitis</u> is a disease in which scarring of the liver and the development of excessive fibrous connective tissue occur. — **(true)** / false — *Cirrhosis*

180

8. Laennec's cirrhosis is associated with heavy, chronic alcoholic intake, usually coincident with poor nutrition. (**true**) / false

9. The surgical shunting of blood from the portal vein to the vena cava is called a <u>splenorenal</u> shunt. true / (**false**) — portacaval

10. The tube used to stop esophageal bleeding is called a <u>Sengstaken-Blakemore</u> tube. (**true**) / false

11. The term <u>cholecystitis</u> may be defined as stones in the gallbladder. true / (**false**) — cholelithiasis

12. The pancreas is an endocrine organ producing the hormone <u>pepsin</u>. true / (**false**) — insulin

II. True or false.

Read each statement carefully and place your answer in the space provided.

T 1. The liver is the largest glandular organ in the body.
F 2. The liver can be palpated in a healthy individual with the inferior edge approximately 2 fingers below the last rib.
F 3. Unlike many blood tests, most liver function tests do not require a period of fasting and, therefore, can be done at any time during the day.
T 4. Cholesterol is synthesized by the liver.
T 5. An esophagoscopy may be done in the assessment of liver disease.
F 6. Jaundice is a form of liver disease.
T 7. A serious complication of advanced cirrhosis is infection.
F 8. The only cause of cirrhosis is excessive alcoholic intake.
T 9. A life-theatening complication of cirrhosis of the liver is bleeding esophageal varices.
F 10. Portal hypertension refers to a tumor of the portal vein causing an increase in pressure in the hepatic artery.

T 11. The bleeding varices of portal hypertension are in the lower esophagus and upper stomach.
F 12. Infectious and serum hepatitis have different symptoms, disease patterns, and incubation periods.
T 13. Patients with hepatitis may become jaundiced.
F 14. Once a patient has completely recovered from hepatitis he can donate blood.
T 15. Patients with hepatitis are usually placed in isolation.
T 16. Exposure to carbon tetrachloride, insecticides, and some drugs and chemicals can cause severe liver damage.
T 17. The liver manufactures approximately 1000 ml. of bile per day.
F 18. Gallstones (cholelithiasis) are more common in men than in women.
T 19. Diagnosis of cholelithiasis is made by cholecystogram.
T 20. The pancreas is an endocrine and an exocrine gland.
T 21. The etiology of acute pancreatitis is unknown.

III. Multiple choice questions.

Select the most appropriate answer and place it in the space provided.

1. Serum enzymes such as SGOT, SGPT and LDH are __a__.
   a. increased in liver disease
   b. decreased in liver disease
   c. unchanged in liver disease

2. Which of the following are tests of liver function? __D__
   1. blood urea nitrogen (BUN)
   2. bromsulphalein time (BSP)
   3. cephalin flocculation
   4. phenylketonuria
   5. thymol turbidity

   a. 1, 2, 3
   b. 1, 4, 5
   c. 2, 3, 4
   d. 2, 3, 5

3. A liver scan utilizes the __a__.
   a. intravenous injection of radioactive substances
   b. swallowing of a special dye
   c. intravenous injection of an iodine dye
   d. swallowing of a radiopaque substance similar to barium

4. Hemolytic jaundice is due to __b__.
   a. an excessive amount of iron in red blood cells which when normally broken down create excess pigment
   b. the overabundance of breakdown products of the blood
   c. intrinsic liver failure

5. Hepatocellular jaundice is due to __b__.
   a. extrinsic liver disease due to a bacterial infection
   b. internal liver disease preventing normal transformation of bile by liver cells
   c. blockage of the common bile duct

6. Obstructive jaundice is due to __c__.
   a. obstruction of the cells in the liver that manufacture bile
   b. the end products of red blood cell breakdown
   c. the inability of normally formed bile to be passed into the intestine

7. If a patient is in hepatic coma an antibiotic such as neomycin is administered to __b__.
   a. prevent secondary infection
   b. decrease intestinal bacteria which produce ammonia from proteins
   c. treat the inflammation present in the liver
   d. decrease intestinal bacteria which break down ammonia

8. Portal hypertension can be relieved by draining blood from the portal vein into an adjacent __a__.
   a. vein
   b. artery

9. The Sengstaken-Blakemore tube has three separate openings __b__.
   1. one inflates the esophageal balloon
   2. one empties the esophagus
   3. one inflates the gastric balloon
   4. one empties the stomach
   5. one empties the duodenum

   a. 1, 2, 3
   b. 1, 3, 4
   c. 2, 3, 4
   d. 2, 4, 5

10. Hepatitis is __c__.
    a. infectious
    b. contagious
    c. both a and b
    d. neither a nor b

11. The blood or blood product that can be made hepatitis virus-free is __b__.
    a. whole blood
    b. albumin
    c. pooled plasma
    d. packed cells

12. Infectious hepatitis can be transmitted by __d__.
    a. insects
    b. animals
    c. both a and b
    d. neither a nor b
13. The gallbladder normally stores approximately __B__ ml. of bile.
    a. 15
    b. 60
    c. 150
    d. 250
14. Bile functions in the __A__.
    a. absorption of fats, fat soluble vitamins, iron, and calcium
    b. release of the gastric enzymes pepsin and ptyaline
    c. synthesis of vitamin K and the digestion of fats and proteins
    d. emulsification of fats and the breakdown of protein and carbohydrates in the stomach and duodenum
15. The function of the gallbladder is to __D__.
    a. manufacture and emulsify bile
    b. inject bile into the jejunum
    c. collect the bile manufactured by the liver
    d. concentrate and store bile
16. Symptoms of chronic cholecystitis probably are the result of temporary obstruction of the outflow of bile and usually occur __B__.
    a. when the stomach is empty
    b. after a meal containing fried and/or fatty foods
    c. in the presence of a meal high in carbohydrates and foods high in cholesterol
    d. when the stomach is full
17. Patients having had a cholecystectomy may have moderately severe discomfort when deep breathing and coughing because __D__.
    a. surgery requires a relatively long time under anesthesia
    b. the diaphragm is usually traumatized during surgery
    c. of the position of the patient during surgery
    d. the incision is high in the abdomen
18. A cholecystectomy may be performed for cholelithiasis. During surgery, a T-tube may be inserted to __B__.
    a. support the T-shaped common bile duct
    b. drain bile from the common bile duct
    c. provide drainage of blood and serous fluid through the incision
    d. aid in the healing of the gallbladder

CLINICAL SITUATIONS

Mr. Jones is a 44-year-old engineer with cirrhosis of the liver. He has a past history of heavy alcohol intake since high school. He has been under the care of a physician; however he does not adhere to his physician's recommendations. Recently he began drinking heavily and became ill. His physician has admitted him to the acute medical service for re-evaluation of his disease.

19. The emphasis in nursing management of patients with liver disease is __B__.
    a. aimed at creating an atmosphere conducive to curing the disease
    b. on physiological support of the patient so that the liver will have a chance to regain adequate function
    c. on psychological support since little can be done to help the physical problems
20. It is noted that Mr. Jones is slightly jaundiced. Jaundice is due to staining of the skin, by an abnormally high concentration of __b__.
    a. bile
    b. bilirubin
    c. icterus
    d. transaminase

21. Jaundiced patients may have bleeding tendencies because the __D__.
    a. bile pigment weakens the walls of the capillaries
    b. outer layer of the skin has been affected by the pruritus, scaling, and jaundice
    c. excess bile pigment has blocked the reticuloendothelial cells
    d. liver manufactures factors needed for blood coagulation

22. Physical findings in advanced cirrhosis include __D__.
    1. weight loss
    2. spider angiomata
    3. enlarged liver
    4. ascites
    5. jaundice
        a. 1, 2, 5
        b. 1, 3, 4
        c. 2, 3, 5
        d. all of these

23. In patients with Laennec's cirrhosis portal hypertension leads to __C__.
    a. gastric ulcers
    b. pancreatitis
    c. esophageal varices
    d. electrolyte imbalance

24. The physician states that Mr. Jones may be in early hepatic coma. Signs of impending hepatic coma include __C__.
    1. hyperglycemia
    2. lethargy
    3. irritability
    4. mental confusion
    5. decrease in serum ammonia levels
        a. 1, 2, 3
        b. 1, 4, 5
        c. 2, 3, 4
        d. all of these

25. If severe hypoproteinemia occurs in Mr. Jones he may be given __A__.
    a. intravenous albumin
    b. intravenous fluids
    c. a high protein diet
    d. a low sodium diet

26. Daily weighings are ordered on Mr. Jones because __b__.
    a. of his anemia and weight loss
    b. there is a tendency toward water and salt retention, weight gain, and edema
    c. he eats poorly, loses weight, and has generalized muscle wasting

27. Mr. Jones' weight has been increasing and edema and ascites noted. His physician orders a diet change which will be __A__.
    a. low in salt
    b. low in albumin
    c. high in carbohydrates
    d. high in vitamins

28. Mr. Jones develops abdominal fluid due to ascites. The abdominal fluid may be removed by __D__.
    a. ligation of the hepatic artery
    b. insertion of a drain in the portal system
    c. thoracentesis
    d. abdominal paracentesis

29. The physician believes Mr. Jones may go into hepatic coma. In an attempt to avoid this he places Mr. Jones on a special diet low in __C__.
    a. ammonia
    b. gluten
    c. protein
    d. carbohydrates

30. The usual method of treating hepatic coma involves __C__.
    a. addition of extra protein to the diet
    b. replacement of sodium and potassium lost through diuresis
    c. the reduction of blood ammonia levels
    d. administration of ammonia

31. Ammonia is __A__.
    a. formed in the intestines by action of intestinal bacteria on proteins
    b. the result of bacterial action on carbohydrates in the small intestine
    c. a byproduct of fat metabolism

Mrs. Clark, a 30-year-old housewife, became suddenly ill on a Saturday morning. Her husband called their family physician who told Mr. Clark to take his wife to the emergency department of the hospital where he is on staff. He promised Mr. Clark he would meet them at the hospital. On arrival, Mrs. Clark is examined by her physician who admits her to the medical service with a diagnosis of acute pancreatitis.

32. In acute pancreatitis, the most *common* complaint is __B__.
    a. nausea, diarrhea
    b. severe middle-upper abdominal pain
    c. diffuse abdominal pain
    d. vomiting, convulsions

33. The next day Mrs. Clark tells you she is nauseated. An hour later she begins to have emesis. What nursing measure is instituted until her physician is notified? __A__
    a. withhold all food and fluids
    b. encourage sips of room temperature ginger ale
    c. offer her tea and dry crackers to minimize the nausea

34. The physician orders intravenous fluids. If vomiting continues he may order a(n) __D__.
    a. Miller-Abbott tube
    b. barium enema studies
    c. emergency surgery to relieve the intestinal obstruction caused by the pancreatitis
    d. nasogastric tube

35. Mrs. Clark begins to improve and after 9 days she is allowed a clear liquid diet. Once solid food is allowed she will probably be given a __C__.
    a. soft diet
    b. low cholesterol, low sodium diet
    c. bland diet progressing to a low fat diet
    d. bland diet progressing to a house diet

36. If Mrs. Clark develops chronic recurrent pancreatitis, it is possible she would lose all or part of her pancreatic function—the __A__.
    1. secretion of the hormone insulin
    2. production of digestive enzymes
    3. manufacture of pepsin
    4. manufacture of bile
        a. 1, 2
        b. 1, 3
        c. 2, 3
        d. 2, 4

IV. Fill-in and discussion questions.

Read each question carefully and place your answer in the space provided.

1. VOCABULARY. Define the following terms.

    a. cholecystectomy: removal of the gallbladder

    b. cholelithiasis: stones in the gallbladder

    c. endocrine gland: ductless gland that secretes its hormones into the bloodstream

    d. endogenous: originating in an organism or cell

e. exocrine: _gland that has ducts_

f. exogenous: _originating outside of an organ_

g. glycogen: _carbohydrate stored in the body particularly in the liver._

h. hormone: _____

i. hypercholesterolemia: _____

j. icterus (adj. icteric): _jaundice_

k. reticuloendothelial cells: _ingest worn out red blood cells + bacteria_

2. List 3 important functions of the liver.
   1. _Excrete & Manufacture bile_
   2. _Store vitamins, glycogen_
   3. _produce fibrinogen & prothrombin_

3. What nursing observations are made after the patient has had a liver biopsy?
   Vital signs
   Abd bleeding & distension
   Severe pain

4. Patients with liver disease may have bleeding tendencies. What might the nurse do to lessen the likelihood of bleeding in these patients? _____

CHAPTER—34

The urologic patient

Patients with disorders of the urinary tract not only suffer from the accompanying physical discomfort, but often from embarrassment and anxiety as well. Disclosure of genitourinary difficulties often involves the sharing of very personal information and the experience of an extensive physical examination of this part of the body. Every effort should be made by the nurse and other personnel to protect the patient's modesty and privacy and to deal matter-of-factly with the problem.

The following questions deal with the contents of Chapter 34.

I. True or false.

Read each statement carefully and place your answer in the space provided.

__T__ 1. The urinary tract is one of several systems by which the body rids itself of the by-products of metabolism.

__F__ 2. Urine is carried from the kidney down the urethra to the bladder.

__T__ 3. The kidneys filter over 50 gallons of plasma every day.

__T__ 4. Certain metabolic disturbances, dyes, and foods may impart a red color to the urine.

__T__ 5. Bowman's capsule is a part of the kidney nephron.

__F__ 6. The convoluted tubule is part of the ureter.

__T__ 7. Failure of the nephron to remove waste products from the blood results in an alteration of blood chemistry.

__T__ 8. An intravenous pyelogram is based on the ability of the kidneys to excrete radiopaque contrast media in the urine.

__T__ 9. Renal arteriograms are used to evaluate the blood vessels of the kidney.

__T__ 10. Some tumors of the bladder can be treated by fulguration.

__F__ 11. A cystoscopy cannot be performed on an outpatient basis as a general anesthesia is necessary for the procedure.

__T__ 12. Mild hematuria may be seen after a cystoscopy or any bladder instrumentation.

__T__ 13. As a general rule, the urologic patient should drink extra fluids to keep the urine dilute.

__T__ 14. The patient with a neurogenic bladder may not completely empty his bladder when he voids.

__F__ 15. Patients who have a tendency to form stones in the urinary tract should limit their fluid intake to prevent recurrence of the stones.

__T__ 16. Patients with gout should limit their purine intake to prevent uric acid stones.

__F__ 17. A catheter size 20 F is larger in

187

___ diameter than a catheter size 24 F.
_T_ 18. Urethral strictures may be treated by dilatation with specially designed instruments, such as bougies and sounds.
_T_ 19. Bladder tumors may be malignant or benign.
_F_ 20. In a cutaneous ureterostomy the ureters are implanted in the posterior wall of the bladder.
_T_ 21. A focus of infection elsewhere in the body may spread to the urinary tract.
_F_ 22. Tuberculosis usually starts in the urinary tract and spreads to the lungs.
_T_ 23. Chronic pyelonephritis may be asymptomatic.
_F_ 24. The urine normally contains a few bacteria.
_F_ 25. Nonspecific urethritis is caused by gonorrhea.
_T_ 26. Another term for nephritis is Bright's disease.
_T_ 27. Treatment of glomerulonephritis is nonspecific and guided by symptoms and their underlying pathology.
_F_ 28. Most patients with chronic glomerulonephritis have a history of acute glomerulonephritis.
_T_ 29. Polycystic disease is a congenital disorder of the kidney.

II. Multiple choice questions.

Select the most appropriate answer and place it in the space provided.

1. Three functions of the kidneys are __B__.
    1. excretion of excess water
    2. production of renin
    3. manufacture of urea
    4. maintenance of acid-base balance
    5. manufacture of epinephrine
        a. 1, 2, 3
        b. 1, 2, 4
        c. 2, 4, 5
        d. 3, 4, 5

2. The most important diagnostic study of the urinary tract is __a__.
    a. urinalysis
    b. blood urea nitrogen
    c. P.S.P. test
    d. concentration and dilution test

3. Deterioration in renal function is manifested chemically by __c__.
    1. decrease in creatinine
    2. rise in creatinine
    3. rise in blood urea nitrogen
    4. decrease in blood urea nitrogen
        a. 1, 3
        b. 1, 4
        c. 2, 3
        d. 2, 4

4. When the kidneys are damaged __a__
    a. the ability to concentrate or dilute urine is impaired
    b. sodium and potassium are no longer excreted in the urine
    c. the ability to conserve the products of metabolism is impaired
    d. the urine becomes concentrated

5. If a patient with renal disease is given phenolsulfonphthalein (P.S.P.) there will be a __B__.
    a. rapid excretion of the dye
    b. delay in excretion of the dye

6. If a patient is admitted to the hospital for an extensive diagnostic workup and is to have barium studies *and* an intravenous pyelogram, the study that should be performed first is the __B__.
    a. barium study
    b. intravenous pyelogram

7. Prior to an intravenous pyelogram, the patient receives nothing by mouth for 12 hours. The reason for this fasting is that it __B__.
   a. dehydrates the patient so the urine and the contrast media will be at maximum concentration
   b. keeps the bowel empty and, therefore, permits better visualization of the kidneys
8. A cystoscope enables the physician to see the bladder and the __A__.
   1. ureter
   2. urethra
   3. kidney pelvis
   4. ureteral orifices
      a. 1, 2
      b. 1, 3
      c. 2, 3
      d. 2, 4
9. When the bladder is filled and the cystoscope passes the internal sphincter at the bladder neck, the patient will __B C__.
   a. experience a severe but brief episode of suprapubic pain
   b. feel a pulling sensation in the lumbar region
   c. feel the urge to void
   d. have the urge to defecate
10. Following cystoscopy the patient should be told to drink extra fluids to __a__.
    a. lessen the irritation of the lining of the urinary tract and dilute the urine
    b. remove the dye from the kidneys, ureter, and bladder and prevent stone formation due to the action of the dye on the urine
11. Following cystoscopy __c__.
    a. the first voiding will be painful because of the dye used during the procedure
    b. voiding is usually painful for a week to 10 days
    c. voiding will be painful for about a day
12. The urologic patient is observed for edema, especially __c__.
    a. peripheral edema
    b. edema of the fingers
    c. periorbital edema
13. If blood calcium is low, the patient is observed for __B__.
    a. nausea and vomiting
    b. hypocalcemic tetany
    c. hypertension
    d. muscle weakness
14. If the urologic patient has an elevated potassium level, he is observed for __B__.
    1. mental confusion
    2. hypertension
    3. tetany
    4. changes in pulse rate and rhythm
    5. listlessness
       a. 1, 2, 3
       b. 1, 4, 5
       c. 2, 3, 4
       d. 2, 4, 5
15. If a patient has an *adequate* fluid intake, the daily urinary output should be more than __c__ ml.
    a. 100
    b. 200
    c. 500
16. The kidney pelvis has a capacity of __a__ of fluid.
    a. 5 to 8 ml.
    b. 10 to 15 ml.
    c. 15 to 30 ml.
    d. 30 to 50 ml.
17. The amount of fluid used in the irrigation of a ureteral catheter is __a B__.
    a. 5 ml.
    b. 15 ml.
    c. 30 ml.
    d. 50 ml.
18. The amount of fluid usually used in the irrigation of a urethral catheter is __c__.
    a. 5 ml.
    b. 15 ml.
    c. 30 ml.
    d. 100 ml.

19. A neurogenic bladder may be __d__.
    a. spastic, preventing the retention of urine
    b. flaccid, preventing the complete expulsion of urine
    c. neither a nor b
    d. both a and b

20. Increasing intra-abdominal pressure may aid the patient with a neurogenic bladder to void. One way of increasing intra-abdominal pressure is __c__.
    a. to place the patient in a supine position
    b. to have the patient stand
    c. gentle manual pressure immediately above the symphasis pubis

21. If a patient has an indwelling catheter for a long period of time, bladder training may be necessary to re-establish normal function. One method of bladder training is __D__.
    a. removing the catheter and reinserting it every 4 hours to empty the bladder
    b. forcing fluids
    c. removing the catheter and having the patient void every 4 hours
    d. alternate clamping and unclamping of the catheter

22. Catheterizing the patient after he has voided may be done to __A__.
    a. remove residual urine
    b. control postvoiding bladder spasms
    c. reduce the pain of voiding usually experienced by the incontinent patient

23. Urea-splitting organisms, such as *Micrococcus ureae* cause urea in the urine to react with water, producing __B__.
    a. uric acid
    b. ammonia
    c. hydro-uric acid

24. When the kidney pelvis is enlarged due to a backflow of urine, the condition is called __A__.
    a. hydronephrosis
    b. ureteral constriction
    c. pelvic expansion

25. Urinary stones often occur in those __D__.
    a. drinking large amounts of fruit juices
    b. eating large amounts of foods high in calcium
    c. not following a regular exercise schedule
    d. on long-term bed rest

26. A malignant hypernephroma __C__.
    a. is usually first diagnosed when the patient complains of lumbar pain
    b. gives rise to early symptoms and, therefore, is easily cured
    c. usually metastasizes early and presents symptoms late in the course of the disease

27. A right or left flank incision may be used for a nephrectomy. The patient will have a great deal of pain when coughing after surgery because this incision is __C__.
    a. large and requires sutures and drains that are painful
    b. small but requires the insertion of several Penrose drains
    c. close to the thoracic cavity
    d. near the rectus abdominus muscle

28. When a portion of the bladder is removed (segmental resection) the __B__.
    a. patient must have an indwelling catheter for the rest of his life
    b. capacity as a reservoir is decreased
    c. patient will be permanently incontinent
    d. capacity of the bladder is increased

29. The most common early symptom of a malignant tumor of the bladder is __C__.
    a. suprapubic pain
    b. fever
    c. painless hematuria
    d. pain on urination

30. Ureterosigmoidostomy is a urinary diversion surgery. In this surgery the __D__.
    a. ureters are re-implanted into the bladder
    b. sigmoid colon is anastomosed to the bladder
    c. ureters are implanted in or near the hepatic flexure of the large intestine
    d. ureters are attached to the sigmoid colon
31. When ureters are implanted in the bowel, there is a danger of __D__.
    a. fluid retention
    b. absorption of urine through the bowel mucosa
    c. high blood urea due to poor absorption of urea in the bowel
    d. microorganisms getting into the ureter and pelves resulting in infection
32. The patient with a cutaneous ureterostomy drains urine __B__.
    a. by means of cutaneous catheters
    b. by means of a collecting appliance similar to that worn by an ileostomate
    c. from a catheter in the bladder
    d. from a suprapubic cystotomy tube
33. An ileal conduit is another form of urinary diversion. In this surgery __C__.
    a. the ureters are implanted into the ileocecal junction
    b. the ureters are implanted into the colon
    c. an isolated segment of ileum is used as a urinary reservoir
    d. a segment of ileum is anastomosed to the bladder and acts as a urinary reservoir
34. Treatment of urinary tract infections usually includes __A__.
    1. placing the patient in the hospital for observation and control of the infection
    2. identification and removal of contributing factors
    3. using appropriate measures to combat infection
    4. increasing fluid intake
        a. all but 1
        b. all but 2
        c. all but 3
        d. all but 4
35. Diagnosis of cystitis is made by __D__.
    1. culture and sensitivity of the offending organism
    2. physical examination
    3. urinalysis
    4. patient history
        a. 1, 2
        b. 1, 3
        c. 2, 3
        d. all of these
36. Cranberry juice may be ordered for the patient with cystitis as it __A__.
    a. acidifies the urine providing a less favorable climate for bacterial growth
    b. soothes the bladder wall because of its analgesic qualities
    c. makes the urine alkaline
    d. changes the urine pH from acid to alkaline providing a medium that makes it impossible for microorganisms to multiply
37. A common cause of urethritis is __A__.
    a. irritation from an indwelling catheter
    b. drinking too much fluid
    c. drinking fruit juices and eating spicy foods
    d. exposure to a cold, damp climate
38. A nursing measure used to avoid urethritis in the female patient, especially if the patient is incontinent of feces, is to __B__.
    a. avoid getting fecal material on or near the urethral meatus by placing a cotton pledget soaked in antiseptic on the urethra
    b. avoid wiping toward the urethra; wipe away from the urethral meatus to the anus in a single stroke.
39. Nephrosis is __C__.
    a. the formation of thrombi in the sclerotic arteries of the kidney

b. a generalized disease of the kidney resulting in renal enlargement
c. a degenerative noninflammatory disease of the renal tubules

40. Any patient thought to have incurred trauma to the kidney is observed for __A__.
    a. anuria
    b. hypo- or hypertension
    c. diuresis
    d. anasarca

CLINICAL SITUATIONS

Mr. Abbott is a 52-year-old truck driver. Several weeks ago he noted pain in his right side radiating to his groin. Most of the time the pain was severe. Two days later the pain disappeared. This morning he experienced chills and fever along with severe flank pain. This time the pain is more severe and he calls his physician. He is examined in the physician's office and referred to a urologist, followed by admission to the hospital with a possible stone in the right ureter.

41. Mr. Abbott is having severe pain which is due to __A__.
    a. violent contractions and spasms as the ureter tries to pass the stone
    b. contraction and spasm of abdominal muscles due to the pain experienced as the stone travels down the ureter
    c. the rough edges of the stone

42. The collicky pain characteristic of a kidney or ureteral stone usually __A__.
    a. comes in waves that may start in the kidney or ureter and radiate to the inguinal region
    b. is a steady, stabbing pain usually beginning in the lumbar region and radiating to the umbilicus

43. To detect the passage of a stone, the physician may order that Mr. Abbott's urine be __B__.
    a. saved for laboratory analysis
    b. strained through gauze and the gauze inspected for a stone
    c. checked for stones by holding the container of urine next to a strong light

44. One way of locating Mr. Abbott's stone is by an abdominal x-ray. Another way is by __C__.
    a. aortic arteriography
    b. cystoscopy
    c. intravenous pyelogram

45. If Mr. Abbott's ureteral stone does not pass it may have to be removed surgically. This surgery is called a __B__.
    a. pyelolithotomy
    b. ureterolithotomy
    c. heminephrectomy
    d. nephrolithotomy

46. Mr. Abbott is found to have several stones in his ureter. Three days after admission he passes one of the stones and a chemical analysis is performed. It was found to be a uric acid stone which sometimes can be prevented by __B__.
    1. low purine diet
    2. acidification of the urine
    3. alkalinization of the urine
    4. low protein diet
        a. 1, 2
        b. 1, 3
        c. 2, 3
        d. 2, 4

47. Mr. Abbott has surgery for the removal of the other stone in his ureter. The surgical approach was by abdominal incision. A ureteral catheter is left in the ureter and connected to a separate drainage bottle. Normally there will be __B__.
    a. no urine draining from the ureteral catheter
    b. urine draining from the ureteral catheter

Josie Phillips, age 17, had an acute upper respiratory infection 3 weeks ago. She now complains of "feeling sick" and states she has a headache. Her mother takes her to their family physician who calls attention to Josie's puffy face and ankle edema. After a complete physical examination the physician decides to admit Josie to the hospital with a tentative diagnosis of acute glomerulonephritis.

48. Acute glomerulonephritis occurs most frequently in __d__.
    a. elderly, debilitated patients
    b. chronically ill patients
    c. those with prior urinary tract infections
    d. children and young adults

49. Laboratory findings in glomerulonephritis include __A__.
    1. slightly elevated blood urea nitrogen
    2. albuminuria
    3. gross or microscopic hematuria
    4. decreased blood urea nitrogen
    5. absence of albumin in the urine
        a. 1, 2, 3
        b. 1, 3, 5
        c. 2, 3, 4
        d. 3, 4, 5

50. If Josie has glomerulonephritis her blood pressure will probably be __A__.
    a. elevated
    b. decreased

51. Josie's fluid intake is limited. This is the usual practice if __C__.
    a. there is any change in the blood pressure, that is hypo- or hypertension
    b. she is eating poorly
    c. there is edema or signs of oliguria or anuria
    d. she is not given sulfonamides for the infection

52. Josie remains in the hospital 2 weeks and then is discharged. The physician explains to Mrs. Phillips that Josie is *not* considered cured until her __A__.
    a. urine is free of albumin and red blood cells for 6 months
    b. blood pressure is normal and her urinary output over 1500 ml. per day
    c. color improves and she looks and feels better

53. Mrs. Phillips asks the physician if Josie will recover. Although nothing definite can be stated, the prognosis of acute glomerulonephritis is usually __A__.
    a. good
    b. fair
    c. poor

Frank Smith, age 25, has chronic glomerulonephritis. He has had 2 severe periods of symptoms followed by latent or quiescent periods of several years. In the past month he has experienced an exacerbation of his disease and is admitted to the hospital with generalized anasarca, hypertension, nocturia, and dyspnea.

54. Generalized anasarca is an indication that Frank is in __A__.
    a. the nephrotic stage
    b. the terminal stage
    c. a non-nephrotic stage
    d. a latent stage

55. Frank's urine will __B__.
    a. not contain albumin
    b. contain albumin

56. The course of chronic glomerulonephritis is highly variable. As a nurse you know that there are many complications associated with this disease, including __C__.
    1. hypotension
    2. anemia
    3. diuresis
    4. congestive heart failure
    5. renal insufficiency
        a. 1, 2, 3
        b. 1, 4, 5
        c. 2, 4, 5
        d. all of these

57. The usual outcome of chronic glomerulonephritis is death from __b__.
    a. anemia
    b. uremia
    c. fluid depletion

58. Because of his generalized edema, Frank is placed on a __a__.
    a. diet limited in sodium and potassium
    b. diet limited in potassium
    c. high protein diet
    d. high protein, low carbohydrate diet

59. Frank's prognosis is good if he responds to therapy. He is placed on bed rest to __a__.
    a. decrease the workload of the heart
    b. aid in the excretion of excess fluid and potassium
    c. help control the anemia and albuminuria

III. Fill-in and discussion questions.

Read each question carefully and place your answer in the space provided.

1. Label the 4 areas identified in the drawing below by filling in the blanks to the right of the drawing. The 4 areas are to be selected from the words given below the drawing.

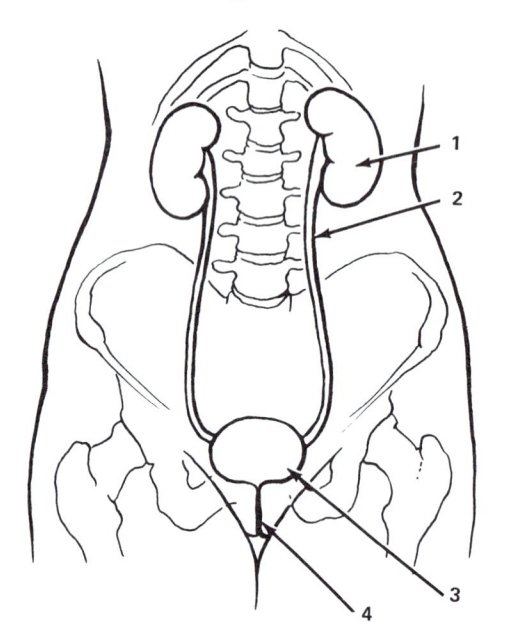

   1. _Kidney_
   2. _Ureter_
   3. _Bladder_
   4. _Urethra_

   ureter   urethra   kidney   bladder

2. Below is a urinalysis report on a patient's chart. Place a check mark (√) in front of the *abnormal* laboratory findings.

____ specific gravity	1.007
____ color	yellow
√ pH	alkaline
√ glucose	3+
____ protein	none
√ red blood cells	50 to 60
____ white blood cells	0 to 2
____ casts	none

3. Cystoscopy is the visual examination of the inside of the bladder. List 3 purposes of a cystoscopy.

   1. _Inspection_ 3. _treatment_
   2. _Biopsy_

4. When a patient must drink extra fluids he should drink several extra glasses of water every day. What other foods/fluids can be given to increase the total fluid intake in a patient who has *no* dietary restrictions? _Ice cream, tea, coffee, cocoa, milk, soda, juice_

5. Some discomforts are very disturbing to the urologic patient. In the spaces below, a discomfort or problem is given. In the space to the right briefly describe how the nurse might manage the problem.

Discomfort	Management
Itching	cut nails
Odor	remove soiled goods, skin care
Dryness of the mouth	lemon, glycerin swabs
Pain or burning on urination	sitz baths
Long-term bed rest	ROM exercises, turn frequently
Embarrassment and fear	Don't expose pt. Let him ventilate

195

6. Name four causes of urinary tract obstruction.
    1. Calculi
    2. Ureteral kink
    3. Ureteral spasm or stenosis
    4. Tumor

7. Give 4 symptoms that may be present if the patient has cystitis.
    1. Frequency
    2. Nocturia
    3. chill, fever
    4. urgency
    pain in perineal & suprapubic areas

UNIT EIGHT
Problems resulting from endocrine imbalance

CHAPTER—35

The patient with an endocrine disorder

The consequences of diseases of the ductless (endocrine) glands are usually due to overproduction or underproduction of the hormones that the glands secrete, causing a disturbance in the delicate balance that the hormones normally maintain. This often results in a widespread chain of events within the body.

The following questions deal with the contents of Chapter 35.

I. True or false.

Read each statement carefully and place your answer in the space provided.

_____ 1. Disorders of the endocrine system usually are due to overproduction or underproduction of the hormones secreted by these glands.

_____ 2. Hyperthyroidism is also called Graves' disease.

_____ 3. The etiology of hyperthyroidism is unknown.

_____ 4. The BMR is the most reliable test for thyroid function.

_____ 5. Thyroid scanning may be used when there is a suspicion of a thyroid malignancy.

_____ 6. Lugol's solution contains a thyroid preparation and is administered to the hypothyroid patient.

_____ 7. Thyroid crisis may occur within the first 12 hours after thyroid surgery.

_____ 8. The thyroid gland requires large amounts of iodine to manufacture thyroid hormones.

_____ 9. Thyroid cancer is suspected when there is an enlarged lump which is hard to the touch.

_____ 10. Hypothyroidism in the adult is called myxedema.

_____ 11. The side effects of thyroid replacement therapy are symptoms of hypothyroidism.

_____ 12. The adrenal medulla manufactures and secretes glucocorticoids.

_____ 13. Glucocorticoids and mineralocorticoids are essential to life.

_____ 14. Glucocorticoids affect body metabolism.

_____ 15. Adrenal crisis is not an acute emergency unless the patient is hypotensive.

_____ 16. Cushing's syndrome is an adrenal malfunction that is the opposite of Addison's disease.

_____ 17. Aldosterone is one of the hormones of the adrenal cortex.

_____ 18. Cushing's syndrome may be due to an adrenal tumor.

_____ 19. Treatment of hyperaldosteronism is surgical, and a bilateral adrenalectomy usually is considered to provide the best chance of a cure.

___ 20. Antidiuretic hormone (ADH) is manufactured and secreted by the anterior lobe of the pituitary gland.

II. Multiple choice questions.

Select the most appropriate answer and place it in the space provided.

1. Simple goiter is _____.
    a. the development of nodes in or near the thyroid gland
    b. an enlargement of the thyroid gland without symptoms of thyrotoxicosis
    c. a decrease in the size of the thyroid gland

2. Simple goiter may be due to _____.
    1. a lack of iodine in the diet
    2. the inability of the thyroid to utilize iodine
    3. a malignancy
    4. a benign tumor
       a. 1, 2
       b. 1, 3
       c. 2, 3
       d. 2, 4

3. Symptoms of a simple goiter include _____.
    1. nervousness, anxiety
    2. severe weight loss
    3. sense of fullness in the throat
    4. enlargement of the gland
       a. 1, 2
       b. 1, 4
       c. 2, 3
       d. 3, 4

4. To generally eliminate simple goiter due to iodine deficiency _____.
    a. sea food should be eaten at least once a month
    b. green leafy vegetables must be eaten regularly
    c. salt manufacturers add iodine to common table salt

5. Treatment of cancer of the thyroid may include _____.
    a. a total thyroidectomy with radical neck dissection
    b. thyroid lobectomy
    c. both a and b

6. In hypothyroidism, tests such as the TSH stimulation test, BMR, and PBI are _____.
    a. increased
    b. decreased

7. The symptoms of hypothyroidism include _____.
    1. warm and flushed skin
    2. masklike face
    3. weight gain
    4. lethargy
    5. tachycardia, insomnia
       a. 1, 3, 4
       b. 1, 4, 5
       c. 2, 3, 4
       d. 2, 3, 5

8. Generally, hypothyroidism is treated by _____.
    a. replacement therapy
    b. administration of antithyroid drugs
    c. inclusion of iodized salt in the diet

9. The parathyroids, usually 4 in number, secrete a hormone regulating the concentration of _____ and _____ in the blood.
    a. sodium   potassium
    b. calcium   phosphorus
    c. phosphorus   sodium
    d. potassium   calcium

10. In patients with hyperparathyroidism there is a(n) _____.
    a. overproduction of parathormone
    b. reduction of calcium in the body
    c. decrease in serum calcium
    d. rise in circulating thyroid hormone

11. Treatment of hyperparathyroidism is ____.
    a. surgical, with removal of hypertrophied gland tissue
    b. surgical removal of all the parathyroids and ⅔ of the thyroid gland
    c. administration of parathormone
    d. administration of calcium by mouth

12. The postoperative management of the hyperparathyroid patient is similar to the management of the patient with a thyroidectomy, including observation for symptoms of ____.
    a. thyroidism
    b. parathormonism
    c. hyperparathyroidism
    d. hypoparathyroidism

13. Problems that may be seen in the untreated hyperparathyroid patient are ____.
    1. goiter
    2. pathological fractures
    3. kidney stones
    4. weight gain
    a. 1, 2
    b. 1, 4
    c. 2, 3
    d. 2, 4

14. Patients with hypoparathyroidism exhibit a(n) ____.
    1. decrease in the excretion of calcium in the urine
    2. decrease of calcium blood levels
    3. increase in calcium blood levels
    4. increase in the excretion of calcium in the urine
    a. 1, 2
    b. 1, 3
    c. 2, 4
    d. 3, 4

15. One sign of severe hypoparathyroidism is tetany. If the facial nerve at the area in front of the ear is tapped the patient's mouth twitches and the jaw tightens. This is known as ____.
    a. Homan's sign
    b. a Hoffman reflex
    c. Chvostek's sign
    d. a Babinski reflex

16. Management of the patient with hypoparathyroidism may include the ____.
    a. weekly to biweekly injection of calcium
    b. administration of vitamin D and calcium
    c. addition of milk and milk products to the diet
    d. administration of vitamins C and E

17. Mineralocorticoids are concerned with the ____.
    a. maintenance of water and electrolyte balance
    b. supression of inflammation
    c. body metabolism
    d. adaptation of the body to stress

18. The patient with hyperaldosteronism has ____.
    1. hypertension
    2. hypokalemia
    3. hypoglycemia
    4. hypercholesterolemia
    a. 1, 2
    b. 1, 3
    c. 2, 3
    d. 2, 4

19. A pheochromocytoma is a tumor of the adrenal medulla causing ____.
    a. an increased secretion of corticosteroids
    b. an increased secretion of epinephrine and norepinephrine
    c. Cushing's syndrome
    d. a decreased production of epinephrine

20. Acromegaly results when the ____.
    a. anterior lobe of the pituitary stops secreting human growth hormone
    b. posterior lobe of the pituitary produces excess ADH
    c. pituitary ceases functioning
    d. anterior lobe of the pituitary produces excess human growth hormone

21. Acromegaly may be treated ____.
    a. surgically
    b. by radiation of the pituitary gland
    c. both a and b
22. Simmond's disease is also called ____.
    a. panhypopituitarism
    b. hyperpituitarism
23. Antidiuretic hormone (ADH) regulates the ____.
    a. reabsorption of water in the kidney tubules
    b. excretion of sodium and potassium
    c. conservation of electrolytes
    d. urea content of the urine
24. The patient with diabetes insipidus ____.
    a. requires insulin for control of the disease
    b. produces copious amounts of urine
    c. is hypoglycemic and, therefore, requires frequent high carbohydrate feedings
    d. will have to restrict his fluid intake until the disease is under control
25. Treatment of diabetes insipidus will include the ____.
    a. administration of vasopressin
    b. removal of the pituitary gland
    c. radiation of the pituitary gland
    d. administration of anterior pituitary extract

CLINICAL SITUATIONS

Diane Higgens, age 27, has had symptoms of hyperthyroidism for 3 years. She is now admitted to the hospital for a thyroidectomy.

26. The thyroid gland has the ability to ____.
    a. manufacture thyroid-stimulating hormone
    b. manufacture iodine from triiodothyronine
    c. concentrate and utilize iodine in the manufacture of thyroid hormones
27. The important active hormones released from the thyroid gland are ____.
    1. iodine
    2. triiodothyronine
    3. thyroid-stimulating hormone
    4. tetraiodothyronine
       a. 1, 2
       b. 1, 3
       c. 2, 3
       d. 2, 4
28. Symptoms of hyperthyroidism may include ____.
    1. weight loss and emotional lability
    2. weight gain and sleepiness
    3. bradycardia and anorexia
    4. tachycardia and intolerance to heat
    5. exophthalmos and excessive sweating
       a. 1, 3, 5
       b. 1, 4, 5
       c. 2, 3, 5
       d. 4 only
29. Diane is to have a radioactive iodine uptake study. The *normal* thyroid gland will remove ____.
    a. all or nearly all of the radioactive iodine in 24 hours
    b. 15 to 20 percent of the radioactive iodine in 24 hours
    c. little if any of the radioactive iodine in 24 to 48 hours
30. The amount of radioactive material used in a thyroid scan and a ^{131}I urine excretion test ____.
    a. requires placing the patient in isolation with radiation precautions
    b. does not require isolation of the patient and radiation precautions
31. Diane has previously had medical treatment for her hyperthyroidism which would have included ____.
    a. a low carbohydrate diet
    b. drugs that block the production of thyroid hormone
    c. the administration of synthetic or semisynthetic thyroid hormones

32. Preoperatively, Diane is given antithyroid drugs in an attempt to establish a euthyroid state to decrease the risk of ____.
    a. hypothyroidism after surgery
    b. iodine intoxication after surgery
    c. a loss of pituitary activity
    d. postoperative thyroid crisis
33. Diane returns from the operating room. Once she is fully awake ____.
    a. the head of the bed will be elevated
    b. the bed will be placed flat and Diane will be turned on her side
34. Pillows are positioned under Diane's head and shoulders. The pillow placed under her head should be ____.
    a. of regular size but placed only behind the head and not the neck
    b. large and soft
    c. small and firm
35. Diane should be instructed not to ____.
    a. move her head up and down until the wound has healed
    b. move her legs since this will encourage the formation of blood clots
    c. swallow unless absolutely necessary
36. Following surgery Diane is observed for symptoms of respiratory obstruction due to ____.
    1. edema in or near the operative area
    2. the surgical dressing
    3. bleeding
    4. enlargement of the remaining part of the thyroid gland
        a. 1, 2
        b. 1, 3
        c. 2, 3
        d. 2, 4
37. Emergency treatment of respiratory obstruction is essential; therefore ____.
    a. oxygen is available at the bedside
    b. the head of the bed is elevated
    c. only a light dressing is applied over the surgical incision
    d. a tracheostomy tray is readily available
38. Diane must also be encouraged to ____.
    a. cough and deep breathe every 2 hours
    b. deep breathe every 2 hours and encouraged to cough only if the physician specifically orders the latter measure
    c. cough and raise mucus from her lungs
39. Diane complains of a feeling of fullness in her throat. On inspection the surgical dressing is dry and intact. Your next step is to ____.
    a. check her chart and administer oxygen if ordered
    b. check for drainage on the bedding or pillow behind her neck
    c. call the physician
    d. turn her on her side and slightly hyperextend her head
40. On occasion the parathyroid glands are inadvertently removed during a thyroidectomy. If this should occur, the patient will develop ____.
    a. hypocalcemic tetany
    b. thyroid crisis
    c. hypothyroid distress

Sam Williams, a 28-year-old factory worker, was discovered to have Addison's disease 2 years ago. He is now admitted to the hospital acutely ill and thought to be in adrenal crisis.

41. Addison's disease is due to ____.
    a. hypofunction of the adrenal cortex
    b. hyperfunction of the adrenal medulla
    c. hyperfunction of the adrenal cortex
    d. hypofunction of the adrenal medulla
42. One test used in the diagnosis of Addison's disease is the ____.
    a. cortisone stimulation test
    b. BSP test
    c. measurement of adrenal cortical response to ACTH

43. Sam has the typical skin manifestations of a patient with Addison's disease and his skin is ____.
    a. abnormally dark and pigmented
    b. ruddy and oily
    c. puffy
    d. pale, dry, and scaly

44. Addison's disease is usually treated with ____.
    a. cortisone
    b. a preparation possessing glucocorticoid and mineralocorticoid properties
    c. ACTH

45. When his vital signs are taken, it is expected that Sam's blood pressure will be ____.
    a. low
    b. high

46. Patients with Addison's disease may develop adrenal crisis when ____.
    1. faced with severe stress
    2. undergoing surgery
    3. taking cortisone
    4. a diet high in sodium and potassium is eaten
    5. suffering from an infection
        a. 1, 2, 4
        b. 1, 2, 5
        c. 2, 3, 4
        d. 3, 4, 5

47. Early signs of acute adrenal crisis are ____.
    1. anorexia
    2. nausea, vomiting
    3. diarrhea, abdominal pain
    4. headache
    5. hypotension
        a. 1, 2, 3
        b. 2, 4, 5
        c. 3, 4, 5
        d. all of these

48. After examination the physician determines that Sam is in acute adrenal crisis. Treatment will now consist of ____.
    a. intravenous administration of corticosteroids, glucose, and normal saline
    b. intravenous administration of ACTH, saline, and potassium
    c. ACTH intramuscularly and glucose intravenously, given at 3-hour intervals
    d. intravenous administration of corticosteroids and potassium

49. No patient should receive a wrong medication. If Sam were given insulin by mistake this would ____.
    a. not be as serious as some medication errors since patients with Addison's disease often require insulin
    b. be serious because the patient with Addison's disease already has hypoglycemia
    c. be serious only because any medication error is serious even though the insulin would not do Sam any real harm

50. The patient with Addison's disease usually has recurrent hypoglycemia which is treated with ____.
    a. insulin
    b. glucose
    c. ACTH

Mrs. Barnes is a 47-year-old housewife with 3 children. She works part time as a clerk in a small dress shop. Three months ago she began to gain weight and noticed other physical changes. Consequently, she visited her family physician. After many clinical tests she was diagnosed as having Cushing's syndrome.

51. Cushing's syndrome is a(n) ____.
    a. overproduction of adrenal cortical hormones
    b. increase in the production of mineralocorticoids
    c. decrease in glucocorticoid production
    d. cessation of pituitary stimulation of the adrenal glands

52. Two typical symptoms experienced by the patient with Cushing's syndrome are ____.
    a. hypoglycemia, mental depression
    b. weight loss, pale face
    c. sodium and water loss, extreme thirst
    d. moon face, buffalo hump

53. Mrs. Barnes has been treated and followed in the endocrine outpatient clinic. The physician orders an abdominal x-ray. The rationale for this procedure is ____.
    a. the adrenal gland enlarges in Cushing's syndrome and an x-ray may show an adrenal mass
    b. patients with Cushing's syndrome often develop a bowel obstruction due to severe constipation
    c. this disease often affects the kidneys as well as the adrenal glands, and the x-ray would reveal the extent of the disease

54. Mrs. Barnes is admitted to the hospital for further treatment. While opinions vary, the 2 methods of treatment of Cushing's syndrome are ____.
    1. hypophysectomy
    2. adrenalectomy
    3. x-ray radiation of the pituitary
    4. administration of corticosteroid preparations
        a. 1, 3
        b. 1, 4
        c. 2, 3
        d. 2, 4

55. If Mrs. Barnes has surgery, she will be treated postoperatively as a patient with ____.
    a. diabetes
    b. panhypopituitarism
    c. Addison's disease
    d. hypoaldosteronism

III. Fill-in and discussion questions.

Read each question carefully and place your answer in the space provided.

1. Label the 8 areas identified in the drawing below by filling in the blanks to the left of the drawing. The 8 areas are to be selected from the words given below the drawing.

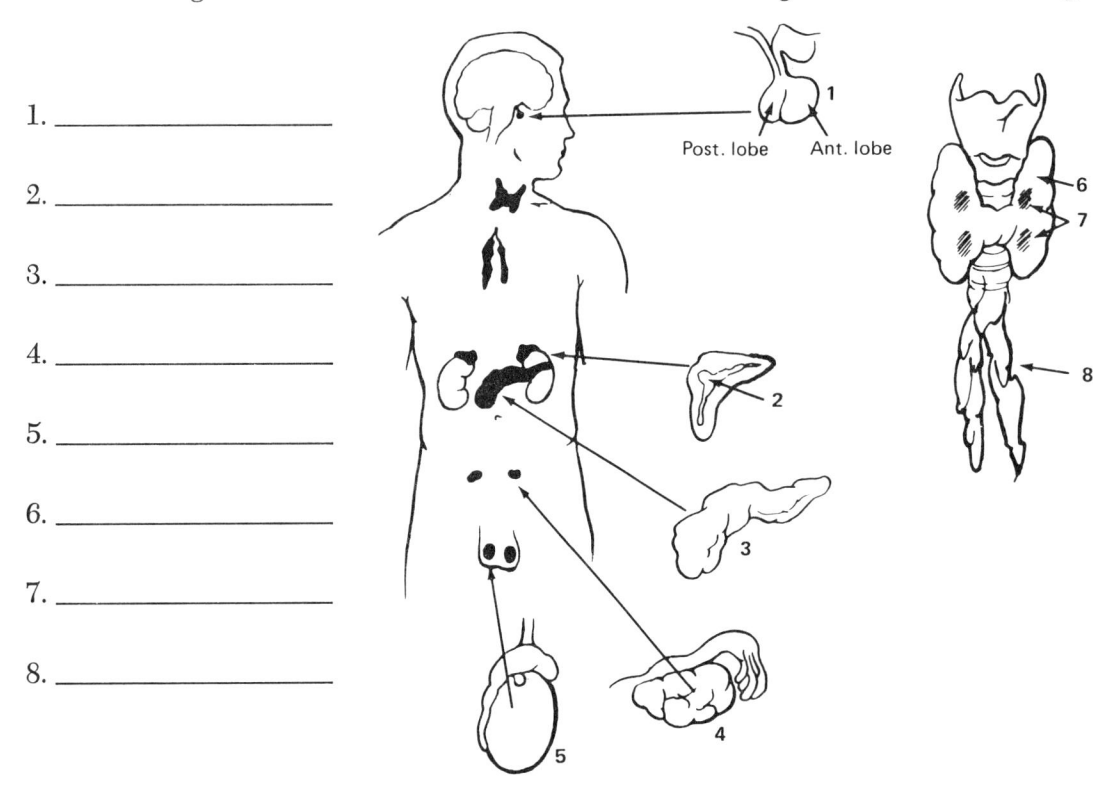

    1. _____
    2. _____
    3. _____
    4. _____
    5. _____
    6. _____
    7. _____
    8. _____

thymus   pancreas   ovary   testis

parathyroid   thyroid   adrenal   pituitary

2. With regard to medications, what points would you include in the discharge teaching of a patient with Addison's disease? _____

CHAPTER—36

The patient with diabetes mellitus

Diabetes mellitus is a metabolic disease in which there is some degree of insulin insufficiency, resulting in an impairment of the body's ability to metabolize carbohydrates, fats and proteins. Because of the lack of insulin or inadequate insulin action, abnormal amounts of glucose accumulate in the bloodstream and are subsequently excreted in the urine. As the condition becomes more advanced, excessive ketone bodies are found in the blood and urine, and virtually every cell in the body is affected by the metabolic derangement.

The following questions deal with the contents of Chapter 36.

I. True or false.

Read each statement carefully and place your answer in the space provided.

_____ 1. Diabetes mellitus is a metabolic disease.
_____ 2. Kussmaul's breathing is common in patients who are acidotic.
_____ 3. Normally, there is no easily detectable glucose or acetone in the urine.
_____ 4. If a patient has glucose in his urine, he is a diabetic.
_____ 5. The diabetic has less glucose in his bloodstream than the nondiabetic.
_____ 6. Treatment of diabetes is carried out for the rest of the patient's life.
_____ 7. Diabetes may be aggravated by excess weight.
_____ 8. Insulin can be given orally; however, the tablet must be enteric-coated to prevent destruction by gastric juices.
_____ 9. The insulin with the most rapid onset of action is Isophane Insulin Suspension, or NPH Insulin
_____ 10. The dose of insulin is expressed in units per milligram.
_____ 11. Exercise, other than brief walks, is not recommended for the diabetic patient taking insulin.
_____ 12. The early symptoms of ketosis may be vague.
_____ 13. An insulin hypoglycemic reaction is less of an emergency than diabetic ketosis.
_____ 14. Diabetics are prone to vascular disturbances.

II. Multiple choice questions.

Select the most appropriate answer and place it in the space provided.

1. After eating a full meal, the blood glucose returns to a fasting level in _____.
   a. ½ to 1 hour
   b. 2 hours
   c. 4 hours
   d. 2 to 4 hours

2. Insulin is secreted into the bloodstream by the ____.
   a. beta cells of the islands of Langerhans in the pancreas
   b. alpha cells located in the head of the pancreas
3. Tes-Tape and Clinitest are methods of testing for ____.
   a. glycogen in the liver
   b. glucose in the urine
   c. acetone in the urine
4. The CO_2 combining power is a general measure of the ____.
   a. amount of carbon dioxide in the blood
   b. amount of carbon dioxide and oxygen in the blood
   c. ability of red blood cells to pick up oxygen from body cells
   d. acidity or alkalinity of the blood
5. If the diabetic patient engages in exercise, his insulin requirement ____.
   a. increases
   b. decreases
6. Oral hypoglycemic agents are prescribed for some diabetics. The sulfonylurea group which includes tolbutamide (Orinase) is only of value if the ____.
   a. patient is young
   b. fasting blood sugar is initially below 100 mg. per 100 ml.
   c. patient is able to produce some insulin
   d. patient is not obese
7. Hypoglycemic reactions ____.
   a. vary somewhat from patient to patient
   b. are the same for nearly all patients
8. The treatment of hypoglycemia includes the administration of ____.
   a. a carbohydrate
   b. insulin
9. A sudden personality change in a diabetic patient might be indicative of ____.
   a. the wrong type of insulin
   b. a hypoglycemic reaction
   c. an impending state of alkalosis
10. When teaching the diabetic, nurses should explain that any slight illness is an indication that the patient should ____.
    a. increase his insulin dose
    b. decrease his insulin dose
    c. eliminate ½ of the carbohydrates in his diet
    d. test his urine more frequently
11. In the diabetic, the area of the body especially vulnerable to vascular changes is (are) the ____.
    a. upper extremities
    b. heart
    c. head and neck
    d. lower extremities
12. The individual best able to control his diabetes is the one who ____.
    a. takes his insulin regularly
    b. does not spill sugar in his urine
    c. understands his disease
    d. is found to be a diabetic while still young
13. If the diabetic develops an infection, the ____.
    1. infection will usually heal slowly
    2. diabetes becomes more severe while the infection persists
    3. patient will require less insulin and more carbohydrates
    4. patient will spill albumin in his urine
       a. 1, 2
       b. 1, 3
       c. 2, 3
       d. 2, 4

CLINICAL SITUATIONS

Mr. West, age 63, is admitted to the hospital for regulation of his diabetes. He has not followed the regimen prescribed by his physician—that is, diet, weight control, and insulin.

On admission he is somewhat lethargic and the physician feels he may be in early diabetic ketosis. Because he is also incontinent, an indwelling catheter is inserted.

14. Signs of diabetic ketosis include ____.
    1. weakness
    2. odor of acetone on breath
    3. skin and mouth are dry
    4. hypertension
    5. absence of acetone in the urine
        a. 1, 2, 3
        b. 1, 3, 4
        c. 2, 3, 4
        d. 2, 4, 5

15. If Mr. West is in early diabetic ketosis, his laboratory tests would show ____.
    1. acetone in his urine
    2. decreased CO_2 combining power
    3. decreased plasma sodium
    4. decreased plasma potassium
        a. 1, 2
        b. 1, 3
        c. 2, 3
        d. all of these

16. You must obtain a urine specimen from Mr. West's catheter. The correct technique would be to ____.
    a. take 15 to 30 ml. from the collecting bag
    b. remove the end of the tubing from the collecting bag and let some fresh urine run into a clean container
    c. clamp the catheter overnight, open it in the morning, and take a specimen
    d. have the patient drink 3 to 4 glasses of water, clamp the catheter for 4 hours, then open and take a specimen

17. Treatment of diabetic ketosis includes ____.
    a. administration of regular insulin
    b. administration of intravenous glucose
    c. administration of long-acting insulin

18. Mr. West responds well to treatment and is going to be reinstructed about diabetes in the hospital's diabetes teaching program. At one point of the instruction he tells you that he didn't understand what was said about the "date of the insulin". Your answer would be ____.
    a. there is a date stamped on every insulin bottle. This date refers to the day, month, and year the insulin was manufactured.
    b. insulin has a data sheet in the package and the sheet explains how to give the drug. There is no "date" on the bottle.
    c. every insulin bottle is stamped with an expiration date. Outdated insulin should *not* be used.

19. Mr. West is able to give his own insulin. Because he has not been reliable in the past it might be of value if ____.
    a. he is given the phone numbers of the community health department or closest hospital
    b. someone checked his urine daily to be sure he is giving himself insulin
    c. someone else in his family also learned the technique of insulin administration

20. Mr. West should be shown rotation sites for insulin injection in order to prevent ____.
    a. hypoglycemia
    b. lipohypertrophy of subcutaneous tissue
    c. an allergic reaction to the insulin

During National Hospital Week, the American Heart Association and the American Diabetes Association conducted a detection service for hypertension and diabetes in a large shopping plaza. Mrs. Young, age 57, decided to have her blood pressure checked. After the procedure the nurse advised Mrs. Young to see her family physician. She decided to have a small sample of blood taken from her finger for a screening test for diabetes. Again she was advised to see her physician. Mrs. Young made an appointment to see her physician and is now admitted to the hospital for medical evaluation.

21. Mrs. Young has a fasting blood glucose drawn. The normal fasting blood glucose is _____ to _____ mg. per 100 ml. of venous blood.
    a. 60   80
    b. 80   120
    c. 100   150
    d. 100   200

22. Mrs. Young is to have a glucose tolerance test. When the nondiabetic is given oral glucose for a glucose tolerance test, his blood glucose level will return to normal in approximately _____ hours(s).
    a. 1
    b. 2
    c. 4
    d. 6

23. Mrs. Young is a diabetic and will participate in the hospital diabetic teaching program. Before beginning to teach the new diabetic, it is important to _____.
    a. be sure the diabetes is severe enough to require participation in the program
    b. see that the patient has accepted her illness before teaching begins
    c. assess how the patient is accepting her illness

24. Mrs. Young will require dietary instruction because what the patient eats is one of the most important factors in controlling diabetes. If her intake of carbohydrates is more than what she can use or store, she will eventually go into _____.
    a. ketosis
    b. alkalosis
    c. hypoglycemia

25. Mrs. Young must also realize the importance of eating all the food on her prescribed diet. If she is taking insulin and eats too little food _____.
    a. hyperinsulinism with resultant hypoglycemia will occur
    b. she will go into diabetic coma
    c. hyperglycemia will occur
    d. hypoinsulinism with resultant hyperglycemia will occur

26. When a diabetic diet is prescribed, the physician takes into consideration the patient's _____.
    1. former dietary habits
    2. age
    3. height and weight
    4. activity and occupation
    5. sex
        a. 1, 2, 3
        b. 1, 3, 4
        c. 2, 4, 5
        d. all of these

27. Mrs. Young asks you if she can eat the dietetic cookies she has seen in the market and if so, are they counted in her diet. Your answer would be _____.
    a. dietetic and diabetic mean the same; therefore, these foods can be eaten
    b. the foods can be eaten providing the fats, proteins, and carbohydrates are counted in the diet
    c. these foods are for people who wish to lose weight and are not intended for diabetics

28. Mrs. Young is presently receiving regular insulin. If she receives 10 units of this insulin at 7:30 A.M., the onset of action would normally be _____.
    a. 8 to 8:30 A.M.
    b. 8 to 10 A.M.
    c. 8:30 to 10:30 A.M.
    d. noon

III. Fill-in and discussion questions.

Read each question carefully and place your answer in the space provided.

1. Fill in the blanks of the following questions with the correct word or words that will complete the statement.

    1. The presence of glucose in the urine is called _____.
    2. The condition of excess glucose in the blood is called _____.
    3. Excessive thirst is called _____.
    4. When fat is metabolized, _____ bodies are formed in the liver.
    5. When there is too much insulin in the bloodstream in relation to the amount of available glucose, _____ results.
    6. Eating large amounts of food is called _____.
    7. Excessive secretion of urine is called _____.
    8. Insulin is manufactured by an endocrine gland called the _____.
    9. The cells that manufacture insulin are the _____ cells of the islands of _____.

2. Place a check mark (√) in front of the foods that usually are excluded from a diabetic diet:

    ____ peas
    ____ chicken
    ____ coffee
    ____ honey
    ____ unsweetened pickles
    ____ pie
    ____ potato
    ____ unsweetened gelatin
    ____ chewing gum
    ____ cranberries
    ____ liver
    ____ soft drinks
    ____ candy
    ____ beets

3. You are doing diabetic teaching and must explain how insulin is stored in the home. List the points you would cover in this explanation. _____

    _____
    _____
    _____
    _____
    _____
    _____

4. List 8 symptoms of a hypoglycemia reaction.

    1. _____   5. _____
    2. _____   6. _____
    3. _____   7. _____
    4. _____   8. _____

UNIT NINE

Disturbances of sexual structures or reproductive function

CHAPTER—37

Introduction: the female reproductive pattern

Besides the basic determination of the patient's physical needs, one of the fundamental requirements of effective nursing care of the gynecologic patient is an ability to listen to the patient's requests for reassurance and information, and recognize manifestations of anxiety. The ability to understand a patient's questions requires sensitive listening because many patients, ashamed of their ignorance, will pose questions in ancedotal forms or attribute them to friends and relatives. A nurse who is listening for such subtleties can often discover the nature of the patient's anxieties and can help by allowing her to verbalize her fears and by supplying facts and advice when necessary.

The following questions deal with the contents of Chapter 37.

I. True or false.

Read each statement carefully and place your answer in the space provided.

_____ 1. Vaginal irrigations are done with clean technique whereas bladder catheterizations require sterile technique.

_____ 2. Douching is usually contraindicated during late pregnancy.

_____ 3. Menstruation usually begins between the ages of 10 and 14.

_____ 4. The menstrual flow normally begins about 4 to 7 days after ovulation.

_____ 5. When conception occurs, the corpus luteum will persist during early pregnancy.

_____ 6. Puberty proceeds at different rates for different individuals.

_____ 7. Physical activity should be limited during menstruation.

_____ 8. Menopause normally occurs between ages 45 and 55.

_____ 9. Dysmenorrhea may be secondary to pathological conditions such as endometriosis.

_____ 10. Basal body temperature is an extremely accurate method of determining when ovulation occurs.

_____ 11. In about ½ of the couples with infertility problems, the difficulty lies with the male.

II. Multiple choice questions.

Select the most appropriate answer and place it in the space provided.

1. To avoid bringing organisms from the anal area to the vagina or urethra, the nurse should _____.

a. always wipe the patient anterior to posterior, using a new cotton ball or sponge with each stroke
   b. always wipe the patient posterior to anterior using a new cotton ball or sponge with each stroke

2. The ovarian follicle matures under the influence of the ____.
   a. hormone progesterone
   b. follicle-stimulating hormone
   c. corpus luteum
   d. luteinizing hormone

3. Ovulation occurs because the mature follicle ruptures with the release of _____ _____ from the anterior pituitary gland.
   a. follicle-stimulating hormone
   b. progesterone
   c. the corpus luteum
   d. luteinizing hormone

4. After the ovum is released, the ruptured follicle is transformed into a small body filled with yellow fluid called the ____.
   a. ovulatory body
   b. corpus luteum
   c. endometrial scar

5. The development of uterine endometrium is governed by _____.
   a. the follicle-stimulating hormone
   b. the posterior pituitary gland
   c. estrogen

6. The corpus luteum produces a hormone called ____.
   a. estrogen
   b. progesterone
   c. luteinizing hormone
   d. follicle-stimulating hormone

7. Primary dysmenorrhea usually is ____.
   a. due to overexertion
   b. hormonal in origin
   c. idiopathic
   d. rare in the teenager or young adult

8. Causes of amenorrhea may be ____.
   1. lack of the hormone progestin
   2. pregnancy
   3. menopause
   4. lactation if the mother is breast-feeding
   5. overproduction of the follicle-stimulating hormone
      a. 1, 2, 3
      b. 1, 4, 5
      c. 2, 4, 5
      d. 2, 3, 4

9. Menorrhagia may be caused by ____.
   1. fibroid tumors
   2. emotional upsets
   3. ovarian cysts
   4. deficiency of luteinizing hormone
   5. lack of a corpus luteum
      a. 1, 2, 3
      b. 1, 3, 4
      c. 2, 4, 5
      d. 3, 4, 5

10. Metrorrhagia may be a(n) ____.
    a. early warning sign of cancer
    b. sign of premature menopause
    c. sign of early menarche

11. For conception to occur, it is necessary for the sperm to travel to the ____.
    a. cervix
    b. vaginal fornix
    c. lower part of the uterus
    d. fallopian tube

12. Conception is most likely to take place ____.
    a. before ovulation
    b. 2 hours before and after ovulation
    c. soon after ovulation
    d. 6 to 9 days after ovulation

13. Tests for infertility include the Sims-Huhner test which is a ____.
    a. microscopic examination of tissue taken from the uterus and cervix
    b. microscopic examination of vaginal and cervical secretions aspirated 6 to 12 hours after intercourse
    c. forcing of carbon dioxide through the uterus into the fallopian tubes

III. Fill-in and discussion questions.

Read each question carefully and place your answer in the space provided.

1. VOCABULARY. Define the following terms.

    a. amenorrhea: _____

    b. dysmenorrhea: _____

    c. endometrium: _____

    d. menarche: _____

    e. menopause: _____

    f. menorrhagia: _____

    g. menses: _____

    h. metrorrhagia: _____

    i. oligomenorrhea: _____

2. Label the 7 areas identified in the drawing below by filling in the blanks to the right of the drawing. The 7 areas are to be selected from the words given below the drawing.

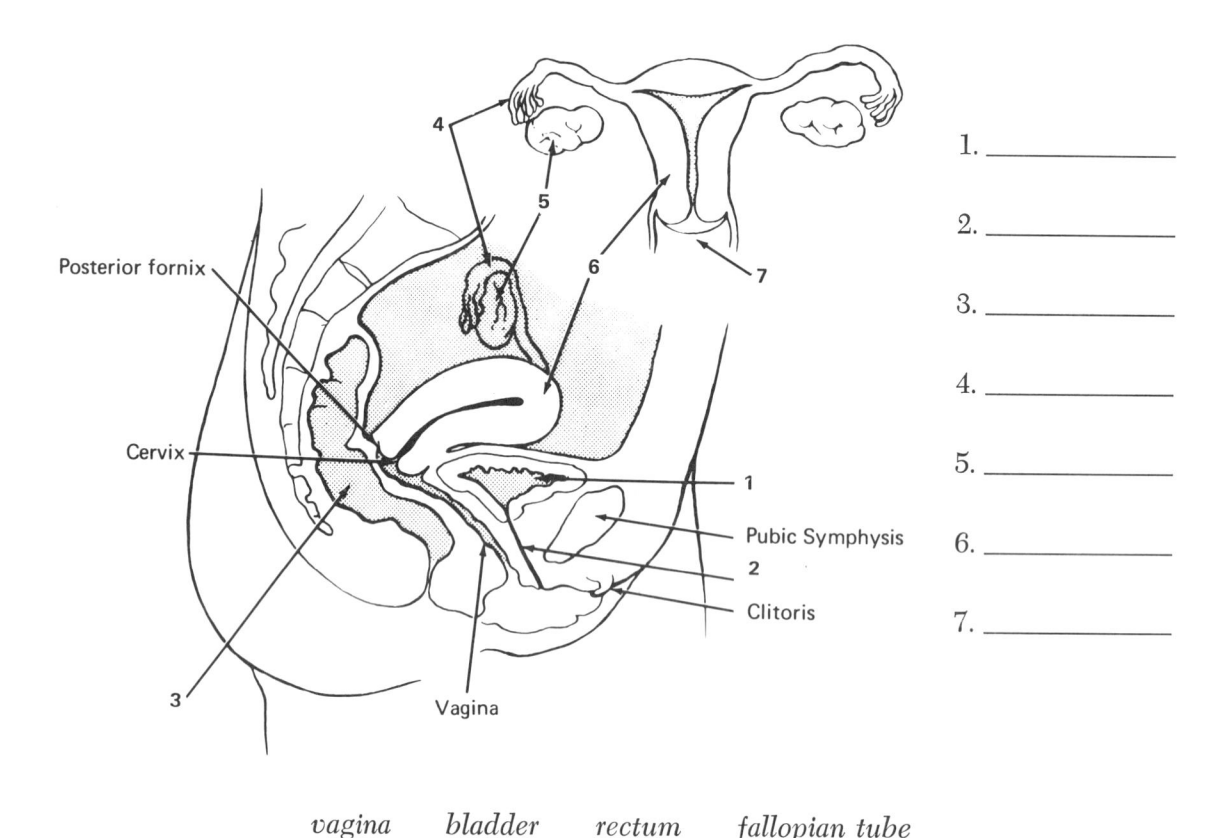

1. _____

2. _____

3. _____

4. _____

5. _____

6. _____

7. _____

vagina   bladder   rectum   fallopian tube

urethra   ovary   uterus

3. A woman may experience many physical and emotional changes during menopause. Name and briefly discuss 2 fears that may be expressed by the woman in menopause.

_____
_____
_____
_____
_____
_____
_____

CHAPTER—38

The woman with a disorder of the reproductive system

Treatment of the gynecologic patient is undertaken with two objectives: to preserve and restore health and to preserve childbearing capacity insofar as possible.

Regardless of when pathology occurs, early diagnosis and medical attention are of the utmost value. The nurse familiar with normal function can often help educate women regarding the importance of regular gynecologic examinations and the time to seek medical help.

The following questions deal with the contents of Chapter 38.

I. True or false.

Read each statement carefully and place your answer in the space provided.

_____ 1. If a patient is 32 years old and has a hysterectomy, she will begin the vasomotor symptoms of menopause immediately after surgery.

_____ 2. In many gynecologic diseases, sexual relations must be suspended and, in some cases, even terminated.

_____ 3. Normally, the patient does not experience pain during a gynecologic pelvic examination unless disease is present.

_____ 4. If the patient has a vaginal discharge, she should douche daily for 3 days before a pelvic examination and Papanicolaou test.

_____ 5. The Papanicolaou test is used to detect cancer by microscopic examination of cells.

_____ 6. If a D and C is performed as part of an investigation for sterility, it is done before menstruation.

_____ 7. Abortion may be defined as a termination of a pregnancy anytime during the 9 months of pregnancy.

_____ 8. Miscarriage is the layman's term for abortion.

_____ 9. Spontaneous abortion may occur in the presence of abnormalities of the fertilized ovum or the placenta.

_____ 10. An incomplete abortion is treated by curettage.

_____ 11. An ectopic pregnancy is the implantation of a fertilized ovum outside the uterus.

_____ 12. Diagnosis of Trichomonas vaginitis is made upon microscopic examination of vaginal secretions.

_____ 13. Pelvic inflammatory disease

219

(PID) is an inflammatory disorder of the uterus.
___ 14. Endometriosis becomes worse during menopause.
___ 15. A myoma is a malignant uterine tumor and is the most common pelvic neoplasm.
___ 16. The most common malignancy of the female reproductive tract is cancer of the cervix.
___ 17. The patient with a vaginal hysterectomy may have some vaginal serosanguinous drainage during the early postoperative period.
___ 18. Vaginal fistulas may either be congenital or occur as a result of surgical or obstetric injury.
___ 19. Surgical repair of a rectocele is called anterior colporrhaphy.

II. Multiple choice questions.

Select the most appropriate answer and place it in the space provided.

1. The diagnosis of endometrial carcinoma is best made by ___.
    a. Papanicolaou smear
    b. blood tests
    c. dilatation of the cervix and curettage of the uterus
2. If a Papanicolaou test is positive or questionable, the physician will usually do a ___.
    a. pelvic examination
    b. cytologic study
    c. cervical biopsy
3. Following a cervical biopsy the patient may notice ___.
    a. a small amount of bleeding which is normal
    b. severe pain for several hours
    c. a heavy sensation in the abdomen
    d. chills and fever which will be controlled with antibiotics
4. Preparation of the patient for a D and C ___.
    a. requires a preoperative sedative because a local anesthetic is used and the patient must remain still during the procedure
    b. is the same as that for any patient receiving a general anesthetic
    c. requires fasting from food and fluids for 4 hours
5. Following a D and C, the menstrual period will ___.
    a. occur almost immediately
    b. most probably be delayed
    c. not occur for 3 to 4 months
6. Perineal care is given to the gynecologic surgical patient ___.
    a. 3 times a day
    b. after a sitz bath
    c. after vaginal or rectal packing is removed
    d. after a bowel movement and after voiding
7. The patient who has an incomplete abortion ___.
    a. still retains some of the products of pregnancy
    b. has expelled the placenta but retained the fetus
    c. has lost blood but not the products of pregnancy
8. The patient with signs of a threatened abortion ___.
    a. always loses the child
    b. sometimes loses the child
9. With a missed abortion ___.
    a. the patient had a threatened abortion but did not lose the child
    b. there was some bleeding which ceased before the products of pregnancy were expelled
    c. the physician thought the patient might abort but did not
    d. the fetus died but was not expelled

10. Habitual abortion(s) is (are) ____.
    a. abortions that occur repeatedly without apparent cause
    b. the term used when a woman has had 6 or more pregnancies, none of which went to full term
    c. when the products of pregnancy are lost twice in a 12 month period of time
    d. the term used when a woman cannot conceive

11. When a patient is admitted to the hospital with a diagnosis of threatened abortion, she is kept on complete bed rest. If large clots are passed the nurse should ____.
    a. leave a large supply of perineal pads with the patient so she can change them frequently
    b. save all clots and tissue for the physician to examine
    c. take vital signs every 4 hours
    d. obtain vaginal packing and keep it at the bedside for emergency insertion should hemorrhage occur

12. The pH of the vagina is normally ____.
    a. acid
    b. alkaline

13. When a douche *and* a suppository are used in the treatment of a vaginal disorder, which is used first? ____
    a. the suppository
    b. the douche

14. Which of the following may be the cause of perineal pruritus? ____
    1. vitamin E deficiency
    2. change of vaginal secretions from a normal alkaline pH
    3. uncontrolled diabetes mellitus
    4. moniliasis
    5. urinary incontinence
        a. 1, 2, 3
        b. 1, 4, 5
        c. 2, 3, 4
        d. 3, 4, 5

15. A prominent symptom of cervicitis is ____.
    a. severe perineal pain
    b. urinary frequency
    c. leukorrhea
    d. vaginal hemorrhage

16. Management of cervicitis may include ____.
    1. douches
    2. electocautery
    3. local or systemic antibiotics
    4. conization
        a. 1, 2
        b. 2, 3
        c. 3, 4
        d. all of these

17. Symptoms of PID (pelvic inflammatory disease) may include ____.
    1. itching
    2. fever
    3. backache
    4. malodorous vaginal discharge
    5. rectal bleeding
        a. 1, 2, 3
        b. 1, 4, 5
        c. 2, 3, 4
        d. 3, 4, 5

18. Treatment of an acute PID usually includes the administration of antibiotics plus ____.
    1. use of a perineal pad and good perineal care
    2. surgery
    3. sitz baths
    4. douches twice a day
        a. 1, 2
        b. 1, 3
        c. 2, 3
        d. 2, 4

19. Endometriosis is a condition in which ____.
    a. there is an overgrowth of functional endometrium resulting in amenorrhea and/or dysmenorrhea
    b. the endometrium becomes thick, spongy, and interlaced with blood vessels resulting in scant menses
    c. tissue that histologically and functionally resembles endometrium is found outside the uterus

20. Drugs used in the treatment of endometriosis include ____.
    1. testosterone
    2. antibiotics
    3. synthetic oral progestins
    4. sulfonamides
       a. 1, 2
       b. 1, 3
       c. 3, 4
       d. all of these

21. Uterine fibroids may be treated by or with ____.
    1. a hysterectomy
    2. a myomectomy
    3. radiation
    4. antibiotics
    5. hormones: estrogens and progestins
       a. 1, 2, 3
       b. 1, 2, 4
       c. 2, 3, 4
       d. 3, 4, 5

22. Cancer of the fundus of the uterus occurs most commonly in ____.
    a. menopausal and postmenopausal women
    b. premenopausal women
    c. women in their late twenties and early thirties
    d. women who have had multiple pregnancies

23. The most common early sign of cancer of the fundus of the uterus is ____.
    a. pain
    b. bleeding
    c. cessation of menses
    d. fever, leukorrhea

24. Treatment of cancer of the fundus of the uterus may include ____.
    a. hysterectomy
    b. deep x-ray therapy
    c. insertion of radium in the uterine cavity
    d. all of the above

25. Cancer of the vulva is a rare malignancy usually occurring in women ____.
    a. prior to menopause
    b. during menopause
    c. past their sixties

26. Cervical carcinoma *in situ* is when the ____.
    a. cellular change is confined to the cervical mucosa
    b. cancer has spread to the fornix
    c. cancer extends into the uterus
    d. biopsy demonstrates metastasis

27. The patient with an inoperable malignancy of the reproductive tract may have severe pain difficult to control with narcotics. In such cases ____.
    a. the dose of the narcotic is doubled
    b. a cordotomy may be done
    c. two narcotics, of normal doses, are administered simultaneously

28. A vesicovaginal fistula results in ____.
    a. fecal incontinence
    b. leakage of urine from the bladder
    c. leakage of fecal material into the vagina
    d. continuous leakage of urine from the vagina

29. Symptoms of relaxed pelvic muscles may include ____.
    1. backache
    2. pelvic pain
    3. a feeling that "something is dropping out"
    4. fatigue
    a. 1, 2
    b. 1, 3
    c. 3, 4
    d. all of these

30. The postoperative care of the patient with an anterior or posterior colporraphy will include ____.
    a. frequent changes of the perineal dressing
    b. perineal care several times a day and each time the patient urinates or defecates
    c. catheterization for residual urine beginning the first postoperative day
    d. reinforcement of the surgical dressing as needed

31. Surgery for relaxed pelvic muscles may not be practical because of the patient's age; therefore, a ring pessary may be inserted. The pessary is usually changed ____.
    a. daily
    b. weekly
    c. every 6 weeks
    d. yearly

CLINICAL SITUATION

Mrs. Sherman, age 44, is admitted to the hospital for a hysterectomy. She has had uterine fibroids for approximately 6 years but has recently started experiencing very heavy menses. She will now require the removal of the fibroids and uterus.

32. The most common symptom of uterine fibroids is ____.
    a. amenorrhea
    b. fever
    c. menorrhagia
    d. pain

33. An indwelling catheter is inserted preoperatively to ____.
    a. measure bladder capacity prior to surgery
    b. measure bladder capacity during surgery
    c. minimize the chance of injuring the bladder during surgery
    d. make it easier for the nurse to measure the urinary output during the postoperative period

34. Following surgery, Mrs. Sherman's indwelling catheter is connected to closed drainage. Intake and output are measured. Should signs of oliguria or anuria occur, the patient may have ____.
    a. renal shutdown due to the sudden hormonal change caused by surgery
    b. a surgical injury to the bladder or a ligated ureter
    c. abdominal edema blocking the flow of urine

35. When Mrs. Sherman's catheter is removed there is an order for catheterization after each voiding to ____.
    a. note the amount of residual urine
    b. check for urinary tract infection
    c. accurately measure all urinary output
    d. none of these

36. Antiembolitic stockings are applied to prevent ____.
    a. leg cramps
    b. thrombophlebitis
    c. footdrop
    d. postoperative varicosities

37. Mrs. Sherman asks you if a hysterectomy will make her begin menopause. As a nurse you know that this surgery ———— produce a surgical menopause.
    a. will
    b. will not

III. Fill-in and discussion questions.
Read each question carefully and place your answer in the space provided.
1. VOCABULARY. Define the following terms.

   a. curettage: _____

   b. cystocele: _____

   c. exfoliate: _____

   d. hysterectomy: _____

   e. leukorrhea: _____

   f. oophorectomy: _____

   g. oophoritis: _____

   h. salpingectomy: _____

   i. salpingitis: _____

   j. rectocele: _____

2. One serious problem in the patient with a vesicovaginal or rectovaginal fistula is excoriation of the skin, due to constant urine or fecal drainage. Give any 2 nursing measures that may lessen skin irritation in these patients.

   1. _____

   2. _____

CHAPTER—39

The man with a disorder of the reproductive system

Embarrassment, fear of impotence, and the feeling of loss of manly self-esteem frequently make a disorder of a reproductive organ difficult for the patient to bear. It is important for the nurse to realize that, although the patient may be more willing to discuss his concerns with the physician, the nurse should show a willingness to listen.

The following questions deal with the contents of Chapter 39.

I. True or false.

Read each statement carefully and place your answer in the space provided.

__T__ 1. The testes produce sperm and the epididymides and vas deferens deliver the sperm to the seminal vesicles and prostate.

__f__ 2. Seminal fluid is produced by the testes and stored in the seminal vesicles.

__f__ 3. Symptoms of benign prostatic hypertrophy usually appear suddenly and with little forewarning.

__f__ 4. The seminal vesicles lie on the anterior surface of the bladder.

__T__ 5. It is not unusual to see some hematuria in the early postoperative period of the patient who has had a prostatectomy.

__f__ 6. Deep black/red blood in the urinary drainage system following a prostatectomy is indicative of arterial bleeding.

__T__ 7. Normal saline is often the preferred irrigating fluid if a large volume is necessary to irrigate the bladder.

__T__ 8. Bladder spasms can be extremely painful.

__T__ 9. Prostatic cancer is most common in men over age 50.

__f__ 10. Symptoms of carcinoma of the prostate occur early in the disease.

__f__ 11. The cure rate of cancer of the prostate is high, even in those discovered when the disease is advanced.

__T__ 12. Failure of the testicle to lie in the scrotum is called cryptorchidism.

II. Multiple choice questions.

Select the most appropriate answer and place it in the space provided.

1. The surgery performed for an undescended testicle is a(n) __B__.
   a. orchiectomy
   b. orchiopexy
   c. orchotomy

2. Symptoms of epididymo-orchitis include __B__.
   1. chills, fever
   2. scrotal pain
   3. hematuria
   4. pyuria
   5. swelling of the testes and epididymis
      a. 1, 2, 4
      b. 1, 2, 5
      c. 2, 3, 4
      d. 3, 4, 5

3. Treatment of epididymo-orchitis will include __C__.
   1. insertion of an indwelling catheter
   2. complete bed rest
   3. scrotal elevation
   4. application of heat to relieve pain and swelling
      a. 1, 2
      b. 1, 3
      c. 2, 3
      d. all of these

4. Torsion of the spermatic cord will require __C__.
   a. immediate application of heat to prevent swelling
   b. application of ice packs and elevation of the scrotum
   c. surgery

5. A large accumulation of fluid between the tunica vaginalis and the testis is called a __A__.
   a. hydrocele
   b. varicocele
   c. orchitis

6. Testicular tumors __A__.
   a. tend to metastasize early
   b. are slow growing tumors
   c. rarely metastasize beyond the scrotal sac

7. Testicular malignancies are usually treated with __D__.
   a. radical surgery
   b. chemotherapy
   c. radiotherapy
   d. all of these

Clinical Situations

Mr. Greene, age 67, is admitted to the hospital for surgical treatment of benign prostatic hypertrophy.

8. Early and typical symptoms of benign prostatic hypertrophy include __D__.
   1. pain on urination
   2. narrowing of the urinary stream
   3. fever
   4. urinary frequency
   5. urgency to void
      a. 1, 2, 3
      b. 1, 4, 5
      c. 2, 3, 4
      d. 2, 4, 5

9. Diagnosis of benign prostatic hypertrophy may be made by __BD__.
   1. digital examination of the prostate gland
   2. cystoscopy
   3. blood chemistries
   4. intravenous pyelogram
   5. measurement of residual urine
      a. 1, 2, 3
      b. 1, 2, 4
      c. 3, 4, 5
      d. all of these

10. According to Mr. Greene's history of symptoms, the physician notes that Mr. Greene has chronic urinary retention. If a catheter is inserted to empty the bladder __B__.
    a. all the urine is let out at one time
    b. the bladder is decompressed slowly over a period of several hours
    c. the urine is slowly drained from the bladder over a period of 3 to 5 minutes

11. The aim of prostatic surgery for benign lesions is the removal of the __A__.
    a. adenoma while leaving the true capsule behind
    b. entire gland and capsule
    c. entire gland and capsule plus the seminal vesicles

12. The operative approaches used for removal of the prostate are __D__.
    1. suprapubic prostatectomy
    2. retropubic prostatecetomy
    3. perineal prostatectomy
    4. transurethral prostatectomy
        a. 1, 2
        b. 1, 4
        c. 2, 3
        d. all of these

13. The easiest of the prostatic surgeries *for the patient* is a __D__.
    a. suprapubic prostatectomy
    b. retropubic prostatectomy
    c. perineal prostatectomy
    d. transurethral prostatectomy

14. The surgery performed on Mr. Greene is a suprapubic prostatectomy. When he returns from surgery the catheters __B__.
    a. are all connected to a drainage bottle which is kept below the level of the bed
    b. are attached to separate containers

15. When measuring Mr. Greene's output at the end of each shift __B__.
    a. all urine is totaled and entered as one figure on the intake and output sheet
    b. the amount from each catheter is measured and recorded separately
    c. urine from the ureteral catheters is totaled and recorded while urine from the other catheter need not be recorded

16. During the first 4 to 5 days after surgery, Mr. Greene's temperature is taken __B__.
    a. rectally, every 4 hours
    b. orally, every 4 hours
    c. rectally every 2 hours

17. To control arterial bleeding after a suprapubic prostatectomy, the surgeon may _____.
    a. place traction on the urethral catheter
    b. clamp the suprapubic catheter every 4 hours
    c. put traction on the ureteral and/or suprapubic catheter

18. Mr. Greene has an order for continuous irrigation of his catheters which is instituted to _____.
    a. prevent clots from forming in the bladder
    b. reduce the possibility of postoperative bladder infection
    c. control the pain caused by urinary retention
    d. prevent a backup of urine in the ureters

19. When continuous irrigation is used, the _____ catheter is usually used for inflow and the _____ tube for outflow.
    a. cystotomy   urethral
    b. urethral   cystotomy
    c. urethral   ureteral
    d. ureteral   urethral

20. After Mr. Greene's cystotomy tube is removed, the suprapubic wound _____.
    a. will bleed for a few hours
    b. will close in 2 to 3 hours
    c. will most likely be painful for several weeks
    d. frequently leak urine for a few days

21. Following removal of the urethral catheter, Mr. Greene may notice _____.
    a. severe pain for 2 to 3 hours and may require a narcotic
    b. some dribbling of urine
    c. bleeding which may persist for 7 to 10 days

22. Mr. Greene is to be discharged from the hospital tomorrow. He tells you that he is retired but wonders if he can do any lifting after he goes home. While this question must be answered by his physician, as a nurse you know that ____.
    a. there are no restrictions on lifting except for extremely heavy objects
    b. generally no lifting or straining is allowed for several weeks
    c. the patient can lift any object that does not cause discomfort

Mr. Wright, age 56, has his yearly physical examination at which time his physician detected a small nodule on his prostate gland. He is admitted to the hospital with a tentative diagnosis of cancer of the prostate.

23. Diagnosis of cancer of the prostate is usually made by ____.
    a. Papanicolaou smear
    b. intravenous pyelogram
    c. cystoscopy
    d. an open perineal biopsy

24. The nodule is found to be malignant and the physician decides to perform a radical perineal prostatectomy. Following surgery special care is taken that the Foley catheter is not dislodged because it ____.
    a. prevents urine from exiting the body through the perineal wound
    b. keeps the suprapubic wound clean and dry
    c. will be used as part of the through-and-through irrigation of the perineal wound
    d. supports the urethral anastomosis to the bladder neck

25. The physician orders perineal irrigations to ____.
    a. keep the wound clean and decrease pain and inflammation
    b. remove any urine draining through the wound

26. Mr. Wright is allowed out of bed on the second postoperative day. He should sit on a(n) ____.
    a. firm even surface
    b. rubber ring
    c. air mattress
    d. cool surface

27. Occasionally the patient with a perineal prostatectomy develops urinary or fecal incontinence. Some patients may be helped to regain bowel control by ____.
    a. eating only soft foods
    b. doing perineal exercises: contracting and relaxing gluteal muscles
    c. increasing fluid intake and eating foods high in roughage
    d. using laxatives

Mr. Brent, age 70, comes to the hospital emergency room in urinary retention. A catheter is inserted with moderate difficulty. Once the initial problem is relieved, Mr. Brent is admitted to the urology service. A perineal biopsy reveals a prostatic carcinoma, but, because of his physical condition and past medical history, he will be treated with drugs.

28. Medical treatment for Mr. Brent will include ____.
    a. estrogens
    b. androgens
    c. estrogen/androgen combinations

29. Mr. Brent has a history of congestive heart failure. During drug therapy for his malignancy he will have to be observed for ____.
    a. the fluid retention associated with androgen therapy
    b. the fluid retention associated with estrogen therapy
    c. a sudden diuresis due to drug therapy, which may cause a severe electrolyte imbalance

30. If estrogens are given in high doses, the patient may experience ____.
    a. nausea, vomiting, hypotension
    b. feminizing changes
    c. hypertension, dizziness, visual difficulties
    d. tumor progression

31. Mr. Brent is discharged from the hospital to be followed up in the urology clinic. He is presently not a candidate for surgery because of his medical problems. If, in the future, his medical status improves, androgen influence on the tumor may be curtailed by a ____.
   a. transurethral prostatectomy
   b. chordotomy
   c. bilateral orchiectomy

32. If Mr. Brent should develop bladder neck obstruction despite drug therapy, he may require ____.
   a. a transurethral prostatectomy
   b. androgen therapy
   c. a chordotomy

III. Fill-in and discussion questions.

Read each question carefully and place your answer in the space provided.

1. Label the 9 areas identified in the drawing below by filling in the blanks to the right of the drawing. The 9 areas are to be selected from the words given below the drawing.

1. _____
2. _____
3. _____
4. _____
5. _____
6. _____
7. _____
8. _____
9. _____

prostate   testis   rectum   urethra   bladder

symphysis pubis   epididymis   penis   seminal vesicle

229

CHAPTER—40

The patient with breast disease

The breast is a complicated glandular organ that produces milk after pregnancy. Considerable space in the breast is devoted to a network of ducts that carry milk to the nipple.

The most common breast disease is cystic disease. In American women, the breast is the most common site of cancer, which often requires radical surgery. Because of the emotional impact of a mastectomy, the care of the patient with a carcinoma of the breast requires special nursing consideration.

The following questions deal with the contents of Chapter 40.

I. True or false.

Read each statement carefully and place your answer in the space provided.

____ 1. It is not unusual for the breasts to become tender and enlarged immediately before menstruation.

____ 2. The chief importance of self-examination of the breasts lies in the early discovery of lumps in the breast.

____ 3. Any discharge from the breast nipple is abnormal and highly suspicious of cancer.

____ 4. Chronic cystic mastitis is an inflammatory breast disorder causing extreme tenderness of breast tissue

____ 5. A radical mastectomy is indicated in those with known metastasis, as removal of the primary tumor source will prevent further metastasis.

____ 6. The patient with a mastectomy will go through a period of grieving following her surgery.

____ 7. The patient should not be encouraged to look at her mastectomy excision because the incisions are often unsightly due to the excessive formation of scar tissue.

____ 8. The emotional significance of a mastectomy varies from patient to patient.

____ 9. There is no one way to treat metastatic breast cancer.

____ 10. Breast abscesses occur most frequently as a postpartal complication.

II. Multiple choice questions.

Select the most appropriate answer and place it in the space provided.

CLINICAL SITUATIONS

Mrs. Howard, age 56, sees her physician because of a lump she discovered in her right breast. She is now admitted to the hospital for a breast biopsy.

1. Breast self-examination is done every month. In the premenopause woman, the examination is performed ____.
   a. immediately after the menstrual period
   b. immediately before menstruation
   c. midway between menstrual periods
2. The survival rate for breast cancer is lower if ____.
   a. the patient is past menopause
   b. the patient is under 40
   c. there is lymph node involvement
   d. there is an associated fibroadenoma
3. Prior to surgery, the physician informs Mrs. Howard that he is not sure if the lump is malignant or benign and will not know for certain until it is examined under a microscope. In preparing Mrs. Howard, the explanation of the surgery should include ____.
   a. an explanation of radical surgery, what it entails, and what structures will be removed
   b. only an explanation of the biopsy procedure, since the lesion may not be malignant
4. Mrs. Howard has a biopsy of the lesion in surgery. The biopsy is performed under ____.
   a. general anesthesia
   b. local anesthesia and, if it is malignant, the patient is given a general anesthesia
5. The pathologist examined the specimen and found it to be malignant. The surgeon decided to perform a radical mastectomy which is the removal of the breast and ____.
   a. adjacent lymph nodes
   b. the pectoralis major
   c. the pectoralis minor
   d. all of these
6. Had a simple mastectomy been selected as the surgery of choice ____.
   a. only a small section of the breast would be removed
   b. the breast is removed but the adjacent structures and lymph nodes are not
   c. half the breast is removed along with the lymph nodes directly adjacent to the section of breast removed
7. If a patient with breast cancer has not gone through menopause, a second surgery may be performed at the time of the mastectomy or shortly thereafter and is called a(n) ____.
   a. adrenalectomy
   b. bilateral oophorectomy
8. When will Mrs. Howard most likely discover that a radical mastectomy has been performed? ____
   a. once she is fully awake, that is, the morning after surgery
   b. when the physician first changes the surgical dressing
   c. when the physician tells her
   d. in the recovery room as she wakes from anesthesia
9. A drain has been inserted in Mrs. Howard's incision and connected to a Hemo-Vac suction. This suction is usually emptied every ____.
   a. hour
   b. 2 hours
   c. 4 hours
   d. 8 hours
10. Mrs. Howard has a second dressing on her thigh, this dressing covers ____.
    a. an incision made to remove some lymph nodes
    b. a distant biopsy site
    c. the skin graft donor site
11. Mrs. Howard has a postoperative hemoglobin and hematocrit ordered with the blood to be drawn 8 hours after surgery. The blood is *not* drawn from her ____.
    a. right arm
    b. left arm
12. The physician orders that Mrs. Howard's right arm be elevated on a pillow. Since she had a skin graft, it is important that her arm not be allowed to ____.
    a. abduct
    b. adduct

13. When you check Mrs. Howard's dressing you should not only inspect the top surgical dressing but also look for hidden drainage ____.
    a. on top of the sheets
    b. underneath the patient's upper body
    c. on the first layers of the surgical dressing

14. Some patients will begin exercises of the operative arm 1 or 2 days after surgery, but the patient with a skin graft must wait until the graft has healed before exercises are begun. The most effective exercises are ____.
    a. active exercises
    b. passive exercises

15. The physician prescribes exercises since he now believes the skin graft and surgical wound have healed. The exercises will be for ____.
    a. the operated side only
    b. the unoperated side only
    c. both arms

16. The physician removes all dressings and bandages. Care of the skin over and around the operative area ____.
    a. should be done only by the nurse
    b. is best done by the patient with help from the nurse
    c. is best done by the patient alone, because she is probably embarrassed by her disfigurement

17. After discharge from the hospital, Mrs. Howard will be able to wear a commercial prosthesis ____.
    a. once the skin has healed
    b. when she can fully move the arm on the operative side
    c. when she psychologically accepts her surgery

18. One of the complications of a radical mastectomy is ____.
    a. sympathetic swelling of the opposite arm
    b. swelling of both arms and shoulders
    c. lymphedema in the arm on the operative side

Two years ago Miss Taylor, age 34, had a right radical mastectomy. She is now admitted to the hospital for treatment of metastatic carcinoma.

19. There are many different methods of treating metastatic cancer. If hormonal therapy is used, the primary reason for the therapy will be to ____.
    a. change the hormonal environment of the body
    b. increase estrogen levels while decreasing progesterone levels
    c. make the tumor hormone dependent

20. Surgery is another method that may be used in the treatment of metastatic carcinoma and may include ____.
    1. oophorectomy
    2. adrenalectomy
    3. hypophysectomy
    4. lymphectomy
       a. all but 1
       b. all but 2
       c. all but 3
       d. all but 4

21. Hormones may also be used to relieve pain. Estrogens are used in some patients but are contraindicated in ____.
    a. premenopausal women
    b. postmenopausal women
    c. women who have had an adrenalectomy

22. If hormone therapy is selected as the treatment of choice, Miss Taylor will be given ____.
    a. estrogen
    b. progestin
    c. ACTH
    d. testosterone

23. While hormonal therapy will not cure Miss Taylor, it may ____.
    a. stop her nausea and vomiting and make her feel better
    b. reduce the possibility of fluid retention and congestive heart failure
    c. make her more comfortable and possibly increase her life span
    d. improve her appetite and reduce the size of the tumor
24. Chemotherapy with antineoplastic drugs may also be selected for some patients with metastatic carcinoma. These drugs are capable of causing ____.
    1. bone marrow depression
    2. anemia
    3. nausea and vomiting
    4. skin reactions
       a. 1, 2
       b. 1, 4
       c. 2, 3
       d. all of these

III. Fill-in and discussion questions.

Read each question carefully and place your answer in the space provided.

1. Self-examination of the breast is an important task for every woman. All nurses should be thoroughly familiar with it and should be able to explain what is done during the examination. In the spaces below, fill in the appropriate information relating to parts of the breast self-examination.

   a. When standing in front of the mirror, what does the patient look for? ____

   b. When lying down to examine the breast, what position is assumed to first examine the right breast? ____

   c. What part of the hand is used to examine the breast? ____

2. Briefly describe the treatment of a breast abscess and describe the nursing management of the patient with regard to the dressings after surgery. ____

CHAPTER—41

The patient with venereal infection

A venereal disease can be described as one that is communicated through sexual intercourse, or close, intimate contact with an infected person. The two most common venereal diseases are syphilis and gonorrhea, which, in some areas of this country, are reaching epidemic proportions.

The following questions deal with the contents of Chapter 41.

I. True or false.
Read each statement carefully and place your answer in the space provided.

__F__ 1. Gonorrhea is a protozoan infection. *bacterial*

__T__ 2. The organism causing gonorrhea does not live on dry surfaces.

__T__ 3. The usual incubation period for gonorrhea is 3 days to 2 weeks after intercourse with an infected person.

__F__ 4. Penicillin is the only drug proven effective in the treatment of gonorrhea.

__T__ 5. Gummas can develop anywhere but appear most frequently in skin, bones, liver, and larynx.

__T__ 6. A cardiovascular complication that may be seen during the tertiary stage of syphilis is an aortic aneurysm.

__T__ 7. Syphilis is a venereal disease that can result in widespread destructive lesions in the body.

__F__ 8. Tabes dorsalis usually appears 1 to 3 years after the original syphilis infection.

__F__ 9. If the patient with syphilis cannot tolerate penicillin, he must go without treatment since no other drug is effective.

__T__ 10. Chancroid is caused by the microorganism *Hemophilus ducreyi.*

__F__ 11. Treatment of a venereal disease almost always requires a short (24 to 48 hours) period of hospitalization.

__T__ 12. One major problem in the control of venereal disease is its prevalence among young people.

II. Multiple choice questions.
Select the most appropriate answer and place it in the space provided.

1. In the male, the first symptom of gonorrheal infection is __a__.
   a. burning and pain on urination
   b. hematuria
   c. chills and fever
   d. perineal and scrotal pain

234

2. In the female, the gonorrheal infection may be __a__.
   a. without symptoms for long periods of time
   b. first apparent with the appearance of hematuria
   c. first noted when a greenish-yellow vaginal discharge becomes apparent

3. In the female, if gonorrhea is not treated, the infection __b__.
   a. might go away after a period of time
   b. may move up into the uterus and fallopian tubes
   c. may enter the bladder and uterus

4. If a male goes without treatment for gonorrhea he may develop __d__.
   a. a reinfection with the microorganisms
   b. an immunity to the microorganisms
   c. ureteritis, pyelonephritis, and nephritis
   d. prostatitis, epididymitis and infection of the seminal vesicles

5. Laboratory diagnosis of gonorrhea in the male is usually made by __c__.
   a. urinalysis and staining of a centrifuged sample
   b. 24-hour urine specimen
   c. stained smear of the urethral discharge
   d. culture and sensitivity of the urine

6. The recommended therapy for treatment of gonorrhea in the male is __a__.
   a. antibiotic therapy
   b. urethral irrigations
   c. local application of heat followed by use of an antibiotic ointment

7. The cause of syphilis is the __a__.
   a. microorganism *Treponema pallidum*
   b. protozoan *Treponema syphilum*
   c. *gonococcus syphilae*

8. Persons with primary syphilis that is successfully treated __a__.
   a. rapidly become noninfectious
   b. remain infectious for approximately 3 months
   c. become noninfectious 1 year after treatment
   d. develop an immunity to the spirochete

9. A definite diagnosis of syphilis is made by __d__.
   a. culture and sensitivity of the discharge
   b. examination of the discharge from the urethra
   c. visual examination of the lesion
   d. dark-field examination of a smear taken from the lesion

10. The first sign of a syphilitic infection—the chancre—is seen approximately __c__ after contact.
    a. 3 days
    b. 1 week
    c. 3 weeks
    d. 6 weeks

11. A syphilitic chancre is a __b__.
    a. cratered lesion which is painful to touch
    b. painless, round lesion
    c. lesion that appears during the secondary stage of syphilis

12. The secondary stage of syphilis begins about __c__ after the initial infection.
    a. 1 week
    b. 3 weeks
    c. 6 weeks
    d. 6 months to 6 years

13. During the secondary stage of syphilis the patient may experience __c__.
    1. a skin rash
    2. leutic plaques
    3. a chancre
    4. loss of hair
       a. all but 1
       b. all but 2
       c. all but 3
       d. all but 4
14. After the secondary stage, syphilis enters a(n) __a__.
    a. latent stage
    b. exacerbation stage
    c. recurrent stage
15. Late and serious complications of syphilis begin to appear at the __c__.
    a. primary stage
    b. secondary stage
    c. tertiary stage
    d. latent stage
16. In congenital syphilis, the fetus contracts the infection from the mother __a__.
    a. through the placenta
    b. during the birth process
    c. through the amniotic fluid
    d. immediately after birth
17. The patient with tabes dorsalis has eye involvements, one of which is __d__.
    a. optic aneurysm
    b. arcus senilis
    c. posterior sclerosis
    d. Argyll Robertson pupil reaction
18. Treatment of early syphilis may include the administration of __b__.
    1. 2.4 million units of long-acting penicillin, X 1
    2. 1 million units of long-acting penicillin every month, X 6
    3. 10 daily injections of 600,000 units of procaine penicillin
    4. 30 daily injections of 100,000 units of crystalline penicillin
       a. 1, 2
       b. 1, 3
       c. 2, 3
       d. 2, 4
19. Therapy in the later stages of syphilis is aimed at __a c__.
    a. eradicating the microorganism from body organs and structures, particularly in the central nervous system
    b. giving a dual course of antibiotic therapy, for example, 5 days of treatment, 2 weeks of rest, and 5 days of treatment
    c. treatment of any damaged area of the body with specific measures dictated by the pathology and symptoms
20. The VDRL is a standard screening test for __b__.
    a. gonorrhea
    b. syphilis
    c. lymphogranuloma inguinale
    d. chancroid
21. The Frei test is used to diagnose __c__.
    a. syphilis
    b. gonorrhea
    c. lymphogranuloma inguinale
    d. none of these
22. Lymphogranuloma inguinale is treated with __b__.
    a. antigens
    b. broad-spectrum antibiotics
    c. antiviral agents

III. Fill-in and discussion questions.
Read each question carefully and place your answer in the space provided.
1. Fill in the blanks of the following questions with the correct word or words that will complete the statement.
   1. The 2 most common venereal diseases are _____ and _____.
   2. The organism responsible for gonorrhea is the _____.

3. Another term for tabes dorsalis is _____.

4. Lymphogranuloma inguinale is caused by a(n) _____.

5. An acute disease characterized by large ulcerations of the genitals is _____.

2. From your general reading and thinking about venereal disease, give some reasons why a person might not wish to reveal his/her contact and possible source of venereal infection. _____

UNIT TEN
Common problems involving disfigurement

CHAPTER—42

The patient with a dermatological condition

Since the skin is in constant contact with the environment, it is usually subject to injury and irritation. Nurses are in a strategic position to help others to maintain a normal healthy skin.

The following questions deal with the contents of Chapter 42.

I. True or false.

Read each statement carefully and place your answer in the space provided.

_____ 1. Skin diseases are rarely serious.
_____ 2. Bacteria, most of which are non-pathogenic, normally exist on the skin.
_____ 3. The sebaceous glands secrete sebum, an oily substance that protects the hair and skin from becoming excessively dry.
_____ 4. Creams and lotions help keep the skin soft and smooth.
_____ 5. Creams containing hormones improve skin tone and, in some instances, remove wrinkles and age spots.
_____ 6. Acne may be improved by exposure to sunlight.
_____ 7. The nurse should wear plastic or rubber gloves when caring for any patient with a skin disorder.
_____ 8. Certain foods may cause a rash or skin eruption.
_____ 9. Dressings applied to open, denuded areas should be sterile.
_____ 10. Acne vulgaris is one of the most common contagious skin conditions.
_____ 11. Another term for blackheads is comedones.
_____ 12. Permanent scarring can occur in cases of severe acne.
_____ 13. The red, round wheals seen in those with urticaria are a result of localized edema due to increased capillary permeability.
_____ 14. Eczema is a chronic skin disorder.
_____ 15. Psoriasis frequently occurs during young adulthood and middle life.
_____ 16. Methotrexate, a drug used in the treatment of malignant diseases, has also been useful in treating severe forms of psoriasis.
_____ 17. Impetigo contagiosa is more common in adults than children and most frequently occurs in middle life.
_____ 18. Herpes zoster is caused by a virus.
_____ 19. When the normal protective functions of the skin are impaired, pathogens existing harmlessly on the skin may cause infection.
_____ 20. Pediculosis capitis can be spread

by shared toilet articles such as combs and brushes.
_____ 21. Pemphigus is a systemic disease with skin manifestations.
_____ 22. Repeated exposure to sunlight can be a predisposing cause of skin cancer.
_____ 23. Malignant growths of the skin are usually metastatic rather than primary lesions.

II. Multiple choice questions.

Select the most appropriate answer and place it in the space provided.

1. If the alkalinity of certain soaps sometimes cause skin irritation in patients, the physician may order a(n) _____.
   a. soap substitute with a neutral pH
   b. acid-base soap
   c. soap that is mildly acid

2. One of the most frequent causes of skin lesions in hospitalized patients is _____.
   a. soaps used to launder hospital linen
   b. humid air
   c. drugs

3. An important nursing measure in preventing the spread of infection is _____.
   a. handwashing
   b. having all patients wash with a germicidal soap that has an alkaline base
   c. the wearing of masks when nursing personnel have respiratory infections

4. A keratolytic lotion or cream is used to _____.
   a. soften skin
   b. dissolve thickened horny skin
   c. stop itching
   d. treat skin infections

5. An example of an emollient is _____.
   a. Desenex cream
   b. calamine lotion
   c. potassium permanganate
   d. lanolin

6. The sensation of itching may be closely related to the sensation of _____.
   a. heat
   b. cold
   c. pain
   d. pressure

7. Wet dressings have a cooling and soothing effect produced by the _____.
   a. evaporation of the moisture
   b. humidification of the surrounding air
   c. contact of the skin with moisture
   d. temperature of the liquid used in the dressing

8. The types of baths used to relieve itching are _____.
   a. sitz baths
   b. colloid baths
   c. warm water baths
   d. emollient baths

9. In acne vulgaris the skin of the affected area is _____.
   a. excessively oily
   b. excessively dry

10. Another term for dandruff is _____.
    a. urticaria
    b. psoriasis
    c. dermatitis venenata
    d. seborrheic dermatitis

11. Treatment of dandruff includes _____.
    1. regular shampooing of hair
    2. exclusion of oily foods from diet
    3. application of a local medication between shampoos
    4. a diet high in B complex vitamins

    a. 1, 3
    b. 1, 4
    c. 2, 3
    d. all of these

12. Mild forms of angioneurotic edema may be treated with ____.
    a. epinephrine (Adrenalin)
    b. starch baths
    c. antihistamines
    d. calamine lotion

13. Eczema typically occurs ____.
    a. in the folds of the elbows and knees, and on the neck and face
    b. on the abdomen and back
    c. on the arms and legs, but rarely above the neck
    d. in the axilla and groin

14. The usual treatment of eczema includes ____.
    1. starch baths
    2. antipruritic ointments
    3. systemic antibiotics
    4. wet dressings
    5. ultraviolet light
        a. 1, 2, 3
        b. 1, 2, 4
        c. 2, 3, 4
        d. 3, 4, 5

15. Psoriasis is characterized by ____.
    a. weeping, excoriated tissue usually appearing on the elbows, knees and scalp
    b. scattered patches of raised, scaly lesions covered with crusts
    c. patches of erythema covered with silvery scales
    d. infection of the outer layer of the skin, resulting in a sloughing of the skin

16. Treatment of psoriasis is individualized and may include ____.
    1. ultraviolet light
    2. tar ointments
    3. oral salicylates
    4. surgical removal of the lesions
        a. 1, 2
        b. 1, 3
        c. 2, 3
        d. 2, 4

17. Contact dermatitis is characterized by ____.
    1. erythema, edema
    2. appearance of silver scales over the lesions
    3. vesicles, itching
    4. deep lesions with raised edges
        a. 1, 2
        b. 1, 3
        c. 2, 3
        d. 3, 4

18. Treatment for contact dermatitis includes ____.
    a. wet compresses
    b. medicated baths
    c. systemic corticosteroids
    d. all of the above

19. Treatment of impetigo contagiosa includes ____.
    a. x-ray therapy with low doses given to the affected area daily for 5 days
    b. treatment with coal tar ointments and ultraviolet light
    c. removal of crusts before local medications are applied

20. Treatment of herpes zoster may include ____.
    a. antibiotics, ultraviolet light
    b. wet soaks, abrading ointments
    c. analgesics, corticosteroids, lotions
    d. coal tar ointments, surgical excision

21. Sebaceous cysts are caused by ____.
    a. obstruction of the duct of an oil gland
    b. a break in the skin causing infection around the hair follicle
    c. poor nutrition, eating greasy and fried foods

22. Scabies is caused by ____.
    a. a virus
    b. infestation with the itch mite
    c. infestation with pediculi
    d. bacteria

III. Fill-in and discussion questions.
Read each question carefully and place your answer in the space provided.

1. In column B place the number identifying the disorder listed in column A.

   COLUMN A   **COLUMN B**
   1. carbuncle   ____ multiple boils
   2. furunculosis   ____ shingles
   3. herpes zoster   ____ pruritus
   4. itching   ____ seborrheic dermatitis
   5. hives   ____ large swollen lesion usually found in back of neck
   6. herpes simplex   ____ cold sore
   7. dermatophytosis   ____ athlete's foot
   8. dandruff   ____ a form of skin cancer
   9. melanoma   ____ urticaria

2. Briefly discuss why a patient with a skin disfigurement (scars, acne, rash, etc.) may undergo a personality change. _____

   _____

   _____

   _____

   _____

   _____

3. Place a check mark (✓) in front of the measures that may be of value in the treatment of acne.
   1. ____ keeping hands away from the face
   2. ____ use of a slightly acid soap
   3. ____ washing hands before applying medications
   4. ____ keeping hair short and away from the face
   5. ____ use of an oil-based soap
   6. ____ short treatments with ultraviolet light (as prescribed by a physician)

CHAPTER—43

The patient undergoing plastic surgery

The terms *plastic surgery* and *reconstructive surgery* are used interchangeably to refer to the surgical repair of defects that may be congenital or acquired.

This highly specialized surgery combines art and medicine. In cosmetic surgery, the aim is not to produce beauty as such, but beauty in the sense that the changed appearance is appropriate for the particular patient and blends unnoticeably into his features, producing a natural appearance.

The following questions deal with the contents of Chapter 43.

I. True or false.

Read each statement carefully and place your answer in the space provided.

_____ 1. A rhinoplasty is a surgical reconstruction of the nose.
_____ 2. Dermabrasion is a technique for removing surface layers of scarred skin.
_____ 3. A mammoplasty may be performed to change the size and shape of the breasts.
_____ 4. A homograft is a skin graft in which the skin is transplanted from one person to another.
_____ 5. Skin cannot be transplanted between identical twins.
_____ 6. When a skin graft is performed there must be a space between the graft and the tissues below so the graft can move freely during the healing process.
_____ 7. A dermatone is used to remove skin from the donor site.
_____ 8. A pedicle flap is a full-thickness graft that is devoid of blood vessels and subcutaneous fat.
_____ 9. One extremely serious problem that may occur after skin grafting is infection.
_____ 10. Skin grafting is usually performed under a local anesthetic.

II. Multiple choice questions.

Select the most appropriate answer and place it in the space provided.

1. Plastic surgery may be performed to _____.
   1. correct congenital deformities
   2. correct deformities due to trauma
   3. correct disfigurement due to malignant disease
   4. improve cosmetic appearance, for example, a face lift

   a. 1, 3
   b. 1, 4
   c. 2, 4
   d. all of these

2. A blepharoplasty is a ____.
    a. plastic surgery reconstruction of the eyelid
    b. reconstruction procedure which involves the nose and cheeks
    c. face lift
    d. plastic surgery on the outer ear
3. An autograft is a skin graft taken from ____.
    a. an animal
    b. one part of the patient's body and used on another part
    c. another individual
4. For a skin graft to "take," there must be ____.
    a. an exact match of color of skin
    b. a sufficient blood supply to the part and an absence of infection
    c. a thickness of more than 0.008 inch but less than 0.030 inch
    d. a firm dressing applied over the graft
5. The 2 basic types of skin grafts are ____.
    a. pinch graft and autograft
    b. slit graft and split graft
    c. full graft and part graft
    d. split-thickness and full-thickness grafts
6. A pinch graft is a small piece of skin ____.
    a. cut from the patient's donor site and placed on his recipient site
    b. cut from the donor (another individual) and placed on the recipient
7. The slit graft is used when ____.
    a. only small areas require grafting
    b. there is a limited area available as a recipient site
    c. there is a limited area available as a donor site
8. The type of graft used to restore function and cosmetic appearance is the ____.
    a. postage stamp graft
    b. pinch graft
    c. full-thickness graft
    d. slit graft
9. When the patient has had a skin graft, care must be taken to ____.
    1. avoid excessive pressure on the recipient site
    2. maintain aseptic technique if wet dressings are applied
    3. protect the donor and recipient sites from injury
    4. never remove a dressing over a skin graft without a specific order
        a. 1, 2
        b. 1, 3
        c. 2, 4
        d. all of these

III. Fill-in and discussion questions.

1. If you had a noticeable deformity or scar would you have plastic surgery? Discuss why you answered yes or no. _____

UNIT ELEVEN
Intensive care nursing

CHAPTERS—44 & 45

Introduction to intensive care nursing and the patient in shock

Intensive care nursing involves a concentration of medical and nursing and allied health personnel specially prepared to observe, assess, and treat critically ill patients. One clinical syndrome—shock—is a common emergency faced by intensive care nursing personnel as well as personnel in all areas of the hospital.

The following questions deal with the contents of Chapters 44 and 45.

I. True or false.

Read each statement carefully and place your answer in the space provided.

___ 1. Intensive care nursing is a blend of expertise in the technical, judgmental, and interpersonal skills exercised in behalf of the patient and family at a time of life-death crisis.

___ 2. The patient's stay in the intensive care unit is almost always long-term, because of the seriousness of the illness.

___ 3. Shock is usually classified according to etiology.

___ 4. A frightened patient is a poor surgical risk.

___ 5. Deep shock can develop in minutes.

___ 6. The blood pressure is an infallible index of shock.

___ 7. Pain can cause as well as enhance shock.

___ 8. The CVP (central venous pressure) can be a critical guide in the management of the patient in shock.

___ 9. An alteration in cerebral function is often the first sign of impaired oxygen delivery to cerebral tissues.

___ 10. Hypovolemic shock is best treated with intravenous glucose in normal saline.

___ 11. Adrenergic drugs may be administered to the patient in shock.

___ 12. When shock is treated adequately and promptly, the patient usually recovers.

II. Multiple choice questions.

Select the most appropriate answer and place it in the space provided.

1. Hematogenic shock is also called ___.
   a. hypovolemic shock
   b. hypervolemic shock

249

2. Hematogenic shock is caused by a reduction in blood volume but may also be due to _____.
   1. severe burns
   2. fright
   3. severe allergic reaction
   4. loss of large amounts of fluid in vomitus and diarrhea

   a. 1, 3
   b. 1, 4
   c. 2, 3
   d. 2, 4

3. Cardiogenic shock is due to _____.
   a. failure of the heart to act as an efficient pump
   b. cardiac arrest
   c. blood loss which causes heart failure

4. Vasogenic shock is a _____.
   a. disproportion between the amount of plasma and the number of red and white blood cells
   b. hypovolemic type of shock
   c. diffuse vasodilatation resulting in an increase in the size of the vascular bed

5. Neurogenic shock results from _____.
   a. a lack of blood supply to the brain and spinal cord
   b. an insult to the nervous system

6. Bacteremic shock usually occurs in _____.
   a. those with staphylococcus infections
   b. the patient who is succumbing to an overwhelming infection
   c. the patient with an infection who is also having an antibiotic (drug) reaction

7. The patient in shock or whose blood pressure is falling may appear to be in pain. If a narcotic is prescribed for pain, the nurse would _____.
   a. give the drug, because pain can influence the blood pressure
   b. give ½ of the dose prescribed since this would sufficiently alleviate the pain without influencing the blood pressure
   c. first check with the physician regarding a possible change in dose and route of administration

8. Central venous pressure (CVP) is the pressure _____.
   a. in the venous circulation as measured in the extremities
   b. of the blood in the right atrium
   c. of venous blood in the center of the body
   d. that is measured by inserting a catheter in the left ventricle

9. Vasoconstriction, the body's physiologic response to shock, contributes to _____.
   a. an increase in urinary output as the body tries to compensate for shock
   b. a decrease in urinary output because of an increase in renal blood flow
   c. a marked reduction in renal blood flow and a decrease in urinary output

10. The physician should be notified if the patient in shock has a urinary output below _____.
    a. 30 ml. per hour
    b. 100 ml. per hour
    c. 500 ml. in 8 hours
    d. 1000 ml. in 8 hours

11. If the patient shows signs of shock, the nurse should contact the physician and _____.
    1. administer oxygen
    2. start an intravenous infusion (if one is not presently running)
    3. assign a nursing assistant to stay with the patient and take his blood pressure
    4. elevate the head of the bed to facilitate breathing

    a. 1, 2
    b. 1, 4
    c. 2, 3
    d. 2, 4

12. If whole blood is needed to treat hemorrhagic shock but is not immediately available, solutions that can be used in the interim include ____.
    1. concentrated albumin
    2. saline
    3. plasma
    4. low molecular weight dextran
       a. 1, 2
       b. 2, 3
       c. 3, 4
       d. all of these
13. When fluids are administered to the patient in shock there is always the danger of fluid overload. If a CVP line is inserted, a rise of over ____ ml. of H_2O indicates the inability of the right side of the heart to accept further fluid load.
    a. 5
    b. 15
    c. 30
    d. 60
14. Unless ordered otherwise, the patient in shock is ____.
    a. kept flat
    b. placed in a supine position with the head of the bed elevated
    c. kept flat with the legs elevated 20 to 30 degrees

III. Fill-in and discussion questions.
Read each question carefully and place your answer in the space provided.

1. The blood pressure of the patient in shock may be difficult to hear. Describe another method of determining the systolic blood pressure level. ____

2. Describe the structures, organs, or phenomena listed below as they appear in the patient in shock.

   a. skin: ____

   b. arterial blood pressure: ____

   c. pulse: ____

   d. pulse pressure: ____

   e. respirations: ____

   f. temperature: ____

CHAPTER 46

Respiratory insufficiency and failure

Regardless of the cause, survival is threatened when there is acute disruption of breathing, with the human organism reacting swiftly and strongly with emergency neural adaptive mechanisms. The major objectives of nursing care of the patient with respiratory distress are to facilitate ventilation and reduce the work of breathing. Competent observation, judgment, technical ministration, and emotional support of the patient are integral parts of the nursing care of these patients.

The following questions deal with the contents of Chapter 46.

I. True or false.

Read each statement carefully and place your answer in the space provided.

True 1. The main function of the respiratory system is to exchange oxygen and carbon dioxide between air and blood.

True 2. Abnormalities in ventilation can lead to hypoxia.

True 3. The normal carbonic acid to bicarbonate ratio is 1:20.

False 4. Blood gas studies are only of value in the pH determination of arterial blood.

True 5. Laboratory values may vary (slightly) from hospital to hospital.

True 6. Catheters used for suctioning must be lubricated with a water-soluble substance.

False 7. Suctioning cannot be carried out when the patient has an endotracheal tube, but can be performed when the patient has a tracheostomy.

True 8. Once inserted, an endotracheal tube must be anchored in place.

False 9. An endotracheal tube can be connected to a respirator, but a tracheostomy tube cannot be conected to either a respirator or ventilator.

True 10. The cuff of the tracheostomy tube should be deflated at regular intervals.

True 11. Ventilators may be pressure cycled or volume cycled.

False 12. Volume-cycled ventilators are never used with cuffed tracheostomy tubes.

True 13. Gastric dilatation and paralytic ileus are two problems that may arise when a patient is on respirator therapy.

True 14. Many patients on respirators are conscious and aware of the machinery and treatments.

False 15. Generally, the longer the patient has received artificial ventilation the easier it will be to wean him from the machine.

II. Multiple choice questions.

Select the most appropriate answer and place it in the space provided.

1. Arterial pH is kept within normal limits by the __d__.
   1. kidneys
   2. lungs
   3. electrolytes
   4. body fluids
   5. body buffer systems
      a. 1, 2, 3
      b. 1, 4, 5
      c. 2 only
      d. all of these

2. Carbon dioxide is present in body fluids primarily as __a__.
   a. sodium bicarbonate
   b. a hydrogen ion
   c. a hydrocarbon
   d. carbonic acid

3. The kidney contributes to the normal pH by __c__.
   a. excreting excess hydroxyl ions
   b. maintaining hydrogen ion levels
   c. maintaining serum bicarbonate levels and excreting excess hydrogen ions

4. Acute respiratory failure is a life-threatening complication in which __a__.
   a. alveolar ventilation becomes inadequate to maintain the body's need for oxygen
   b. tissue hypoxia occurs because of hypocapnia
   c. the respiratory rate rises in an attempt to decrease hypercapnia

5. Symptoms of acute respiratory failure include __c__.
   1. increased PaO_2
   2. decreased $PaCO_2$
   3. severe dyspnea
   4. apprehension
   5. marked use of accessory muscles of respiration
      a. 1, 4, 5
      b. 2, 3, 4
      c. 3, 4, 5
      d. all of these

6. The major mechanism for clearing the tracheobronchial tree of mucus is __c__.
   a. deep breathing
   b. inspiration of humid air
   c. coughing
   d. proper exercise and fresh air

7. Aids in the prevention of the drying of respiratory secretions are __a__.
   1. position change every hour
   2. increased fluid intake
   3. semi-Fowler's position
   4. humidification of surrounding air
   5. addition of milk and other vitamin-enriched foods to the diet
      a. 1, 2, 4
      b. 1, 3, 5
      c. 2, 3, 4
      d. 3, 4, 5

8. An endotracheal tube cannot be connected to a respirator unless __a__.
   a. the cuff is inflated
   b. an endotracheal tube a size larger than the trachea is used
   c. an endotracheal tube a size smaller than the trachea is used

9. An endotracheal tube can become obstructed by __a__.
   1. air
   2. the patient biting down on the tube
   3. secretions
   4. kinking of the tube
      a. all but 1
      b. all but 2
      c. all but 3
      d. all but 4

10. *Accidental* removal of an endotracheal tube can result in __a__.
    1. laryngeal edema
    2. respiratory arrest
    3. decrease in respiratory rate
    4. decrease in $PaCO_2$
       a. 1, 2
       b. 1, 3
       c. 1, 4
       d. 2, 4

253

11. Usually, a decision to remove the patient's endotracheal tube is made when the patient's __b__.
    a. color improves
    b. vital capacity is adequate
    c. respiratory rate and rhythm are normal
    d. blood gas studies are within 20 percent of the normal range

12. After an endotracheal tube is removed, the patient is placed in a semi-Fowler's position to __c__.
    a. lessen apprehension as he breathes on his own
    b. make it easier to reinsert the endotracheal tube should he have difficulty breathing
    c. promote chest expansion and optimal alveolar ventilation

13. The frequency of suctioning depends upon __c__.
    a. whether cyanosis is or is not present
    b. arterial blood gas studies
    c. the amount of secretions present

14. Giving the patient too much oxygen __b__.
    a. is not dangerous
    b. can depress the respirations
    c. is not dangerous if the patient has lung disease such as emphysema

15. A respirator is usually necessary if conventional therapy is not sufficient to maintain oxygenation above __b__.
    a. 40 mm Hg.
    b. 60 mm Hg.
    c. 80 mm Hg.
    d. 90 to 95 mm Hg.

16. A respirator forces air into the lung to __a__.
    a. give the patient adequate tidal volume
    b. bypass obstructions to breathing
    c. inflate all the alveoli
    d. dilate the bronchi

17. In controlled ventilation by use of a respirator, the inspiration is initiated by the __d__.
    a. patient when he feels light-headed
    b. machine when the patient has not inspired air for 8 seconds
    c. patient when he feels a need for oxygen
    d. machine at a preset rate

18. Positive pressure breathing does not adequately ventilate the entire lung unless __d__.
    a. it is turned to the "maximum pressure" setting
    b. the patient is sitting upright
    c. the patient learns how to use the machine properly
    d. secretions are moved from the distal air passages to the main bronchi

19. If a patient is on a respirator, hyperventilation can result in __b__.
    a. respiratory acidosis
    b. respiratory alkalosis

20. Oral feedings may be allowed in patients with a(n) __a__.
    a. tracheostomy tube
    b. endotracheal tube

21. A patient with a tracheostomy tube connected to a respirator __b__.
    a. can talk, but must do so with great effort
    b. cannot talk while connected to the respirator

22. What should be kept at the patient's bedside in case of mechanical breakdown of a respirator or a power failure? __c__
    a. a portable battery pack to operate the respirator until power is restored
    b. a spare respirator
    c. a manual device such as an Ambu bag
    d. an alarm system warning of a power failure

23. During the period of weaning from a respirator the patient may be given __c__.
    1. respiratory stimulant drugs
    2. mild sedation
    3. humidified oxygen
    4. narcotics to control dyspnea
       a. 1, 2
       c. 2, 3
       b. 1, 3
       d. 2, 4

III. Fill-in and discussion questions.
Read each question carefully and place your answer in the space provided.
1. VOCABULARY. Define the following terms.
    a. diffusion: _process by which O_2 & CO_2 are exchanged across alveolar capillary membranes_
    b. hypercapnia: _Excess CO_2 in body fluids_
    c. hypocapnia: _decrease of CO_2 in body fluids_
    d. hypoxemia: _reduced oxygen in body fluids_
    e. hypoxia: _diminished availability of oxygen to cells in the body_
    f. ventilation: _The movement of air in & out of the lungs_

CHAPTER—47

The patient with heart disease: cardiac arrhythmias

To pump blood, the heart must alternately relax and contract, allowing blood to enter the atria (or upper chambers) during the relaxation phase and forcing it out during the contraction phase. The alternate contraction and relaxation is provided by an inherent rhythmicity of the cardiac muscle.

The following questions deal with the contents of Chapter 47.

I. True or false.

Read each statement carefully and place your answer in the space provided.

_____ 1. An electrical impulse arising in any single cardiac fiber eventually spreads over the membranes of all cardiac fibers.

_____ 2. The normal cardiac muscle cell has more negative than positive ions inside the cell membrane.

_____ 3. Only the sympathetic nervous system has an effect on the cardiovascular system.

_____ 4. Vasovagal syncope is due to a predominance of vagal reflexes with a slowing of the heart rate.

_____ 5. Cardiac arrest almost always occurs without previous electrocardiographic warning.

_____ 6. Continued sinus tachycardia while at rest may add an intolerable workload to the heart already damaged by a myocardial infarction.

_____ 7. In normal sinus rhythm, the A-V node is the pacemaker.

_____ 8. In sinus bradycardia, the rate is below 60 and the pacemaker site is the S-A node.

_____ 9. In patients with a myocardial infarction, sinus bradycardia may be serious.

_____ 10. In the healthy individual without heart disease, PVC's are usually harmless.

_____ 11. Cardioversion is used to convert slow cardiac rhythms, such as bradycardia, to a normal sinus rhythm.

_____ 12. Elective cardioversion is a planned cardioversion, which means that a definite time is preselected for the procedure.

_____ 13. Digitalis is withheld before an elective cardioversion because it may increase the chance of the development of a death-producing arrhythmia after the procedure.

_____ 14. A pacemaker generator may be inserted as a temporary measure to suppress rapid arrhythmias.

_____ 15. Following insertion of a pacemaker, the patient is placed on a cardiac monitor.

_____ 16. An external pacemaker apparatus is usually anchored to the patient's bedside stand.
_____ 17. The use of a pacemaker will aid in the regeneration of the diseased myocardium.
_____ 18. Pacemaker generators are sensitive to such outside electrical interference as diathermy and microwave ovens.
_____ 19. Cardiac arrest is the sudden cessation of effective cardiac output.
_____ 20. Dilatation of the pupils begins about 45 minutes after cardiac arrest.
_____ 21. Endotracheal intubation is necessary for an adequate airway during cardiopulmonary resuscitation.
_____ 22. For effective cardiac compression during cardiopulmonary resuscitation, the patient must be on a soft, flexible surface.
_____ 23. Rhythmic pressure applied over the lower half of the sternum results in the compression of the heart.
_____ 24. External cardiac compression is contraindicated in crushing chest injuries.

II. Multiple choice questions.

Select the most appropriate answer and place it in the space provided.

1. The sino-atrial (S-A) node is normally located in the _____.
   a. posterior wall of the left atrium
   b. posterior wall of the right atrium
   c. anterior wall of the left atrium
   d. atrial septum

2. The S-A node has a rhythmic rate of approximately _____.
   a. 40 beats per minute
   b. 60 beats per minute
   c. 72 beats per minute
   d. 90 beats per minute

3. Which progression is correct? _____
   a. S-A node → A-V node → bundle of His → Purkinje fibers
   b. A-V node → S-A node → Purkinje fibers → bundle of His
   c. bundle of His → A-V node → S-A node → Purkinje fibers
   d. Purkinje fibers → bundle of His → A-V node → S-A node

4. The heart can increase the amount of blood that it pumps by _____.
   1. closing heart valves early in the cardiac cycle
   2. closing heart valves completely at the end of the cardiac cycle
   3. increasing the volume pumped with each beat
   4. beating faster
      a. 1, 2
      b. 2, 3
      c. 3, 4
      d. all of these

5. Cardiac rhythm and conduction can be disturbed by _____.
   1. anxiety
   2. pain
   3. electrolyte imbalance
   4. disturbance in body fluid pH
      a. 1, 2
      b. 3, 4
      c. all but 2
      d. all of these

6. If the pulse rate rises to 108 after running up a flight of stairs, this is a(n) _____.
   a. abnormal physiologic response
   b. normal physiologic response

7. Bradycardia may be seen in patients with _____.
   1. hypothyroidism
   2. digitalis toxicity
   3. panhypopituitarism
   4. excessive sympathetic nervous system stimulation
   5. increased intracranial pressure
      a. 1, 2, 4
      b. 1, 2, 5
      c. 2, 3, 4
      d. 3, 4, 5

8. Sinus tachycardia _____.
   a. is never serious
   b. is a result of irritability of the A-V node
   c. can increase the work of the heart and be initial evidence of cardiac failure

9. In atrial fibrillation the _____.
   1. atrial rate is usually 350 to 800
   2. ventricular rate is always over 125
   3. ventricular rate varies and is usually irregular
   4. atrial rate is lower than the ventricular rate
      a. 1, 2
      b. 1, 3
      c. 2, 4
      d. 3, 4

10. In complete heart block the _____.
    1. atria and ventricles beat independently of each other
    2. atrial rate is one half the ventricular rate
    3. ventricular rate is 40 or below
    4. ventricular rate is extremely irregular
       a. 1, 3
       b. 1, 4
       c. 2, 3
       d. 2, 4

11. Treatment of complete heart block usually includes _____.
    1. use of an electronic pacemaker
    2. drug therapy such as isoproterenol (Isuprel)
    3. adequate ventilation to control hypoxia
    4. treatment of associated clinical conditions
       a. 1, 2
       b. 1, 3
       c. 3, 4
       d. all of these

12. PVC's that occur in patients with an acute myocardial infarction may be a precursor of _____.
    a. congestive heart failure
    b. a lethal arrhythmia
    c. a reversion to normal rhythm
    d. pulmonary edema

13. Treatment of cardiac arrhythmias is aimed at _____.
    1. conversion to normal sinus rhythm if possible
    2. producing maximum physiologic improvement
    3. prevention of acute life-threatening arrhythmias
    4. curing atherosclerotic-type heart disease
       a. all but 1
       b. all but 2
       c. all but 3
       d. all but 4

14. Mechanical means of slowing the heart include _____.
    1. carotid sinus pressure
    2. eyeball pressure
    3. closed chest massage
    4. Valsalva maneuver
       a. all but 1
       b. all but 2
       c. all but 3
       d. all but 4

15. Drug therapy for cardiac arrhythmias includes drugs acting _____.
    1. solely on the bundle of His
    2. primarily on nerves controlling the S-A node
    3. on the autonomic nervous system
    4. primarily on tissues within the heart
       a. 1, 2
       b. 1, 3
       c. 2, 3
       d. 3, 4

16. Restoration of normal cardiac rhythm may be accomplished by the use of drugs as well as by electrical therapy such as ____.
    1. fibrillation
    2. use of a pacemaker
    3. defibrillation
    4. cardioversion
       a. all but 1
       b. all but 2
       c. all but 3
       d. all but 4
17. The treatment for ventricular fibrillation is ____.
    a. administration of atropine
    b. immediate insertion of a pacemaker
    c. administration of adrenergic drugs which promptly act on the autonomic nervous system
    d. immediate defibrillation
18. A pacemaker generator is used to ____.
    a. maintain the patient's ventricular rate at a minimum level for effective cardiac output
    b. keep the pulse rate over 50 but under 100
    c. control cardiac output
    d. decrease cardiac volume
19. A demand type pacemaker is ____.
    a. cheaper than a synchronous pacemaker
    b. operational when the patient's pulse falls below a preset rate
    c. used only as an external temporary measure until an internal pacemaker can be inserted
    d. used only in the treatment of digitalis toxicity
20. Symptoms of Stokes-Adams syndrome include ____.
    1. irregular pulse
    2. convulsions
    3. fainting
    4. severe bradycardia
    5. tachycardia
       a. 1, 2, 3
       b. 1, 2, 4
       c. 2, 3, 4
       d. 3, 4, 5
21. When an external or internal pacemaker is used to maintain the heart rate at a given rate, the pacemaker lead is inserted into the ____.
    a. left atrium
    b. right atrium
    c. left ventricle
    d. right ventricle
22. Two complications of a temporary external pacemaker are ____.
    1. battery failure
    2. localized phlebitis
    3. pacemaker lead can wear out
    4. cellulitis
       a. 1, 2
       b. 1, 4
       c. 2, 3
       d. 2, 4
23. An internal pacemaker runs on batteries and ultimately the batteries become nonfunctional and the entire unit must be replaced. Symptoms of battery failure may include ____.
    1. weakness
    2. dizziness
    3. change in pulse rate
    4. unconsciousness
       a. 1, 2
       b. 1, 3
       c. 3, 4
       d. all of these
24. When there are two rescuers performing cardiopulmonary resuscitation, one breath is given for every ____ chest compressions.
    a. 2
    b. 5
    c. 10
    d. 15
25. Artificial ventilation may cause ____.
    a. distention of the stomach
    b. rupture of the alveoli
    c. intestinal puncture
    d. cardiac arrest

26. During resuscitation, effort will be made by the physician to combat acidosis with the administration of ____.
    a. epinephrine
    b. calcium chloride
    c. sodium bicarbonate
    d. vasopressors

III. Fill-in and discussion questions.

Read each question carefully and place your answer in the space provided.

1. Fill in the blanks of the following questions with the correct word or words that will complete the statement.

    1. The _____ node is called the pacemaker of the heart.
    2. Complete heart block is also called _____ degree heart block.
    3. When more positive than negative ions appear inside the cell membrane of cardiac muscle, this is called _____.
    4. When the ions realign themselves to their original position, this is called _____.
    5. Stimulation of the _____ nervous system speeds the heart rate whereas stimulation of the _____ nervous system slows the heart rate.
    6. A ventricular ectopic beat is called a _____.
    7. The special conduction system carrying impulses throughout the ventricles is called the _____.

2. The ABCDE's are extremely important points in cardiopulmonary resuscitation. Below identify and briefly explain the meaning behind these letters.

	STANDS FOR	BRIEF COMMENT OR EXPLANATION
A		
B		
C		
D		
E		

CHAPTER—48

The patient with acute myocardial infarction

In myocardial infarction, the interference with the blood supply to a portion of the muscle of the heart is so severe that necrosis of a part of the heart results. This may be precipitated by the occlusion of a coronary artery, from capillary hemorrhage within an atherosclerotic plaque or by the formation of a thrombus on one of the plaques. Myocardial infarction may also occur without the occlusion of an artery when there is a sudden reduction in the blood supply to the heart.

The following questions deal with the contents of Chapter 48.

I. True or false.

Read each statement carefully and place your answer in the space provided.

_____ 1. The pain experienced at the time of a myocardial infarction is usually more severe and of longer duration than the pain experienced in angina pectoris.

_____ 2. The patient with an acute myocardial infarction may display symptoms of shock.

_____ 3. The majority of deaths from myocardial infarction occur 2 to 3 weeks after the infarction during the recovery phase.

_____ 4. On admission, patients who are dyspneic or cyanotic are usually given oxygen.

_____ 5. Giving oxygen in a high concentration can result in respiratory arrest.

_____ 6. In the patient with a myocardial infarction, pain usually results in prolonged periods of hypertension.

_____ 7. Cardiac monitors are considered as aids to, but not substitutes for, nursing care.

_____ 8. Carbonated beverages, providing they are served at room temperature, are allowed in the diet of a patient with a recent myocardial infarction.

_____ 9. An electrocardiogram may be repeated several times to establish the diagnosis of myocardial infarction.

_____ 10. Serum enzyme studies will show a decrease if the patient has had a recent myocardial infarction.

_____ 11. An elevated erythrocyte sedimentation rate and white blood cell count are evidence of tissue necrosis in myocardial infarction.

_____ 12. Prolonged bed rest favors the development of many complications which can prove to be serious.

_____ 13. The area of a myocardial infarction heals by the formation of scar tissue.

_____ 14. The patient may expend less en-

ergy when using a bedside commode than when getting on and off a bedpan.
_____ 15. The patient with cardiogenic shock, if properly treated, has an excellent recovery rate.
_____ 16. Rupture of a ventricular aneurysm is almost always fatal.
_____ 17. Transfer out of the CCU may produce varying forms of anxiety as the patient worries about his progress and fate in a less specialized area of the hospital.
_____ 18. The nurse can be of help during the rehabilitation period by being a good listener.
_____ 19. The prognosis of a myocardial infarction is good, with many patients returning to full-time employment.

II. **Multiple choice questions.**

Select the most appropriate answer and place it in the space provided.

CLINICAL SITUATION

Mr. Mason, a 52-year-old sales representative, is admitted to the coronary care unit with a diagnosis of probable myocardial infarction. He became ill at work during a sales meeting, at which time he experienced severe pain, nausea, and diaphoresis. An electrocardiogram (ECG) was performed in the emergency department.

1. The emphasis in a coronary care unit is on _____.
   a. educating nurses in the care of patients with coronary artery disease
   b. providing sophisticated electronic equipment for patient care
   c. prevention of the need for resuscitation measures by detecting early changes in the patient's condition

2. Upon admission, Mr. Mason's pulse rate is 58, which could mean _____.
   a. he is not excited and has confidence in his physician and the nursing personnel
   b. the involvement of the S-A or A-V node or a marked vagal tone
   c. he was probably given a cardiac drug prior to admission and he is showing signs of drug toxicity

3. Mr. Mason is *slightly* dyspneic and cyanotic. Before giving him oxygen, the nurse should _____.
   a. wait until his symptoms are more pronounced
   b. check to see if the physician has examined the patient and written admitting orders
   c. check with him or his family to see if he has chronic obstructive lung disease

4. Mr. Mason's physician orders morphine sulfate 10 mg. to be administered stat. After the drug is given, Mr. Mason should be observed for _____.
   1. respiratory depression
   2. nausea
   3. arrhythmias
   4. hypotension
      a. 1, 3
      b. 2, 4
      c. 3, 4
      d. all of these

5. The advantage of placing Mr. Mason on a cardiac monitor is that _____.
   a. changes in cardiac rate and rhythm can be detected early
   b. it frees the nurse to care for other patients
   c. the monitor is able to detect changes in the blood pressure with more accuracy than nursing personnel

6. The physician orders an intravenous infusion of 5% glucose in water to keep the vein open. This is a usual procedure so that _____.
   a. in an emergency, drugs can be given quickly with no time wasted looking for a vein or performing a cutdown

b. drugs can be administered by the intravenous route without disturbing the patient and causing discomfort each time the drug is given
c. drugs can be administered by the intravenous route because most patients with a myocardial infarction have severe nausea

7. A 12-lead electrocardiogram was taken on Mr. Mason shortly after he was admitted to the CCU. This will serve as a ____.
   a. basis for intravenous fluid therapy
   b. basis for later comparison and immediate arrhythmia treatment
   c. screening test, looking for past cardiac problems

8. The diet for patients with a myocardial infarction who are newly admitted to the CCU is usually a ____.
   a. full liquid diet
   b. soft diet
   c. soft bland diet
   d. house diet with moderate sodium restrictions

9. Ice water or iced beverages are contraindicated because they are ____.
   a. gas-producing fluids
   b. cardiac depressants
   c. cold enough to lower the body temperature and, therefore, produce an arrhythmia
   d. vagal stimulants

10. The physician orders an oral temperature every 4 hours while the patient is awake. A rectal temperature is usually not taken on the cardiac patient because of the ____.
    a. anxiety caused by this procedure
    b. inaccuracy of rectal temperatures in these patients
    c. danger of tachycardia and dyspnea
    d. danger of vagal stimulation and cardiac slowing

11. Serial ECG's are ordered to determine the area of infarction. The most frequent site of a myocardial infarction is in the ____.
    a. right atrium
    b. left atrium
    c. right ventricle
    d. left ventricle

12. The prime objective of Mr. Mason's treatment will be ____.
    a. keeping him comfortable and explaining the importance of complete physical and mental rest so that further cardiac damage does not occur
    b. promoting a healthy outlook and understanding of heart disease
    c. reducing the workload of the heart to prevent further cardiac damage and promote healing

13. Sudden death from a myocardial infarction is usually attributed to ____.
    a. atrial fibrillation
    b. ventricular fibrillation
    c. first- or second-degree heart block
    d. sinus tachycardia

14. One of the hazards of bed rest is the Valsalva maneuver which might happen when a patient ____.
    1. sighs
    2. strains to defecate or void
    3. tries to lift himself up in bed
    4. coughs, vomits or gags
       a. all but 1
       b. all but 2
       c. all but 3
       d. all but 4

15. Performance of the Valsalva maneuver is dangerous in the cardiac patient because ____.
    a. a reflex bradycardia can occur which may be fatal to the patient with a damaged heart
    b. there is a decrease in intrathoracic pressure causing an overdistention of the ventricles
    c. there is an increase in venous pressure which may cause a tachycardia

16. Mr. Mason begins to object to his restricted activities. At this point the nurse should ____.
    a. explain to Mr. Mason that he must rest
    b. talk to Mrs. Mason and have her impress on her husband the importance of following the physician's orders
    c. discuss this problem with Mr. Mason's physician who may permit more flexibility in what Mr. Mason is allowed to do

17. Mr. Mason's physician orders a tranquilizer for anxiety. The nurse should check Mr. Mason to be sure ____.
    a. he is not disturbed for any reason during the time (3 to 4 hours) the medication is taking effect
    b. he does not become so somnolent that he no longer initiates deep-breathing or leg exercises or movement in bed
    c. the medication is reducing internal anxiety

18. Venous thrombosis is one of the complications of a myocardial infarction. A drug that may be administered to decrease the likelihood of this complication is ____.
    a. an anticoagulant
    b. vitamin K
    c. a cardiotonic preparation
    d. an antispasmodic

19. Another complication that could develop in Mr. Mason is pulmonary embolism, which usually arises from ____.
    a. clots formed in the aorta
    b. clots formed in the superior vena cava
    c. arterial clots in the lower extremities
    d. venous clots in the lower extremities

20. Another complication is a clot in the left ventricle which has formed over the infarcted area. This is known as a ____.
    a. mural thrombus
    b. cardiac embolus
    c. ventricular embolus

21. Other complications of a myocardial infarction include ____.
    1. atherosclerosis
    2. ventricular aneurysm
    3. ventricular rupture
    4. congestive heart failure
    a. all but 1
    b. all but 2
    c. all but 3
    d. all but 4

22. Mr. Mason is doing well and after 9 days in the coronary care unit he is transferred. Ideally, Mr. Mason should be transfered to a(n) ____.
    a. area fully equipped and exactly like the CCU but with other patients who are also going through a transition period
    b. general hospital area so that he can learn to be without his monitor and other electronic hardware
    c. postcoronary division where specially trained personnel can help him through this period of transition

III. Fill-in and discussion questions.

Read each question carefully and place your answer in the space provided.

1. List the symptoms that may be experienced by the patient with a myocardial infarction. _____

2. An admission history is an important nursing task when a patient is admitted to the coronary care unit. If you were assigned to take an admission history, what questions would you ask of the patient and/or his family? _____

3. The patient with a myocardial infarction may have many fears. Briefly discuss some of the fears and worries this patient may have. _____

CHAPTER—49

Cardiac surgical nursing

The patient deciding to have surgery performed on his heart is taking a calculated risk for a longer and more healthy life. Patients enter the hospital with varying degrees of emotional readiness to face such an operation. The preoperative period is very important because it helps the patient to feel secure in the hospital situation, provided that the physicians and nurses demonstrate competence and concern.

The following questions deal with the contents of Chapter 49.

I. True or false.

Read each statement carefully and place your answer in the space provided.

_____ 1. In the patient undergoing cardiac surgery there are 2 physiologic systems of the body that have been affected, the cardiac and the respiratory systems.

_____ 2. Severely damaged aortic, mitral, or tricuspid valves can be replaced by artificial valves.

_____ 3. Insufficient or incompetent heart valves result in blood regurgitating backward through the valve.

_____ 4. The closed repair of a stenotic valve is the suturing of the valve in a closed position to improve valve function.

_____ 5. Open repair of damaged cardiac valves includes using cardiopulmonary bypass.

_____ 6. The most common surgical method of treatment of coronary atherosclerosis is the saphenous vein revascularization procedure.

_____ 7. Atherosclerotic deposits or clots obstructing the coronary arteries usually involve a large portion of the artery.

_____ 8. Surgical removal of an atherosclerotic plaque is called a veinotomy.

_____ 9. An aneurysm of the wall of the ventricle is the most lethal complication among patients surviving the acute stage of a myocardial infarction.

_____ 10. Patients undergoing cardiac surgery are almost always given a house diet before surgery because they will have severe dietary restrictions afterwards.

_____ 11. Some patients develop a temporary psychoticlike reaction after cardiovascular surgery.

II. Multiple choice questions.

Select the most appropriate answer and place it in the space provided.

1. Acquired lesions of the valves of the heart are most frequently due to _____.
   a. rheumatic fever
   b. pneumonia
   c. drugs

2. A stenosed heart valve opens on contraction of the ventricles but the reduced size of the lumen ____.
   a. causes no problem unless the patient develops an arrhythmia or sinus tachycardia
   b. prevents contraction of the ventricles
   c. limits the amount of blood that can flow through the valve

3. The leading type of heart disease in the United States is ____.
   a. myocardial infarction
   b. valvular heart disease
   c. atherosclerosis
   d. cardiac insufficiency

4. In an atrial-septal defect the blood flows from the ____.
   a. right atrium to the left atrium
   b. left atrium to the right atrium

5. Following a nonpenetrating chest injury blood may accumulate in the pericardial sac, causing ____.
   a. myocardial ischemia
   b. pulmonary embolus
   c. cerebral anoxia
   d. cardiac tamponade

6. Signs of blood accumulating in the pericardial sac may include ____.
   1. hypertension
   2. flushing of the face
   3. dyspnea
   4. distention of neck veins
   5. paradoxical pulse
      a. 1, 2, 3
      b. 1, 3, 4
      c. 2, 4, 5
      d. 3, 4, 5

CLINICAL SITUATION

Jim Park is a 20-year-old college student with a history of an acquired heart lesion—mitral stenosis. He has been admitted for open heart surgery on the mitral valve.

7. In preparation for cardiac surgery, cardiopulmonary evaluation may include ____.
   1. x-rays
   2. pulmonary function studies
   3. laboratory blood studies
   4. cardioangiography
      a. 1, 2
      b. 2, 3
      c. 3, 4
      d. all of these

8. For several days prior to cardiac surgery, the skin over or near the operative area is prepared by ____.
   a. scrubbing with a bacteriostatic soap
   b. washing or showering with a bactericidal soap
   c. application of a bactericidal ointment

9. Following cardiac surgery, Jim's blood pressure may be monitored and recorded directly and continuously by means of a(n) ____.
   a. blood pressure cuff that continuously inflates and deflates
   b. polyethylene catheter placed in the femoral artery
   c. electrode placed on a neck vein

10. To evaluate the effectiveness of the respirator and Jim's response to the respirator the nurse can use a(n) ____.
    a. Ambu bag
    b. Bird or Bennett respirator
    c. respirometer
    d. rebreathing bag

11. Central venous pressure measurements are used as a(n) ____.
    a. indication of a decrease or increase in serum electrolytes
    b. indication of edema
    c. guide to fluid needs or fluid replacement
    d. measurement of blood gasses

12. Jim has a Foley catheter that was inserted prior to surgery. On arrival in the intensive care unit his urinary output increased during the first several hours. This is probably due to the ____.
    a. administration of blood during surgery
    b. action of diuretics given prior to surgery
    c. saline intravenous fluids given during surgery
    d. administration of osmotic diuretics during surgery
13. Jim's indwelling catheter is to be irrigated to prevent clogging. To ensure an accurate output determination, the amount of the irrigating solution is ____.
    a. added to the total output
    b. subtracted from the total output
    c. added to the intake and subtracted from the output
14. After Jim's endotracheal tube is removed he will probably complain of ____.
    a. being unable to swallow
    b. a sore throat
    c. chest pain
15. Oral fluids can be started after the endotracheal tube is removed. The diet will probably consist of ____.
    a. clear liquids
    b. full liquid diet
    c. restricted sodium liquid diet
16. When Jim is finally ready for discharge it is important to collaborate with the physician to help the family learn ____.
    a. exactly what type of surgery was performed
    b. what Jim can and cannot do when he goes home
    c. how to give skilled nursing care once Jim is home

III. Discussion question.

Read the following question carefully and place your answer in the space provided.

1. Preoperative teaching of the patient undergoing cardiac surgery is very important. List and describe any 4 points you would include in a preoperative teaching plan.

    1. _____

    2. _____

    3. _____

    4. _____

CHAPTER—50

The patient in renal failure

Renal failure, acute or chronic, is a serious inability of the kidneys to carry out the normal functions necessary to eliminate the end products of metabolism from the body. When kidney function is insufficient and such products as urea, other nonprotein nitrogens, creatinine, and uric acid accumulate in the blood, a state of azotemia is present. If not corrected, the patient experiences the signs and symptoms of uremia, such as lethargy, irritability, and anorexia in the early stage and progressively more ominous ones as uremia advances.

The following questions deal with the contents of Chapter 50.

I. True or false.

Read each statement carefully and place your answer in the space provided.

__T__ 1. In some patients, renal failure can be prevented by planning a routine of oral fluid intake, especially in those who may be too old or too weak to take fluids on their own.

__T__ 2. In renal failure the quantity of urine can be normal or even increased in volume.

__F__ 3. Hypotension commonly accompanies renal failure.

__T__ 4. The patient with uremia is often very ill and may even be comatose.

__F__ 5. Most patients in uremia are placed on a forced fluid regimen.

__T__ 6. Accurate measurement of intake and output is an essential element of the nursing management of the patient in renal failure.

__F__ 7. The uremic patient with an accumulation of uric acid crystals on his skin should have a bath with copious amounts of soap which will be necessary to remove the crystals.

__T__ 8. Most instances of acute renal failure develop as a complication of a major medical or surgical problem.

__T__ 9. Hemodialysis permits the replacement of substances such as calcium and bicarbonate as well as the removal of substances such as urea and potassium.

__T__ 10. The hemodialysis procedure usually lasts from 4 to 8 hours.

__F__ 11. The patient must fast 12 hours prior to a hemodialysis procedure.

__T__ 12. The special chemical bathing solution used in dialysis procedures is called the dialysate.

__F__ 13. The equipment used in peritoneal dialysis is more complicated than the equipment used in hemodialysis.

__T__ 14. Peritoneal dialysis is the use of a

dialysate that flows into and out of the peritoneal cavity.

_F_ 15. The patient undergoing peritoneal dialysis must remain in a supine position at all times.

_T_ 16. The patient undergoing peritoneal dialysis may usually eat and drink.

II. Multiple choice questions.

Select the most appropriate answer and place it in the space provided.

1. Renal failure can result from _d_.
   1. severe and prolonged episodes of hypotension
   2. acute renal tubular necrosis
   3. polycystic disease
   4. chronic glomerulonephritis
      a. 1, 2
      b. 2, 3
      c. 3, 4
      d. all of these

2. Oliguria is a _a_.
   a. decrease in normal urinary output
   b. cessation of urinary output
   c. the secretion of urine with a low specific gravity

3. Laboratory blood studies that are indicative of renal failure include a(n) _c_.
   1. decrease in blood urea nitrogen
   2. rise in serum creatinine
   3. elevated uric acid
   4. hypocalcemia
   5. increased number of platelets
      a. 1, 2, 3
      b. 1, 4, 5
      c. 2, 3, 4
      d. 2, 4, 5

4. To prevent uremia in acute and chronic renal failure, a substitution for kidney function may be employed. An example of a substitute for kidney function is _B_.
   a. drug therapy with agents to acidify the urine
   b. hemodialysis
   c. cardiopulmonary bypass
   d. aortic-renal artery bypass

5. A urinary output below _A_ ml. in 24 hours is significant and must be reported to the physician.
   a. 500
   b. 750
   c. 1000
   d. 1200

6. The type of foods that may be restricted in patients in renal failure are _B_.
   a. carbohydrates
   b. proteins
   c. fats

7. The patient in acute renal failure may reach a diuretic phase of his disease at which time _c_.
   1. urinary output increases
   2. anorexia begins to occur
   3. nausea and vomiting subside
   4. excess sodium is retained
   5. excess sodium is lost
      a. 1, 2, 3
      b. 1, 3, 4
      c. 1, 3, 5
      d. 5 only

8. Anemia is a common problem of patients in renal failure and contributes to _D_.
   a. the appearance of uremic frost
   b. numbness and tingling of the extremities
   c. edema of the extremities
   d. general weakness and lethargy

9. Exposure to infection may be serious for the patient with renal failure as an infection __A__.
   a. increases protein catabolism
   b. decreases protein catabolism

10. Another name for hemodialysis is __a__.
    a. peritoneal dialysis
    b. intrarenal hemodialysis
    c. diffusional dialysis
    d. extracorporeal hemodialysis

11. Substances which may be removed from the patient's blood during hemodialysis are __D__.
    1. urea
    2. potassium
    3. creatinine
    4. bacteria
       a. all but 1
       b. all but 2
       c. all but 3
       d. all but 4

12. The patient's blood pressure and pulse are sometimes taken frequently during a hemodialysis procedure. Taking the pulse may detect a cardiac arrhythmia which may occur if __C__.
    a. not enough bicarbonate is returned to the bloodstream
    b. the patient loses blood during the procedure
    c. too much potassium is removed
    d. not enough sodium is removed

13. The patient on hemodialysis will receive heparin and therefore must be observed for __A__.
    a. bleeding
    b. numbness and tingling
    c. convulsions
    d. muscle twitching

14. After hemodialysis, fluid and dietary restrictions are __B__.
    a. lifted
    b. regulated according to the degree of recovery of renal function

15. When peritoneal dialysis is instituted, a solution is allowed to flow into the patient and is __C__.
    a. immediately drained out of the patient
    b. permanently left in the patient
    c. allowed to remain in the patient for a designated period of time, usually 30 to 45 minutes
    d. left in the patient 24 hours and then allowed to slowly drain out over a period of 12 hours

16. The usual amount of dialysate used for one peritoneal dialysis exchange (or cycle) is ____ ml. __c__
    a. 500
    b. 1000
    c. 2000
    d. 5000

17. Which of the following conditions would warrant a delay in the next dialysis exchange until the physician has been notified? __B__
    a. the patient has become restless and bored
    b. the patient complains of pain and you note abdominal distention
    c. the dialysate took 15 minutes to drain from the peritoneal cavity
    d. the dialysate took 20 minutes to drain into the peritoneal cavity

18. A major complication of peritoneal dialysis is __B D__
    a. hypernatremia
    b. hypercalcemia
    c. hypertension
    d. peritonitis

271

III. Discussion question.
Read the following question carefully and place your answer in the space provided.
1. List 6 general outward signs and symptoms of renal failure.

    1. Edema - eyes & ankles

    2. Pruritis

    3. halitosis

    4. pale

    5. ulceration of oral mucosa

    6. slowed mental processes

CHAPTER—51

The burned patient

Suddenly a well person sustains serious burns, and is confronted with problems resulting from pain, mutilation, fear of death, disfigurement, separation, immobilization, helplessness, and possible abandonment. Along with his injuries and problems he may experience guilt over the cause of the accident and anger that the catastrophe should have happened to him.

The burned patient requires intensive physical and psychological care because he will have a long battle with prevention of infection, continuing pain from dressing changes, surgery, scarring, financial burdens and many other problems.

The following questions deal with the contents of Chapter 51.

I. True or false.

Read each statement carefully and place your answer in the space provided.

_____ 1. The diagnosis of the depth of a burn is easy after the area has been properly cleaned of debris.

_____ 2. A second-degree burn is also a partial-thickness burn.

_____ 3. The "Rule of Nines" is one method of estimating how much of the patient's skin surface has been burned.

_____ 4. Immediately after a burn, the sodium level may decrease because the ions leave the body along with the fluids lost from the burned areas.

_____ 5. The burned patient requires close monitoring and skilled observation because, if changes are not immediately recognized and corrected, irreversible shock can occur.

_____ 6. The severely burned patient is given oral fluids soon after admittance to the intensive care unit in an effort to replace lost fluids.

_____ 7. The crust over a second-degree or partial-thickness burn forms in 6 to 8 weeks after the injury.

_____ 8. The hard, leathery crust which forms over the area of a third-degree burn is called eschar.

_____ 9. When drugs are applied to burned areas, clean rather than sterile technique is used because the skin is not sterile.

_____ 10. Bacteria present in the air, on the skin and on objects in the environment are capable of causing serious infections in burn wounds.

_____ 11. First-degree burns heal with no problems but second-degree burns will require skin grafting.

_____ 12. Good granulation tissue is necessary for successful skin grafting.

273

_____ 13. Active or passive exercises are not performed on or by the burned patient until all skin grafting is complete and healing has occurred.
_____ 14. An increase in body temperature may be the first indication that the burned patient has developed an infection.
_____ 15. Contractures develop in the burned patient because of the pull of tightening scar tissue.

II. Multiple choice questions.

Select the most appropriate answer and place it in the space provided.

CLINICAL SITUATION

Hal Brock was cleaning and repairing his car in his garage. In one corner he had an open can of gasoline. Working in a closed area caused a build-up of fumes and an explosion and fire occurred, apparently caused by a spark. Hal was finally able to get out of his burning garage when the fire department arrived. His clothing was on fire and the firemen immediately rushed to his aid.

1. If the clothing is on fire the victim should be _____.
    a. placed on the ground and rolled in a blanket
    b. rolled in a blanket and kept standing if possible
    c. sprayed with water or flame-retardant foam

2. If the victim has been burned around the face or neck, or has inhaled smoke, steam or flames, he should be closely watched for _____.
    a. excessive salivation
    b. respiratory difficulty
    c. excessive fluid loss
    d. bleeding

3. Upon admission Hal was weighed on a bed scale. His admission weight is important and will be used to determine _____.
    a. the percent of the body that has been burned
    b. whether he should go to a burn intensive care unit
    c. the type of drugs that will be administered
    d. fluid loss and gain

4. After a burn, fluid _____.
    a. contained in body cells is rapidly excreted by the kidneys
    b. from outside of the body cells moves into the body cells
    c. from the body moves toward the burned area
    d. moves away from the burned area removing needed electrolytes and plasma from the burn

5. After a burn, fluid is also lost _____.
    a. from the burned area in the form of water vapor and seepage
    b. by way of the kidneys due to a decrease in urinary output immediately after the accident
    c. from the lungs

6. Hal's initial blood studies show an increase in his hemoglobin and hematocrit. This is due to a(n) _____.
    a. decrease in plasma volume
    b. increase in plasma volume
    c. pooling of blood in the extremities

7. Since both of Hal's arms are burned, his blood pressure ____.
   a. cannot be taken
   b. can be taken by wrapping the cuff around the thigh and listening over the popliteal artery
   c. can be taken by wrapping the cuff around the calf and listening over the femoral artery

8. Hal is given a narcotic analgesic intravenously for severe pain. Severe pain can cause ____.
   a. respiratory difficulty
   b. unconsciousness when the patient must be alert to cooperate in his initial treatment
   c. hypotension

9. With regard to Hal's burned area, the *first* task that must be performed is ____.
   a. cleaning of the burned area
   b. application of an antibiotic to the burned area
   c. application of sterile dressings
   d. removal of all clothing

10. Body hair around the perimeter of Hal's burns is shaved because it ____.
    a. will hinder any attempt at skin grafting
    b. has been singed by the burn and looks unsightly
    c. is a source of bacterial wound contamination

11. Occlusive dressings are applied to Hal's burned areas. Another method of treatment is the ____.
    a. unsterile method
    b. isolation method
    c. open or exposure method

12. Hal's dressings must not be applied too tightly, as constriction would cause ____.
    a. circulation impairment
    b. a squeezing out of the drug applied to the dressing
    c. a rupture of the blisters over the third-degree burn area

13. During the acute phase, the urine of a burn patient is tested hourly for ____.
    1. specific gravity
    2. glucose
    3. acetone
    4. protein
    a. 1, 2
    b. 2, 3
    c. 1, 4
    d. all of these

14. Proper positioning of the extremities will be an extremely important measure in the prevention of ____.
    a. contractures
    b. pneumonia
    c. eschar formation
    d. crust formation

15. If silver nitrate is selected for the treatment of Hal's wounds it will be applied ____.
    a. twice a day
    b. by the continuous wet dressing technique
    c. each time the dressing is changed

16. One disadvantage of silver nitrate is ____.
    a. its expense
    b. it does not prevent infection
    c. the pain caused by its application
    d. the loss of sodium and potassium from body fluids

17. If mafenide (Sulfamylon) is selected to treat burns, the previous applications of the drug are removed by ____.
    a. using a tongue blade to scrape off the cream
    b. tubbing—usually in a Hubbard tank
    c. wiping the area with sterile gauze
    d. dissolving the cream with a weak alkali solution

18. Complaints of stinging or a burning sensation when the mafenide cream is first applied is _____.
    a. abnormal and the physician must be contacted before the cream is reapplied
    b. normal
19. Hal is treated with mafenide but begins to develop acidosis shortly after its use. His physician attributes the acidosis to the mafenide and orders silver sulfadiazine 1 percent ointment. This drug _____.
    a. does not disturb electrolyte or acid-base balance
    b. is less effective than mafenide
    c. has more side effects but does not cause acidosis
    d. has little or no antibacterial action
20. The purpose of skin grafting during the *management* stage of burn treatment is to _____.
    1. lessen the possibility of infection
    2. minimize fluid loss by evaporation
    3. prevent loss of function
    4. prevent scarring
    a. all but 1
    b. all but 2
    c. all but 3
    d. all but 4
21. One of the major causes of death in burn patients is _____.
    a. anemia
    b. hypertension
    c. edema
    d. infection
22. After many weeks of treatment, Hal is scheduled for skin grafts. If skin from another area of Hal's body is used for the graft it is called a(n) _____.
    a. autograft
    b. homograft (or allograft)
    c. heterograft (or xenograft)
23. When skin from another human is used in skin grafting it is called a(n) _____.
    a. autograft
    b. homograft (or allograft)
    c. heterograft (or xenograft)
24. If the material for a skin graft is obtained from an animal or is of a synthetic material it is called a(n) _____.
    a. autograft
    b. homograft (or allograft)
    c. heterograft (or xenograft)
25. Grafts which are *not* permanent are _____.
    a. autografts
    b. homografts and heterografts
26. Discharge planning for Hal should begin _____.
    a. approximately 1 week before discharge
    b. after the skin grafts have begun to take
    c. once Hal begins to get out of bed
    d. as soon as the acute phase is over

III. Fill-in and discussion questions.

Read each question carefully and place your answer in the space provided.

1. With very little to occupy their minds except the hospital routine, their treatments and their personal welfare, nurse-patient relationships and communication are essential components of the care plan for burn patients. How might a nurse make an effort to provide mental stimulation and contact with the outside world to the patient who is in relative isolation because of an infection of his burns? _____

2. List 5 complications that might be seen in a severely burned patient.

   1. _____
   2. _____
   3. _____
   4. _____
   5. _____

CHAPTER—52

The patient with neurological disease

Injuries to the brain and skull and tumors of the brain are serious events requiring nursing management by a skilled and competent nursing staff. Because changes are often subtle, patients with these neurological disorders require close observation and documentation of any change in their condition or symptoms.

The following questions deal with the contents of Chapter 52.

I. True or false.

Read each statement carefully and place your answer in the space provided.

_____ 1. Coughing increases intracranial pressure.
_____ 2. Papilledema may be seen in increased intracranial pressure.
_____ 3. Treatment of increased intracranial pressure is always surgical.
_____ 4. A cerebral concussion is more serious than a cerebral laceration or contusion.
_____ 5. The bleeding of an epidural hematoma occurs slowly; therefore, it is often many days before symptoms are apparent.
_____ 6. Bleeding is more rapid in an epidural hematoma than a subdural hematoma.
_____ 7. Symptoms of a subdural hematoma may occur immediately or may not be evident for several days.
_____ 8. Many skull fractures heal without causing problems.
_____ 9. Patients admitted to the hospital with traumatic brain pathology often have multiple injuries.
_____ 10. Opiates and sedatives are avoided in patients with neurological disorders because these drugs mask changes in the level of consciousness.
_____ 11. Since benign tumors are easily removed and do not metastasize, only malignant brain tumors are serious.
_____ 12. A meningioma is a tumor of the meninges.
_____ 13. The symptoms of a brain tumor are often characteristic of the location of the tumor.
_____ 14. Given sufficient time, brain tissue will regenerate.
_____ 15. The presence of cerebral edema may prompt the physician to limit or restrict fluids.

II. Multiple choice questions.

Select the most appropriate answer and place it in the space provided.

1. A concussion results from ____.
   a. bleeding within cerebral tissue
   b. a violent jarring of the brain
   c. edema of the brain, either due to injury or disease

2. An epidural hematoma is usually caused by ____.
   a. arterial bleeding between the dura mater and pia mater
   b. venous bleeding between the pia mater and arachnoid membrane
   c. arterial bleeding on top of the dura
   d. intracerebral hemorrhaging

3. One of the first signs of increasing intracranial pressure due to arterial bleeding is ____.
   a. a sudden increase followed by a slow drop in the pulse rate
   b. nausea and projectile vomiting
   c. Cheyne-Stokes respirations
   d. drowsiness rapidly progressing to coma

4. Subdural hematoma is usually caused by ____.
   a. arterial bleeding on top of the dura
   b. arterial bleeding below the arachnoid membrane and dura mater
   c. venous bleeding between the dura mater and arachnoid membrane

5. In a depressed skull fracture the bone fragments are ____.
   a. pushed outward
   b. pushed into cerebral tissue
   c. kept out of cerebral tissue by the tough dura mater

6. A sign of bleeding into the meninges is ____.
   a. double vision
   b. nuchal rigidity
   c. bleeding from the nose or ear
   d. dyspnea

7. Bleeding from the ears most often occurs when the patient has a ____.
   a. basal skull fracture
   b. meningeal bleeding
   c. depressed skull fracture of the frontal-temporal lobe

8. One of the essentials in the management of a patient with a head injury is to keep him ____.
   a. comfortable
   b. pain free
   c. quiet
   d. symptom free

9. The physician requests an evaluation of a patient's level of consciousness q ½ h. It is now midnight and the patient is asleep. Should he be aroused to check his level of consciousness? ____
   a. yes
   b. no

10. Your answer to the last question is based on ____.
    a. the fact that nurses always follow the directions of the physician without questioning the rationale
    b. there could be a change in the patient's neurological status while he is asleep which would go undetected if he were not wakened every ½ hour
    c. the patient needs his rest as rest is important in the healing process
    d. an observation every ½ hour is to be performed only while the patient is awake

11. When an inoperable tumor obstructs the flow of cerebrospinal fluid, the fluid may be shunted out of the cranial cavity by ____.
    a. a permanent opening or "window" between a ventricle and the outside
    b. a polyethylene tube between the left and right ventricles
    c. a polyethylene tube inserted into the lateral ventricle and draining into another structure such as a large vein

Clinical Situations

Mrs. Brook, age 60, is admitted to the acute medical service with a diagnosis of a possible expanding lesion of the brain and signs of increased intracranial pressure.

12. If Mrs. Brook continues to show signs of increased intracranial pressure it would be expected that her blood pressure will ____.
    a. increase
    b. decrease
    c. remain the same

13. Vital signs are ordered every ½ hour. If Mrs. Brook continues to show signs of increased intracranial pressure her pulse rate will probably ____.
    a. rise and then decrease
    b. increase
    c. widely fluctuate

14. Which nursing measure may tend to reduce intracranial pressure? ____
    a. a back rub
    b. elevating the head of the bed
    c. application of an ice pack or cold cloth to the forehead
    d. application of a heating pad to the head and back of the neck

15. Mrs. Brook is conscious though lethargic. She can move all four extremities. Asking her to move her extremities is a check for paralysis as well as a check of her ____.
    a. desire to get well
    b. willingness to cooperate with nursing personnel
    c. personality
    d. ability to respond to and follow commands

16. Patients with signs of increased intracranial pressure are kept NPO (nothing by mouth) to decrease the risk of ____.
    a. vomiting or hiccoughing which would increase intracranial pressure
    b. electrolyte imbalance which will then make the treatment of this disorder more difficult
    c. congestive heart failure
    d. peripheral edema

17. Mrs. Brook is kept on complete bed rest. The nurse should ____.
    a. turn, cough and deep breathe her every 2 hours
    b. not encourage coughing
    c. encourage deep breathing and coughing only

18. Patients with increased intracranial pressure have the head of the bed ____.
    a. elevated
    b. kept flat at all times
    c. kept lower than the foot of the bed

19. Since Mrs. Brook may develop seizures the physician orders a(n) ____.
    a. tranquilizer such as Librium
    b. analgesic such as Tylenol
    c. anticonvulsant such as Dilantin

Mr. Kelly, age 50, is admitted to the hospital with the diagnosis of a possible brain tumor. After a series of tests and x-rays a tumor of his right temporal lobe is identified. Surgery for removal of the tumor has been scheduled.

20. Symptoms of a brain tumor usually include ____.
    1. signs of increased intracranial pressure
    2. headache
    3. vomiting
    4. papilledema
    a. 1, 2
    b. 1, 3
    c. 2, 4
    d. all of these

21. On occasion the bone flap is not replaced after surgery for a brain tumor. This is done to ____.
    a. allow the brain room to expand when the tumor could not be totally removed
    b. make it easier to repeat the surgery should it be necessary to remove future tumor growths
    c. prevent future tumor growth
    d. allow for close observation of cerebral tissue during the postoperative period

22. Mr. Kelly's bone flap was not replaced. Two days after surgery a bulging of the scalp over the operative area is noted. This is ____.
    a. normal postoperative fluid collection under the incision
    b. probably a sign of increased intracranial pressure
    c. due to the muscle sutured over the opening and is of no real concern

23. The physician requests observation of Mr. Kelly's motor function. If there is a disturbance of this function it might indicate an injury to the ____.
    a. brain stem
    b. ventricles
    c. frontal lobe
    d. pyramidal tracts

24. On return from surgery there is an order to keep the head of Mr. Kelly's bed elevated to ____.
    a. prevent cerebral edema
    b. more easily change his surgical dressing
    c. help him recover from anesthesia more quickly

25. You note that Mr. Kelly does not blink and that his eyes are open most of the time. If left untreated, Mr. Kelly could develop ____.
    a. double vision
    b. scleral ulcerations resulting in blindness
    c. drying of the cornea and corneal ulcers
    d. conjunctivitis

26. Rehabilitation of Mr. Kelly should begin ____.
    a. approximately a week before discharge
    b. as soon as Mr. Kelly appears alert, responsive, and interested in his surroundings
    c. when Mr. Kelly's family are ready to accept his diagnosis
    d. as soon as he returns from the operating room

III. Fill-in and discussion questions.

Read each question carefully and place your answer in the space provided.

1. Fill in the blanks of the following questions with the correct word or words that will complete the statement.

1. Cerebrospinal fluid is produced in the _____ and absorbed in the _____.

2. Edema of the optic nerve at the point at which it enters the eyeball is called _____.

3. The area between the dura mater and the skull is called the _____ space.

4. The area between the dura mater and the arachnoid membrane is called the _____ space.

5. A surgical incision through the skull is called a(n) _____.

2. Below are the areas or measurements that may show changes when the patient has increased intracranial pressure. To the right of each, describe the change that will have occurred.

   a. Pulse rate

   b. Blood pressure

   c. Respirations

   d. Pupils

   e. Level of consciousness

APPENDIX:

CHAPTER 1

I. True or false

1. true (p. 1)
2. true (p. 2)
3. false (p. 3)
4. true (p. 5)
5. false (p. 5)
6. false (p. 6)
7. true (p. 7)
8. false (p. 7)
9. true (p. 11)
10. true (p. 11)

II. Multiple choice

1. c (p. 2)
2. a (p. 3)
3. d (p. 4)
4. a (p. 4)
5. b (p. 8)
6. b (p. 12)
7. c (p. 17)
8. a (p. 4)
9. b (p. 7)
10. c (p. 8)

III. Fill-in and discussion

1. Answers may vary but may include encourage self-confidence, convey the belief to the patient that he can learn; find out about the patient's past experience and relate new ideas to it; proceed slowly and allow extra time for the patient to think about and respond to new ideas (p. 15).
2. Answers may vary according to the specific individual(s) considered. Guidelines will be found in the text: teeth (pp. 12-13); height and weight (p. 7); speed of reaction (pp. 4, 12); vision (pp. 4, 7, 12); hair (p. 12); hearing (pp. 4, 8); physical growth (pp. 4, 6, 12); eating habits (pp. 19-20).
3. Answers may vary but may include personal feelings of guilt; reluctance to acknowledge declining abilities of the parent (pp. 8-9).
4. Answers will vary but may include loss of employment; financial problems; inability to care for himself as he used to (pp. 9-10).
5. Emotional, social and economic factors; feelings of guilt; other answers are acceptable (p. 10).
6. Check the patient frequently during the night; attempt to discover the cause of the confusion and eliminate it; reality orientation; other answers may be acceptable (pp. 18-19).

CHAPTER 2

I. True or false

1. true (p. 22)
2. false (p. 23)
3. true (p. 23)
4. true (p. 23)
5. true (p. 23)
6. false (p. 25)
7. true (p. 25)
8. false (p. 26)
9. false (p. 30)
10. true (p. 30)
11. false (p. 31)

II. Multiple choice

1. b (p. 23)
2. a (p. 23)
3. a (p. 23)
4. d (p. 24)
5. c. (p. 24)
6. b (p. 24)
7. d (p. 24)
8. a (p. 25)
9. b (p. 30)
10. b (p. 31)

III. Fill-in and discussion

1. The answer to this question will vary, according to the feelings of the student (see also p. 25).
2. Concentrate on what the patient is going through; establish physical contact and eye contact; have equipment handy, neat and in good condition; be alert to both the patient's physiological and emotional reactions; other answers may also be acceptable (pp. 25-26).

CHAPTER 3

I. True or false

1. true (p. 36)
2. false (pp. 36-37)
3. true (p. 38)
4. false (p. 39)
5. false (p. 39)
6. true (p. 39)
7. false (p. 40)
8. true (p. 40)
9. true (p. 40)
10. false (p. 40)
11. true (p. 41)
12. false (p. 41)
13. false (p. 44)
14. false (p. 45)
15. true (p. 48)
16. false (pp. 49-50)
17. false (p. 51)
18. false (p. 51)
19. true (p. 51)
20. true (p. 52)

II. Multiple choice

1. d (p. 36)
2. a (pp. 37-38)
3. c (p. 38)
4. c (p. 38)
5. a (p. 38)
6. b (p. 39)
7. c (p. 39)
8. d (pp. 39-40)
9. d (p. 41)
10. c (p. 41)
11. b (pp. 42-43)
12. a (p. 44)
13. d (p. 44)
14. c (p. 45)
15. a (p. 47)
16. c (p. 47)
17. b (p. 48)
18. d (p. 49)
19. c (p. 52)
20. a (p. 52)

III. Fill-in and discussion

1. Vomitus, urine, diarrhea, perspiration, blood, wound drainage, secretions from the GI tract (p. 42).
2. Chills, fever, dyspnea, cyanosis, sudden sharp pain in the lumbar region (p. 44).
3. (1) **Skin:** protects the body from invading organisms.
   (2) **Rib cage:** protects the thoracic organs from injury.
   (3) **Skull:** protects the brain.
   (4) **Autonomic nervous system:** provides the ability for the body to adjust to its environment and prepares the body for emergency (p. 45).
4. Swelling, pain, redness, heat (p. 46).
5. (1) **Actively acquired immunity:** immunity to a specific disease because of a previous infection by the same microorganism.
   (2) **Artificially acquired immunity:** created when an antigen that has been killed or attenuated is injected into the body.
   (3) **Passive immunity:** achieved through the use of antibodies produced by another person (pp. 50-51).
6. Withhold the drug, contact the physician, chart the incident (p. 51).
7. (1) **Skin:** is pale, diaphoretic.
   (2) **Blood pressure:** falls sharply.
   (3) **Pulse:** weak, rapid—may not be perceptible.
   (4) **Conscious state:** consciousness is lost (p. 53).

CHAPTER 4

I. True or false

1. false (p. 55)
2. true (p. 56)
3. true (p. 56)
4. true (p. 56)
5. false (p. 57)
6. false (p. 58)
7. true (p. 58)
8. true (p. 58)

II. Multiple choice

1. a (p. 57)
2. d (p. 57)
3. a (p. 58)
4. c (p. 59)

III. Fill-in and discussion

1. (1) **Lights:** keep dim, room should be softly lighted.
   (2) **Noise:** keep to minimum.
   (3) **Tone of voice:** speak quietly and slowly.
   (4) **Explanations:** brief, simple, specific and repetitive (p. 58).
2. (1) The prefix "psycho" may imply mental illness with the patient having no physical illness.
   (2) The illness is imaginary.
   (3) The patient may be a malingerer (pp. 56-57).

CHAPTER 5

I. True or false

1. true (p. 60)
2. true (p. 61)
3. false (p. 61)
4. true (p. 62)
5. false (pp. 61-62)

II. Multiple choice

1. d (p. 61)
2. a (p. 62)
3. b (p. 63)
4. b (p. 63)
5. a (p. 63)

III. Fill-in and discussion
1. Sharp, dull, knifelike, throbbing, steady, severe, deep, superficial, mild, bearable, unbearable, burning (other descriptions also acceptable) (p. 61).
2. (1) Administer analgesics promptly.
   (2) Create a position of comfort.
   (3) Provide distraction or diversion.
   (4) Reduce or eliminate noise and disturbance.
   (5) Be gentle in giving care.

Additional measures for the relief of pain are listed in Table 5-2 of the text (p. 62).

CHAPTER 6

I. True or false

1. true (p. 66)	5. false (p. 67)	9. true (p. 71)	13. false (p. 71)	17. false (p. 72)
2. false (p. 66)	6. false (p. 67)	10. true (p. 71)	14. false (pp. 71-72)	18. true (p. 73)
3. true (p. 67)	7. true (p. 68)	11. false (p. 71)	15. false (p. 72)	19. true (p. 73)
4. true (p. 66)	8. false (p. 70)	12. true (p. 71)	16. true (p. 72)	

II. Multiple choice

1. b (p. 66)	4. b (p. 69)	7. a (p. 70)	10. d (p. 72)
2. a (p. 66)	5. c (p. 69)	8. b (p. 71)	11. b (p. 73)
3. d (pp. 67-68)	6. c (p. 70)	9. a (p. 72)	

III. Fill-in and discussion
1. Hangovers increase in intensity, nausea, vomiting, misses work frequently, periods of blackouts, sneaks drinks, does not admit to having a drinking problem. Other answers may also be acceptable (p. 68).
2. Loss of income, tension between alcoholic and spouse, separation or divorce, strained relationships with children, social stigma (p. 69).
3. A form of escape, a substitute for affection, a search for meaning or values, a way of life, a way of relieving loneliness, a way of belonging to a group, peer pressure, curiosity. Other answers may also be acceptable (pp. 70-71).
4. Nausea, vomiting, diarrhea, apprehension, restlessness, repeated yawning, alternating feelings of hot and cold, pilomotor response ("goose flesh"), elevated temperature, pulse and respirations, anorexia, headache, muscle twitching, severe abdominal cramps, possibly coma and physical collapse (p. 72).
5. Cancer of the lung, chronic cough, emphysema, chronic bronchitis, cancer of the oral cavity (pp. 73-74).
6. Weight gain, constipation, irritability, hunger, slowing of the pulse (p. 74).

CHAPTER 7

I. True or false

1. false (pp. 76-77)	3. false (p. 77)	5. true (p. 77)	7. true (p. 78)
2. false (p. 77)	4. true (p. 77)	6. false (p. 77)	8. true (p. 78)

II. Multiple choice

1. a (pp. 76-77) 2. c (p. 77) 3. b (p. 77) 4. d (pp. 78-79)

III. Fill-in and discussion
1. Answers will vary. Sample answers include the following:
   (1) **Denial:** patient may believe that the biopsy report is in error.
   (2) **Anger:** patient may become angry with nurses and will refuse to believe that this is happening to her.
   (3) **Bargaining:** made in secret—patient may promise to do something if she gets better such as being a better wife and mother.
   (4) **Depression:** patient mourns the fact that the breast is removed and not believe she is a whole woman.
   (5) **Acceptance:** patient is detached, quiet, speaks little (p. 77).
2. Try to find a place for the family to have some privacy; make family physically comfortable—provide chairs, etc.; make frequent contacts with the family if they show they wish this contact; show concern for the family's welfare and comfort; listen to the family member's concerns regarding the patient; listen to problems if they are expressed openly (p. 79).

CHAPTER 8

I. True or false

1. false (p. 81)
2. false (p. 81)
3. true (p. 82)
4. true (p. 82)
5. false (p. 82)
6. true (p. 83)
7. false (p. 83)
8. false (p. 83)
9. false (pp. 84-85)
10. true (p. 84)
11. true (p. 85)
12. true (p. 85)
13. false (p. 86)
14. true (p. 87)

II. Multiple choice

1. a (p. 83)
2. d (p. 83)
3. d (p. 84)
4. b (pp. 84-85)
5. b (p. 85)
6. c (p. 85)
7. d (p. 85)
8. a (p. 86)

III. Fill-in and discussion

1. Severe hemorrhage, acute respiratory difficulty, shock, severe chest pain, multiple injuries, high fever, coma. Other answers may also be acceptable (p. 87).
2. (1) **Hemorrhage:** look for bleeding and stop it quickly, apply direct and continuous pressure on the wound, elevate the extremity involved, apply a tourniquet if unable to stop bleeding by pressure and elevation (p. 82).
   (2) **Shock:** place or keep the patient flat with feet elevated 8 to 12 inches, keep warm, give nothing by mouth (p. 83).
   (3) **Wounds—small:** leave uncovered until examined by a physician (p. 83).
   (4) **Snakebite:** keep patient quiet, immobilize affected part, apply tourniquet above and below the area of the bite, apply cold if available (p. 83).
   (5) **Drug/chemical poisoning:** give syrup of ipecac according to the directions on the container (pp. 84-85).
   (6) **Heatstroke:** cool body with wet, cold towels; apply towels to entire body; move the patient to an area out of the sunlight (p. 85).
   (7) **Frostbite:** immerse affected part in (comfortable) warm water for 10 minutes, blot skin dry, apply sterile dressing using sterile gauze to separate skin surfaces, elevate affected area (pp. 85-86).
   (8) **Fainting:** prevent patient from falling, place the patient flat, loosen tight clothing from around the neck and waist (p. 86).
   (9) **Bite by tick:** kill tick with a few drops of turpentine or a hot needle, then carefully remove with a tweezers, scrub the area around the bite with soap and water (p. 86).
   (10) **Sting by hornet, wasp, bee:** remove stinger with a sterile needle or tweezers, apply ice or a paste made of baking soda (p. 86).

CHAPTER 9

I. True or false

1. true (p. 90)
2. false (p. 90)
3. true (p. 91)
4. true (p. 91)
5. true (p. 91)
6. false (p. 93)
7. false (p. 93)
8. true (p. 95)
9. true (p. 96)
10. false (p. 96)
11. true (p. 97)
12. false (p. 97)
13. true (p. 97)
14. true (p. 98)
15. false (p. 99)
16. false (p. 100)
17. false (p. 101)
18. true (p. 101)
19. true (p. 102)
20. true (p. 104)

II. Multiple choice

1. b (p. 90)
2. c (p. 90)
3. a (p. 92)
4. b (p. 96)
5. b (pp. 96-97)
6. a (p. 99)
7. d (p. 99)
8. d (p. 100)
9. b (p. 100)
10. d (p. 101)
11. c (p. 102)
12. d (p. 103)

III. Fill-in and discussion

1. VOCABULARY (See Glossary or medical dictionary.)
   a. **Atelectasis:** a collapse of the lung which may involve a small or large area
   b. **Dehiscence:** a separation of all layers of a wound or surgical incision
   c. **Embolus:** a solid, liquid or gaseous mass carried in the bloodstream or lymphatic vessel
   d. **Evisceration:** separation of wound edges with protrusion of internal organs
   e. **Flatus:** gas
   f. **Hypostatic pneumonia:** pneumonia resulting from lying in one position for a prolonged period of time
   g. **Hypoxia:** lack of an adequate amount of oxygen
   h. **Phlebothrombosis:** a clot in the vein
   i. **Thrombophlebitis:** inflammation of a vein
2. (1) **Having the patient void before surgery:** prevent injury to the bladder during abdominal surgery (p. 93).

(2) **Remove plastic or metal objects from the hair:** these objects could cause injury if the patient were restless during or immediately after surgery (p. 93).
(3) **Removal of makeup and nail polish:** color of face, lips, and nailbeds are observed during surgery by the anesthetist for changes in color (p. 94).
3. (1) Wait one hour after the administration of a narcotic before getting her out of bed (p. 97).
(2) Change of position, use of a small pillow to support the back and shoulders, massaging areas subject to pressure (p. 97).
(3) Change her position frequently; have her cough, turn and deep breath frequently; suction mucus from her nose and mouth while she is unconscious (p. 103).
4. Ambulate, take to the bathroom, offer warm or hot liquids (p. 94).
5. Offer a mouth rinse, place a cool wet cloth or ice chips on his lips (p. 98).
6. Use a pillow or (the nurse's) hand to support the incision, give a narcotic approximately 45 to 60 minutes before deep-breathing and coughing exercises (p. 98).

CHAPTER 10

I. True or false

1. true (p. 109)   3. false (p. 113)   5. false (p. 114)   7. false (p. 114)   9. false (p. 115)
2. true (p. 111)   4. true (p. 113)   6. false (p. 111)   8. true (p. 116)   10. true (p. 116)

II. Multiple choice

1. d (p. 109)   4. b (p. 114)   6. a (p. 114)   8. d (p. 114)   10. a (p. 115)
2. a (p. 111)   5. b (p. 114)   7. c (p. 114)   9. d (p. 114)   11. b (p. 115)
3. c (p. 113)

III. Fill-in and discussion

1. VOCABULARY. Definitions may vary slightly according to the reference consulted. (See Glossary or medical dictionary.)
   a. **Alopecia:** baldness, loss of hair
   b. **Antineoplastic:** inhibiting the growth and reproduction of malignant cells
   c. **Chemotherapy:** treatment by the use of chemicals (drugs)
   d. **Isotope:** an element having the same atomic number as another but a different atomic mass, thereby giving it a different number of neutrons. Many isotopes are radioactive, as example ^{131}I (isotope of iodine)
   e. **Leukemia:** in lay terms—"cancer of the blood." A malignant disease of the bone marrow, spleen and lymph nodes characterized by a rapid and abnormal manufacture of lymphocytes.
   f. **Leukopenia:** a decrease in the number of white blood cells, more specifically leukocytes
   g. **Leukoplakia:** thick, white patches on the lips, gums, tongue and inner cheek. Leukoplakia have a tendency to become malignant
   h. **Metastasis:** spread of a disease from one part or organ to another. Adjective: metastatic
   i. **Radioactivity:** the emission of radiation due to disintegration of a radioactive element. The emissions include alpha particles, beta particles, gamma rays.
   j. **Stoma:** an opening
   k. **Stomatitis:** inflammation of the mucous membrane of the mouth
2. Malignant tumors grow more rapidly, are rarely encapsulated and are more likely to recur after removal. Other answers are acceptable (p. 109, Table 10-2).
3. Smoking, excessive exposure to sunlight, exposure to certain chemicals, leukoplakia, environmental factors, social factors, exposure to x-ray and radioactive elements. Other answers may also be acceptable (pp. 110, 116).
4. A sore that does not heal, a lump or thickening in the breast or elsewhere, unusual bleeding or discharge, any change in a wart or mole, persistent indigestion or difficulty in swallowing, persistent hoarseness or cough, any change in normal bowel habits (p. 110).
5. X-rays, biopsy of tumor and/or lymph nodes, blood samples, bone marrow samples, urine samples, smears, bronchial washings (p. 111).
6. Surgery, radiation, chemotherapy (p. 111).
7. Answer will depend on respondents' feelings regarding the subject.

CHAPTER 11

I. True or false

1. true (p. 118)   3. false (p. 119)   5. false (p. 121)   7. true (p. 122)   9. false (p. 123, Table 11-2)
2. true (p. 119)   4. true (p. 120)   6. true (p. 121)   8. false (p. 122)   10. true (p. 123)

II. Multiple choice

1. c (p. 119)
2. a (p. 118)
3. b (p. 120)
4. d (p. 121)
5. a (p. 120, Table 11-1)
6. c (p. 123)
7. b (p. 121)

III. Fill-in and discussion

1. VOCABULARY. Definitions may vary slightly according to reference consulted. (See Glossary or medical dictionary.)
   a. **Antiemetic:** a drug used in the treatment of nausea and vomiting
   b. **Radioisotope:** a radioactive form of an element
   c. **Radiologist:** a specialist in radiology—the branch of medicine concerned with the use of x-rays
   d. **Radiotherapy:** the therapeutic application of ionizing radiation from x-ray machines or radioactive materials
2. Pick up the applicator with long-handled tongs and quickly place it in the shielded lead container kept in the room. This action is followed by a call to the radiologist or radiation safety officer (p. 123, Table 11-2).
3. Keep skin dry, clean; protect skin against extremes of heat and cold; do *not* apply unprescribed ointments and creams; do *not* remove the skin markings; wear loose clothing to avoid irritation; use corn starch powder over radiated areas where two skin surfaces are in contact (p. 121).
4. (1) **TIME:** the length of exposure. The less time spent in the vicinity of radioactive substances the less radiation received.
   (2) **DISTANCE:** the distance from the radioactive source. The farther away from the source of radiation, the less amount of radiation reaching an individual.
   (3) **SHIELDING:** the placement of a shielding material such as lead between the radiation source and an individual to lessen the amount of radiation reaching that individual (pp. 121-122).
5. (1) **TIME:** spend as little time in the room as possible — work quickly — avoid unnecessary steps.
   (2) **DISTANCE:** stand in doorway to communicate—only approach the bed to give nursing care.
   (3) **SHIELDING:** if longer exposures are necessary, contact the radiation safety officer about advisability of wearing a lead apron—use room wall as a shield (p. 123, Table 11-2).

CHAPTER 12

I. True or false

1. true (p. 127)
2. true (p. 128)
3. false (p. 128)
4. true (p. 128)
5. false (p. 129)
6. false (p. 130)
7. true (p. 131)
8. true (p. 132)
9. true (p. 132)
10. true (p. 133)
11. false (p. 134)
12. false (pp. 134, 138)
13. false (p. 137)
14. true (p. 137, Fig. 12-6)
15. true (p. 137)
16. true (p. 137)
17. false (p. 139)
18. true (p. 139)
19. false (p. 140)
20. true (p. 142)
21. true (p. 145)

II. Multiple choice

1. a (p. 128)
2. c (p. 128)
3. c (p. 129)
4. b (p. 129)
5. b (p. 137)
6. a (p. 137)
7. b (p. 137, Fig. 12-7)
8. b (p. 139)
9. c (p. 143)
10. d (p. 143)
11. d (p. 131)
12. d (p. 133)
13. a (p. 134)
14. a (p. 136)
15. b (p. 131)
16. d (p. 136)
17. d (p. 132)
18. c (p. 136)
19. d (p. 137)
20. c (p. 137)
21. a (p. 138)
22. c (p. 138, Table 12-3)
23. a (p. 138, Table 12-3)
24. d (p. 140)
25. c (p. 140)
26. a (p. 141)
27. a (p. 142)
28. b (p. 142)
29. b (p. 142)
30. c (p. 142)
31. b (p. 142)

III. Fill-in and discussion

1. VOCABULARY. Definitions may vary slightly according to reference consulted. (See Glossary or medical dictionary.)
   a. **Abduction:** to move or draw from a center or midline
   b. **Adduction:** to move toward the center or midline
   c. **Acetabulum:** the cup-shaped cavity of the innominate bone which receives the femur
   d. **Axilla (plural axillae):** the armpit
   e. **Blanching:** to become pale
   f. **Brachial plexus:** a network of nerves supplying the arm, forearm, and hand
   g. **Clavicle:** the collarbone

h. **Closed reduction:** manipulation of a fracture with a return to normal position followed by immobilization with a bandage, cast, traction, or internal fixation
i. **Dislocation:** displacement of a bone from its normal position in a joint, with the articular surfaces no longer in contact
j. **Ecchymotic:** adjective for ecchymosis—the escape of blood into the tissues causing a blue-black discoloration which later changes to green/brown or yellow
k. **Femur:** the large bone in the thigh
l. **Mandible:** the lower jaw bone
m. **Necrosis:** death of a cell or group of cells
n. **Open reduction:** surgical alignment of a fracture under direct vision
o. **Osteomyelitis:** inflammation of the bone usually caused by a pathogenic organism
p. **Sprain:** injury to the ligament(s) surrounding a joint
2. Slippery bathtubs, scatter rugs, highly polished floors, dark stairways, toys or objects on stairs. Other answers also acceptable (p. 128).
3. Pain, loss of function, deformity, edema, spasm, false motion (pp. 128-129).
4. Padded wood splints, inflatable plastic splints, metal splints (p. 130).
5. Handle cast carefully using palm of hand rather than fingertips; leave cast uncovered; elevate cast on pillow; cast dryer may be ordered (pp. 131-132).
6. Check all edges for smoothness once cast is dry; check extremities for any change in color or skin temperature; look for drainage: note color and amount; check cast for unusual odors; investigate any complaint the patient may have; check pulse in extremity and report any absence immediately; check for movement or lack of movement and report any lack of movement immediately (p. 133, Table 12-1).
7. Question the patient about his pain then call his physician. Pain is expected for a few days, but its presence 8 days after the application of a cast should arouse suspicion (p. 134).
8. Circle the area with a pencil, ballpoint pen, fiber-tipped pen (p. 134).
9. The object could injure the skin underneath the cast and cause an infection. The object could also be lost in the cast and cause further irritation (p. 134).
10. Go to bed for 24 hours; keep arm elevated on a pillow; when out of bed use a sling to support arm; move fingers for several minutes every ½ hour; if cast becomes tight, or numbness, swelling, or a change of color occurs return to the hospital immediately (p. 135, Table 12-2).
11. Blanching of the skin; reddened areas; pain or discomfort over pressure points (p. 135, Table 12-3).
12. Foam rubber supports, alternating pressure mattress, flotation pads, sheepskin pads. Other answers also acceptable (p. 138, Table 12-3).
13. Blanching or discoloration of extremity; skin feels cool; peripheral pulses absent (p. 138, Table 12-3).
14. Compress mattress with one hand and slip the other under the patient's back. Apply a small amount of lotion and massage a small area at a time (p. 139).
15. Bony prominences, elbows, sacrum, heels are usual sites (p. 138, Table 12-3).
16. Column B answers in correct order: 6, 3, 1, 7, 2, 5, 4 (p. 128).

CHAPTER 13

I. True or false

1. true (p. 148)
2. true (p. 149)
3. false (p. 150)
4. true (p. 150)
5. true (p. 150)
6. false (p. 150)
7. true (p. 154)
8. true (p. 154)
9. true (p. 152)
10. false (p. 154)
11. false (p. 155)
12. false (p. 155)
13. true (p. 157)
14. true (p. 157)
15. true (p. 158)

II. Multiple choice

1. d (p. 149)
2. b (p. 150)
3. a (p. 151)
4. b (p. 152)
5. b (p. 153, Table 13-1)
6. a (p. 153, Table 13-1)
7. c (p. 153, Table 13-1)
8. d (p. 153, Table 13-1)
9. c (p. 150)
10. b (p. 150)
11. a (p. 151)
12. d (p. 155)
13. d (p. 155)
14. b (p. 155)
15. a (p. 155)
16. c (p. 155)
17. b (p. 156)
18. d (p. 156)
19. c (p. 157)
20. b (p. 157)

III. Fill-in and discussion

1. VOCABULARY. Definitions may vary slightly according to reference consulted. (See Glossary or medical dictionary.)
   a. **Arthritis:** inflammation of a joint
   b. **Arthroplasty:** fashioning of a new joint with artificial materials
   c. **Fibrous ankylosis:** abnormal immobility of a joint
   d. **Hyperuricemia:** an accumulation of uric acid in the blood
   e. **Osseous ankylosis:** bony union of a joint
   f. **Ossify:** to turn to bone
   g. **Osteotomy:** an artificial angling of the bone through a surgical fracture
   h. **Salicylism:** toxic condition caused by overdose of salicylates

i. **Synovectomy:** removal of the diseased lining of a joint
   j. **Synovitis:** inflammation of the synovial membrane surrounding a joint
   k. **Tinnitus:** a noise in the ears, usually described as ringing, roaring or buzzing sound
   l. **Tophi (plural of tophus):** a deposit of urates (crystals) in the tissues around joints. May also be found on the pinna of the ear.
2. High fever, chills, rapid pulse, tenderness and/or pain over the affected area, swelling, redness (p. 158).
3. Sandbags, trochanter rolls, footboard, sheepskin pads, alternating pressure mattress, splints, pillows (p. 158, Table 13-2).
4. Headache, nausea, vomiting, tinnitus, increased pulse, increased respiratory rate, drowsiness, mental confusion (p. 159).
5. Elevated temperature, calf tenderness, pain, warmth or redness in the extremity (p. 154).
6. Answers will vary.

CHAPTER 14

I. True or false

1. true (p. 162, Fig. 14-1)
2. true (p. 163)
3. false (p. 165)
4. true (pp. 164, Fig. 14-2; 166, Table 14-1; 168)
5. true (p. 167)
6. true (p. 167)
7. false (p. 167)
8. true (p. 167)
9. false (p. 168)
10. false (p. 169)
11. true (p. 170)
12. false (p. 170)

II. Multiple choice

1. b (p. 166, Table 14-1)
2. b (p. 166, Table 14-1)
3. d (p. 166, Table 14-1)
4. c (p. 166, Table 14-1)
5. c (p. 164)
6. b (pp. 167-168)
7. a (p. 166, Table 14-1)
8. b (p. 166, Table 14-1)
9. b (p. 164)
10. d (p. 168)
11. d (p. 170)
12. b (p. 169)

III. Fill-in and discussion

1. Answers may vary but may include the following: employment concerns, invalidism, loss of locomotion, change in a way of living, limitation of certain activities, others expressing pity and so on (p. 162).
2. Accidental extensive violence to extremity; death of tissues due to vascular insufficiency; malignant tumors; thermal injuries; a useless limb that is objectionable to the patient; congenital abnormality; conditions which may endanger the life of the patient (p. 162).
3. a. Yes
   b. It varies, perhaps months to decades
   c. Yes (pp. 164-165)
4. a. Lay a drainage pad lightly over the top of the stump to prevent soiling of top covers. Secure the top sheet around the unoperated side.
   b. It can be upsetting and cause unnecessary worry to the patient and his visitors (p. 167).
5. Inspect stump twice a day for irritation, skin breakdown, redness; wash stump twice a day; wash stump sock daily; discard stump socks when they tear or stretch; do not mend or darn stump socks (p. 170).

CHAPTER 15

I. True or false

1. false (p. 175)
2. true (p. 175)
3. true (p. 175)
4. false (p. 177)
5. false (p. 177)
6. false (p. 179)
7. true (p. 180)
8. true (p. 179)
9. false (p. 183)
10. true (p. 183)
11. true (p. 184)
12. true (p. 185)
13. false (p. 185)
14. false (p. 186)
15. true (p. 187)
16. true (p. 188)
17. true (p. 188)
18. false (p. 191)

II. Multiple choice

1. b (p. 179)
2. a (p. 179)
3. d (p. 184)
4. b (pp. 187-188)
5. d (p. 188)
6. c (p. 188)
7. a (p. 182)
8. b (pp. 181-182)
9. c (p. 183)
10. c (p. 181)
11. a (p. 175)
12. c (p. 176)
13. b (pp. 179-180)
14. d (p. 182)
15. a (p. 184)
16. b (p. 174)
17. d (p. 176)
18. a (p. 177)
19. c (p. 177, Table 15-3)
20. b (pp. 186-187)
21. b (p. 186)
22. a (p. 187)
23. b (pp. 184-185)
24. a (p. 185)
25. d (p. 185)
26. b (p. 185)
27. c (p. 185)
28. a (p. 193)
29. d (p. 193)
30. a (p. 189)
31. d (p. 190)
32. c (p. 190)
33. d (p. 192)
34. b (pp. 192-193)

III. Fill-in and discussion
1. VOCABULARY. Definitions may vary slightly according to reference consulted. (See Glossary or medical dictionary.)
    a. **Brachial plexus:** a group of nerves in the lower part of the neck and axilla supplying the arm, forearm, and hand
    b. **Cerebrospinal fluid:** a fluid circulating around and protecting the brain
    c. **Cisternal puncture:** insertion of a spinal needle between the cervical vertebrae into the base of the brain. Purpose is to inject a drug or withdraw spinal fluid.
    d. **Clonic:** alternate contraction and relaxation of the muscles resulting in jerking movements and excessive thrashing of the arms
    e. **Diplopia:** double vision
    f. **Endentulous:** without teeth
    g. **Encephalopathy:** any dysfunction or disorder of the brain
    h. **Gingivitis:** inflammation of the gums
    i. **Hypostatic pneumonia:** pneumonia caused by a pooling of secretions in the lungs and occurring when the position remains unchanged for a long period of time
    j. **Idiopathic:** having an unknown cause
    k. **intrathecal (synonym—intraspinal):** within the spinal cord. Drugs given by this route are injected into the subarachnoid space by means of a spinal needle.
    l. **Meningitis:** inflammation of the meninges
    m. **Nuchal rigidity:** stiffness of the neck; considered a sign of irritation of the meninges
    n. **Nystagmus:** involuntary movement of the eyeball
    o. **Sequelae:** conditions following or resulting from a disease
    p. **Tonic:** a rigid muscular contraction
    q. **Vesicles:** blisterlike elevations
2. 1. *cerebellum;* 2. *cerebrum;* 3. *pituitary;* 4. *pons;* 5. *medulla* (p. 174, Fig. 15-1).
3. 1. *motor area;* 2. *cutaneous and muscular sensory area;* 3. *visual;* 4. *hearing;* 5. *speech* (p. 174, Fig. 15-1).
4. Flashlight, ophthalmoscope, tongue depressor, cotton-tipped applicators, tuning fork, stethoscope, sphygmomanometer, percussion hammer, tape measure, cotton balls, sterile needles (p. 174, Table 15-1).
5. Cerebral angiogram (arteriogram), ventriculogram, pneumoencephalogram, myelogram (p. 176).
6. Slight hyperextension of the head; keep the head of the bed slightly elevated (p. 180).
7. May cause contracture of the neck and shoulder muscles; can make breathing difficult (p. 181).
8. Dura mater—outermost layer and lines the skull; arachnoid—middle layer; pia mater—innermost layer and covers the brain (p. 183).
9. Wear clothing loose; avoid wool or rough materials next to the skin; avoid anything that might cause itching (p. 184).
10. Phase may last minutes to hours; patient experiences vague emotional changes such as depression, anxiety or nervousness (p. 187).
11. Aura may be sensory (odor or sound) or a sensation such as numbness or weakness. In those that experience an aura it is usually the same and may be related to the anatomical origin of the seizure (p. 187).
12. (1) Turn patient on his side; (2) remove oral secretions if possible by suction; (3) remove any objects that may obstruct breathing (pillow, etc.); (4) loosen restrictive clothing if possible; (5) protect from injury (p. 188, Table 15-6).
13. The importance of medication; the seriousness of stopping or omitting medications; the side effects of medications (may need physician approval for this); necessity of routine visits to physician's office or clinic; hazards of operating a motor vehicle or performing potentially dangerous tasks until under control with medication; wearing of a Medic-Alert or other identification tag (p. 189).
14. Answers may vary: employment may be difficult to obtain; may worry about having other attacks; may not want friends to know of his seizure disorder; may be ashamed of the disorder; may wonder what people will think, and so on (p. 189).

CHAPTER 16

I. True or false

1. true (p. 195)	5. true (p. 199)	9. true (p. 200)	13. false (p. 201)	16. false (p. 204)
2. true (p. 196)	6. false (p. 199)	10. false (p. 200)	14. false (p. 201)	17. true (p. 205)
3. true (p. 197)	7. false (p. 199)	11. true (p. 200)	15. false (p. 202, Table 16-2)	18. true (p. 205)
4. true (p. 199)	8. false (p. 200)	12. true (p. 201)		19. false (p. 207)

II. Multiple choice

1. c (p. 199)	5. b (p. 198)	9. d (p. 202, Table 16-3)	13. c (p. 202, Table 16-2)
2. a (p. 200)	6. a (p. 199)	10. c (p. 201)	14. c (p. 201)
3. c (p. 200)	7. a (p. 199)	11. a (p. 202, Table 16-2)	15. b (pp. 201-202)
4. d (p. 196)	8. c (p. 202, Table 16-3)	12. a (p. 202, Table 16-2)	

III. Fill-in and discussion

1. VOCABULARY. Definitions may vary slightly according to reference consulted. (See Glossary or medical dictionary.)
   a. **Aphasia:** the loss of the ability to use or understand spoken and written language
   b. **Ateriosclerosis:** a loss of elasticity of the artery and the thickening of the intima of the artery
   c. **Atherosclerosis:** fatty plaques (atheroma) gradually deposited on the intima of the artery causing the lumen to become narrowed and in some instances occluded
   d. **Hemianopsia:** seeing with only half of a normal visual field
   e. **Infarction:** an area or part of an organ or structure which undergoes death of tissue (necrosis) because of a cessation of blood supply
   f. **Intima:** innermost lining
   g. **Sequelae:** conditions following or resulting from a disease or disorder

2. Rupture of a cerebral aneurysm; hemorrhagic disorders; tumors of the brain (p. 198).
3. Change in level of consciousness; blood pressure elevated; symptoms of shock; severe headache; nausea; vomiting; difficulty in breathing; paralysis; speech disturbance; memory impairment; fatigue; weakness; numbness; tingling of extremity (pp. 198-199).
4. Rise in blood pressure; slowing of pulse; pulse is full and bounding; change in level of consciousness; headache; vomiting with or without nausea; change in pupil size and reaction to light; decrease in respiratory rate (p. 202, Table 16-2).
5. Repeat words used to identify objects; be patient in listening and wait for answers; do not treat patient like a child but as an adult; do not shout (problem is not with his hearing); praise success; involve the family; minimize distractions. Other answers may also be accepted (pp. 207-208).

CHAPTER 17

I. True or false

1. false (pp. 210-211; Fig. 17-1, p. 211)
2. false (p. 211)
3. true (p. 211)
4. true (p. 211)
5. false (p. 212)
6. true (p. 212)
7. true (p. 212)
8. false (p. 213)
9. true (p. 214)
10. false (pp. 213-214)
11. true (p. 214)
12. true (p. 216)
13. false (p. 216, Table 17-2)
14. true (p. 218)
15. false (p. 218)
16. false (p. 220)
17. false (p. 220)

II. Multiple choice

1. c (pp. 211, 216, Table 17-2)
2. a (pp. 211, 216, Table 17-2)
3. c (pp. 211-212)
4. d (pp. 219-220)
5. c (p. 179)
6. b (p. 212)
7. a (p. 212)
8. a (p. 212)
9. b (p. 212)
10. d (p. 213)
11. c (p. 213)
12. a (pp. 213, Table 17-1; 214)
13. c (p. 214)
14. d (p. 213, Table 17-1)
15. a (p. 216)
16. c (p. 211)
17. a (p. 216, Table 17-3)
18. c (p. 216, Table 17-3)
19. c (p. 216, Table 17-3)
20. d (p. 217)
21. b (p. 223)

III. Fill-in and discussion

1. VOCABULARY. Definitions may vary according to reference consulted. (See Glossary or medical dictionary.)
   a. **Flaccid paralysis:** paralysis with the muscles relaxed or flabby and lacking muscle tone
   b. **Hemiplegia:** paralysis of one side of the body
   c. **Laminectomy:** an excision of the posterior arch of a vertebra usually performed to relieve symptoms of a ruptured intervertebral disc or a removal of a tumor of the spinal cord
   d. **Nucleus pulposa:** spongy center of an intervertebral disc
   e. **Paraplegia:** paralysis of both lower extremities
   f. **Quadriplegia:** paralysis of all four extremities
   g. **Spastic paralysis:** paralysis with the muscles rigid

2. Bed is put in the flat position, patient's body is stiff and kept straight, arms are at the side, patient is rolled in one motion without bending the spine. A turning sheet may be used. Use pillows between the legs to keep them straight. Turn gently (p. 214).
3. Answers will vary.
4. Encourage patient to drink plenty of fluid; provide foods that produce bulk (vegetables, bran, fruit); help the patient to the bathroom at a time convenient to him; allow patient privacy and sufficient time in the bathroom; enemas and suppositories may be needed to establish regularity (pp. 220-221).

CHAPTER 18

I. True or false

1. true (p. 225)
2. false (p. 225)
3. false (p. 226)
4. true (p. 226)
5. false (p. 228)
6. true (p. 231)
7. false (p. 231)
8. true (p. 232)
9. false (p. 233)
10. true (p. 233)
11. true (p. 234)
12. false (p. 235)
13. true (p. 235)
14. false (p. 240)
15. true (p. 240)
16. false (p. 242)
17. true (p. 242)
18. false (p. 245)
19. false (p. 245)
20. false (p. 245)

II. Multiple choice

1. d (pp. 226-227)
2. a (p. 227)
3. d (p. 227)
4. b (p. 231)
5. a (p. 233)
6. b (p. 234)
7. d (pp. 234-235)
8. c (p. 239)
9. b (p. 239)
10. a (p. 242, Table 18-3)
11. a (pp. 239, Fig. 18-8; 242)
12. c (p. 243)
13. d (p. 243)
14. b (p. 243)
15. b (p. 244)
16. b (p. 245)
17. d (p. 245)
18. a (p. 232)
19. a (p. 232)
20. c (pp. 232-233)
21. d (p. 233)
22. d (p. 233)
23. b (p. 233)
24. a (p. 242)
25. b (p. 243)
26. b (p. 243)
27. d (p. 243)

III. Fill-in and discussion

1. VOCABULARY. Definitions may vary according to reference consulted. (See Glossary or medical dictionary.)
   a. **Accommodation:** the ability of the eye to focus
   b. **Astigmatism:** a distortion of vision due to unequal curvature of the cornea or lens
   c. **Cerumen:** wax in the outer ear
   d. **Hyperopia:** farsightedness
   e. **Iridectomy:** a surgical removal of a portion of the iris
   f. **Mastoiditis:** inflammation of the mastoid bone air cells
   g. **Miotic:** a drug that constricts the pupil of the eye
   h. **Myopia:** nearsightedness
   i. **Myringotomy:** an incision of the eardrum for the release of fluid trapped in the middle ear
   j. **Oculist:** same as ophthalmologist
   k. **Ophthalmologist:** a physician who has special training in the diagnosis and treatment of eye diseases including refraction and the prescription of glasses
   l. **Optician:** one who fills eyeglass prescriptions
   m. **Optometrist:** one who has special training in testing vision for refractive errors and in prescribing and fitting glasses to correct such errors
   n. **Otosclerosis:** a progressive deafness caused by ankylosis of the stapes which interferes with the vibration of the stapes and thus the transmission of sound to the inner ear
   o. **Photophobia:** intolerance to light
   p. **Presbyopia:** decreased ability to accommodate to near vision
   q. **Valsalva maneuver:** a pinching of the nostrils while at the same time trying to blow air through the nose. Done to equalize pressure on both sides of the eardrum.
2. Column B answers in correct order: 3, 7, 2, 6, 4, 1 (p. 235).
3. 1. *sclera*; 2. *choroid*; 3. *retina*; 4. *optic nerve*; 5. *vitreous body*; 6. *lens*; 7. *iris*; 8. *cornea*; 9. *anterior chamber*; 10. *posterior chamber* (p. 225, Fig. 18-1).
4. At mealtime tell him where food is on the plate, likening the location to the face of a clock; place food on the tray in the same place for each meal; help him with food, e.g., opening milk cartons, buttering bread, etc. until he masters these tasks; let him gradually assume responsibility for his own grooming; tell him when something has been moved; leave doors open or closed; keep his personal articles in the same place. Additional answers may also be acceptable (p. 228).
5. Answers will vary.
6. Call him by name when in a group; tell him who you are when first addressing him; touch him on the sleeve or elbow so he will realize you are there (p. 230).
7. (1) maintain proper bowel habits; (2) avoid heavy lifting or straining; (3) avoid emotional upsets; (4) avoid crying (this increases intraocular pressure); (5) limit activities that make the eyes feel strained or fatigued; (6) keep an extra supply of (eye) drugs on hand; (7) avoid all drugs containing atropine; (8) carry identification stating he has glaucoma so that necessary treatment can be instituted if he is sick or hurt (p. 234).
8. (1) Move from cart to bed *gently*; (2) keep call light within easy reach and touch if both eyes covered; (3) visit patient frequently and talk to him to prevent disorientation if both eyes are covered; (4) feed patient if his head remains immobile (p. 238).
9. Automobile horns, human voice, sound of traffic, sirens. Other answers may also be acceptable (p. 240).
10. Speak somewhat loudly but do not shout, speak slowly and distinctly, try not to show impatience (pp. 240-241).

CHAPTER 19

I. True or false

1. true (pp. 249-250)
2. true (p. 250)
3. false (p. 250)
4. false (p. 250)
5. true (p. 250)
6. true (p. 251)
7. true (pp. 251-252)
8. true (p. 253)
9. false (p. 254)
10. false (p. 254)
11. true (p. 254)
12. true (pp. 256-257)
13. true (p. 257)
14. true (p. 257)
15. true (p. 258)

II. Multiple choice

1. c (p. 250)
2. a (p. 250)
3. a (p. 251)
4. d (p. 252)
5. b (p. 252)
6. c (pp. 255, Table 19-1; 254)
7. a (p. 258, Figure 19-6)
8. d (p. 255)
9. c (p. 255, Table 19-1)
10. b (p. 255, Table 19-1)
11. c (p. 255, Table 19-1)
12. b (p. 257)
13. a (pp. 256, Fig. 19-5; 257)
14. b (p. 257)
15. d (p. 255)
16. a (p. 258)
17. b (pp. 258-259)
18. c (p. 259)
19. d (p. 259)
20. a (p. 259)

III. Fill-in and discussion

1. 1. *uvula*; 2. *epiglottis*; 3. *larynx*; 4. *esophagus*; 5. *trachea*; 6. *nasal septum*; 7. *frontal sinuses*; 8. *ethmoid sinus*; 9. *maxillary sinus*; 10. *sphenoid sinus* (p. 250, Fig. 19-1).
2. Fill in:
    1. submucous resection (p. 252)
    2. antrotomy (p. 251)
    3. larynx (p. 253)
    4. laryngectomy (p. 254)
    5. dysphagia (see Glossary)
    6. tracheostomy (synonym—tracheotomy) (see Glossary)
    7. epistaxis (p. 253)
    8. laryngoscopy (p. 253)
    9. epiglottis (p. 254, Fig. 19-3)
    10. esophageal speech (pp. 254-255)
3. Smoking; overuse of voice; alcohol; industrial pollutants; heredity (p. 254).
4. Answers will vary but may include talking on the telephone, talking person to person, yelling or calling to someone at a distance, talking into a tape recorder, singing, etc.
5. Inner tube; outer tube; obturator (pp. 257-258).

CHAPTER 20

I. True or false

1. true (p. 263)
2. false (pp. 263-264)
3. false (p. 264)
4. true (p. 265)
5. false (p. 265)
6. true (p. 266)
7. true (pp. 266-268)
8. false (p. 269)
9. true (p. 271)
10. true (p. 272)

II. Multiple choice

1. d (p. 264)
2. c (p. 264)
3. a (pp. 270-271)
4. c (p. 271)
5. d (p. 272)
6. a (p. 272)
7. b (p. 272)
8. c (p. 272)
9. c (p. 272)
10. c (p. 267)
11. d (p. 268)
12. a (p. 268)
13. c (p. 268)
14. b (p. 269)

III. Fill-in and discussion

1. VOCABULARY. Definitions may vary slightly according to reference consulted. (See Glossary or medical dictionary.)
    a. **Bronchoscopy:** insertion of a bronchoscope for visual examination of the trachea and bronchi
    b. **Empyema:** pus in the pleural space
    c. **Hemothorax:** blood in the pleural space
    d. **Pleurisy:** inflammation of the pleura
    e. **Pneumothorax:** air in the thoracic cavity
    f. **Thoracentesis:** entry into the thoracic cavity to remove fluid
2. (p. 263, Fig. 20-1).
    1. *right upper lobe*; 2. *middle lobe*; 3. *right lower lobe*; 4. *diaphragm*; 5. *heart*; 6. *left lower lobe*; 7. *bronchiole*; 8. *left upper lobe*; 9. *bronchus*; 10. *trachea*; 11. *larynx*.
3. (1) Aspirin or acetaminophen (Tylenol, Datril)
   (2) Steam or cool vapor inhalation
   (3) Physician may order codeine or cough medicine
   (4) Extra fluids, frequent feedings
   (5) Bed rest (pp. 271-273)
4. (1) Early in the morning, on rising
   (2) To remove saliva and old food particles
   (3) Color, consistency, odor (if any), quantity of sample
   (4) Waxed sputum cup, wide-mouthed bottle (pp. 265-266)

CHAPTER 21

I. True or false

1. true (p. 275)
2. false (p. 275)
3. true (p. 276)
4. true (p. 276)
5. false (p. 278)
6. true (p. 279)
7. false (p. 280)
8. true (p. 280)
9. true (p. 280)
10. true (p. 282)
11. false (p. 282)
12. true (p. 282)
13. true (p. 283)
14. false (p. 284)
15. true (p. 286)
16. false (p. 286)
17. false (p. 287)
18. false (pp. 287-288)
19. true (p. 288)
20. true (p. 291)
21. true (p. 291)
22. false (p. 291)
23. false (p. 292)
24. false (p. 292)
25. true (p. 294)

II. Multiple choice

1. a (p. 275)
2. c (p. 275)
3. a (p. 280)
4. d (p. 280)
5. d (p. 280)
6. a (p. 281)
7. c (p. 285)
8. d (p. 286)
9. c (p. 287)
10. b (p. 289, Table 21-1)
11. c (p. 276)
12. c (p. 277)
13. a (p. 294)
14. a (p. 294)
15. b (p. 277)
16. c (p. 279)
17. c (pp. 278-279)
18. c (pp. 281-282)
19. a (p. 282)
20. d (p. 282)
21. d (p. 283)
22. b (p. 283)
23. b (p. 283)
24. b (p. 283)
25. b (p. 284)
26. a (pp. 284-285)
27. d (p. 288)
28. a (p. 289, Table 21-1)
29. b (pp. 294-295)
30. c (p. 289)
31. d (p. 289)
32. a (p. 290)
33. a (p. 290)
34. d (pp. 292-293)
35. d (p. 293)
36. c (p. 293)

III. Fill-in and discussion

1. VOCABULARY. Definitions may vary according to reference consulted. (See Glossary or medical dictionary.)
   a. **Allergen:** a substance that produces an allergy; may be food, an inhalant, drugs, animals, and so on.
   b. **Allergic rhinitis:** the reaction of the nasal mucosa to various allergens commonly found in the environment
   c. **Attenuated:** to weaken, to reduce the virulence of a pathogenic microorganism
   d. **Bronchitis:** inflammation of the mucous membrane lining of the bronchi
   e. **Bronchodilator:** a drug producing bronchodilatation or dilatation of the bronchi
   f. **Bronchospasm:** spasm of the bronchus resulting in a narrowing of the lumen, thus decreasing the amount of air reaching the lung
   g. **Bulla:** a blister or bleb
   h. **Crepitation:** a crackling or grating sound
   i. **Dyspnea:** labored or difficult breathing
   j. **Extrinsic:** coming from without
   k. **Humidification:** supplying moisture to the air
   l. **Malaise:** discomfort, uneasiness, a feeling of illness
   m. **Mucopurulent:** consisting of mucus and pus
   n. **Suppuration:** the formation of pus
   o. **Thorax:** the chest cavity
2. Chronic bronchitis; smoking; repeated pulmonary infections; industrial pollutants of coal dust, asbestos, cotton fibers and so on; aging process; exposure to molds and fungi; heredity (p. 282).
3. (1) tube #2
   (2) tube #2
   (3) tube #1 (p. 288, Fig. 21-4)
4. (1) tube #1
   (2) tube #2
   (3) bottle A (p. 288, Fig. 21-5)
5. (1), (2), (3) fatigue; anorexia; weight loss; slight nonproductive cough. Other answers may also be acceptable. (p. 292)
6. These symptoms can be attributed to other causes as example poor nutrition, working too hard, smoking too much, etc. (p. 292).

CHAPTER 22

I. Correct the false statements.

1. true (p. 298)
2. false—macrocytic (p. 298)
3. true (p. 299)
4. true (p. 303)
5. false—decreased (p. 306)
6. true (p. 306)
7. false—increase (p. 306)
8. false—decreased (p. 307)
9. true (p. 307)
10. false—lymphocytes (p. 308)

II. True or false

1. true (p. 298)
2. false (p. 299)
3. false (p. 299)
4. true (p. 300)
5. false (p. 300)
6. true (p. 300)
7. true (p. 301)
8. true (p. 302)
9. false (p. 303)
10. true (p. 303)
11. true (p. 305)
12. false (p. 306)
13. true (p. 307)
14. false (p. 308)
15. true (p. 308)

III. Multiple choice

1. c (p. 298)	8. b (p. 300)	15. c (p. 305)	22. d (p. 308)
2. a (p. 299)	9. c (p. 301)	16. b (p. 306)	23. c (p. 303)
3. c (p. 299)	10. b (p. 301)	17. a (p. 307)	24. a (p. 302)
4. d (p. 299)	11. a. (p. 302)	18. a (p. 307)	25. b (p. 304)
5. b (p. 299)	12. a (p. 302)	19. c (p. 307)	26. c (p. 303)
6. d (p. 299)	13. c (p. 302)	20. d (p. 307)	27. d (p. 303)
7. b (p. 300)	14. d (p. 303)	21. a (p. 307)	28. a (p. 303)

IV. Fill-in and discussion

1. VOCABULARY. Definitions may vary according to reference consulted. (See Glossary or medical dictionary.)
   a. **Anemia:** a decrease in the number of red blood cells and a lower than normal hemoglobin
   b. **Erythrocytes:** red blood cells
   c. **Hemolysis:** destruction of red blood cells
   d. **Hyperchromic:** more hemoglobin than normal
   e. **Hypochromic:** less hemoglobin than normal
   f. **Macrocytic:** larger than normal size of a red blood cell
   g. **Microcytic:** smaller than normal size of a red blood cell
   h. **Normocytic:** normal size of a red blood cell
   i. **Petechiae:** small hemorrhagic spots
   j. **Phlebotomy:** removal of blood from a vein
   k. **Purpura:** small hemorrhagic areas in the skin, mucous membrane, or subcutaneous tissues
   l. **Splenomegaly:** enlargement of the spleen
   m. **Viscous:** thick
2. Chronic blood loss; rapid blood loss; hemolysis; inadequate production of red blood cells (pp. 299-302)
3. Fatigue; anorexia; faintness; pallor; shortness of breath; weakness (p. 299)
4. Lymphocytes; monocytes; granulocytes (p. 302)
5. Answers will vary.
6. Chills; cyanosis; fever; dyspnea; orthopnea; pain in lumbar region; restlessness; urticaria (p. 305)

CHAPTER 23

I. True or false

1. true (p. 311)	4. true (p. 313)	7. true (p. 316)	9. false (pp. 316-317)
2. true (p. 311)	5. true (p. 315)	8. false (p. 316)	10. true (p. 317)
3. false (p. 312)	6. false (p. 315)		

II. Multiple choice

1. b (pp. 311, Figure 23-1; 312)	3. a (p. 314)	5. c (p. 316)	7. b (p. 316)
2. d (p. 313)	4. d (p. 316)	6. c (p. 316)	8. a (p. 317)

III. Fill-in and discussion

1. VOCABULARY. Definitions may vary slightly according to reference consulted. (See Glossary or medical dictionary.)
   a. **Atria:** chamber or cavity, the upper chambers of the heart
   b. **Bradycardia:** slow pulse rate; usually below 60
   c. **Cheyne-Stokes respirations:** irregular respirations; slow, shallow respirations that increase in rate and depth, then decrease in intensity and followed by a period of apnea
   d. **Chordae tendineae:** cords which connect edges of atrioventricular valves to papillary muscles
   e. **Diastole:** period of the cardiac cycle when the atria and ventricles fill. Also called the period of relaxation in the cardiac cycle.
   f. **Electrocardiogram (ECG):** a graphic recording of the electrical activity of the heart
   g. **Endocardium:** serous membrane on inner surface of the heart
   h. **Hypoxia:** same as anoxia—lack of adequate oxygen in inspired air
   i. **Myocardium:** muscle (middle) layer of the heart
   j. **Orthopnea:** difficulty breathing in any but a sitting or standing position
   k. **Pericardium:** the outer layer of the heart—the fibroserous sac enclosing the heart
   l. **Systole:** the contraction phase of the cardiac cycle
   m. **Tachycardia:** rapid pulse rate; usually over 100
   n. **Tachypnea:** rapid respiratory rate
   o. **Ventricles:** the lower chambers of the heart
2. Pulse rhythm; pulse quality (p. 313)
3. The numerical difference between the apical rate and the radial rate (p. 313)

CHAPTER 24

I. True or false

1. false (pp. 318-319)
2. true (p. 319)
3. true (p. 319)
4. true (p. 320)
5. false (p. 319)
6. true (p. 322)
7. false (p. 322, Table 24-1)
8. false (p. 322, Table 24-1)
9. false (p. 322, Table 24-1)
10. true (p. 323)
11. true (p. 324)
12. true (p. 324)
13. false (pp. 324, 328)
14. true (p. 325)

II. Multiple choice

1. c (p. 318)
2. c (p. 320)
3. a (p. 320)
4. d (p. 321)
5. a (p. 320)
6. b (p. 321)
7. b (p. 321)
8. c (p. 322)
9. d (p. 322)
10. a (p. 322)
11. d (p. 322)
12. b (p. 322)
13. c (p. 323, Table 24-2)
14. b (p. 325)
15. c (p. 325)
16. a (p. 325)
17. a (p. 325)
18. d (p. 325)
19. d (p. 326)
20. c (p. 326)
21. b (pp. 326, Figure 24-2; 327)
22. b (p. 326)
23. c (p. 327)

III. Fill-in and discussion

1. Rheumatic fever; myocardial infarction; inflammation of the pericardium; hypothyroidism. Other answers may also be acceptable (p. 319).
2. Muscle cramps; muscle weakness; cardiac arrhythmias; postural hypotension; malaise; anorexia; vomiting; abdominal distention; thirst; shallow respirations (p. 323, Table 24-2).
3. Oliguria; anuria; decreased skin turgor; hypotension; dry mucous membrane; tachycardia; apprehension (p. 323, Table 24-2).
4. Necessity of limiting salt intake; avoid foods high in sodium; avoiding all drugs not prescribed or approved by the physician; limitation of activities as recommended by the physician; daily weights at same time each day and with (approximate) same clothing; only use salt substitutes approved by the physician; take drugs exactly as prescribed by the physician (pp. 323-325).

CHAPTER 25

I. True or false

1. true (p. 329)
2. false (p. 330)
3. true (p. 331)
4. true (p. 331)
5. false (p. 333)
6. false (p. 333)
7. true (p. 334)
8. true (p. 334)
9. true (pp. 334-335)
10. false (p. 335)
11. true (p. 336)
12. true (p. 337)

II. Multiple choice

1. a (p. 330)
2. d (p. 330)
3. c (p. 330)
4. a (p. 330)
5. d (p. 332)
6. a (p. 332)
7. a (p. 332)
8. b (pp. 332-333)
9. c (p. 333)
10. d (p. 334)
11. b (p. 336)
12. a (pp. 336-337)
13. c (p. 338)
14. d (p. 338)

III. Fill-in and discussion

1. VOCABULARY. Definitions may vary slightly according to reference consulted. (See Glossary or medical dictionary.)
   a. **Bacteremia:** bacteria in the blood
   b. **Chorea:** uncontrollable, uncoordinated, purposeless movement
   c. **Familial:** occurring or affecting members of a family
   d. **Myocarditis:** inflammation of the heart muscle (myocardium)
   e. **Pericarditis:** inflammation of the sac (pericardium) enclosing the heart
   f. **Polyarthritis:** arthritis in several joints
   g. **Stenosis:** narrowing
   h. **Tamponade:** pressure or compression of a part or organ
2. Give drug on time; give as ordered; observe patient carefully for toxic reactions; rotate injection sites (pp. 336-337).

CHAPTER 26

I. True or false
1. true (p. 340)
2. true (p. 341)
3. true (p. 341)
4. false (p. 341)
5. true (pp. 341-342)
6. true (p. 342)
7. false (p. 342)
8. true (p. 343)
9. false (p. 343)
10. true (p. 343)
11. true (p. 343)
12. true (p. 344)
13. false (p. 344)
14. true (p. 345)
15. true (p. 346)
16. false (p. 346)
17. true (p. 346)
18. false (p. 347)
19. false (p. 347)
20. true (p. 345)

II. Multiple choice
1. c (p. 341)
2. c (p. 341)
3. a (p. 341)
4. a (p. 342)
5. d (p. 342)
6. d (p. 342)
7. d (p. 342)
8. b (p. 343)
9. b (p. 343)
10. c (p. 343)
11. d (p. 343)
12. a (p. 343)
13. b (p. 344)
14. c (p. 344)
15. b (p. 344)
16. a (p. 345)
17. c (p. 345)
18. a (p. 345)
19. c (pp. 345-346)
20. b (p. 347)
21. d (p. 347)
22. c (p. 345)
23. b (pp. 347-349)

III. Fill-in and discussion
1. Age; sex; hypertension; smoking; obesity; rise in serum cholesterol and triglyceride levels; lack of physical activity; stress; personality patterns; other diseases such as gout and diabetes (p. 342).
2. Sudden substernal chest pain or pressure; pain may radiate to shoulders, arms, jaws, teeth, neck. Instead of pain a tight squeezing, choking feeling in the upper chest or throat may be noted. Patients may also describe symptoms of indigestion (p. 342).
3. (1) primary hypertension — unknown etiology
   (2) secondary hypertension — hypertension due to a known cause such as a tumor of the adrenal gland, pregnancy, etc. (pp. 345-346).
4. Headache; dizziness; fatigue; insomnia; nervousness; epistaxis blurred vision; spots before eyes; angina shortness of breath (p. 346).

CHAPTER 27

I. True or false
1. true (p. 352)
2. false (p. 352)
3. false (p. 353)
4. true (p. 353)
5. false (p. 353)
6. true (p. 353)
7. false (p. 354)
8. true (p. 354)
9. false (p. 358)
10. true (p. 358)
11. false (p. 358)
12. false (pp. 358-359)
13. true (p. 359)
14. false (p. 360)
15. true (p. 360)
16. true (p. 360)
17. true (p. 360)
18. false (p. 361)
19. true (p. 361)
20. true (p. 362)
21. true (p. 364)
22. true (p. 364)
23. true (p. 365)
24. false (p. 367)

II. Multiple choice
1. d (p. 353)
2. a (p. 353)
3. a (p. 353)
4. a (pp. 353-354)
5. d (p. 354)
6. c (p. 354)
7. d (p. 355)
8. d (p. 355)
9. b (p. 361)
10. d (p. 361)
11. a (p. 361)
12. d (p. 362)
13. a (p. 362)
14. b (p. 362)
15. b (p. 362)
16. c (p. 363)
17. b (p. 363)
18. d (p. 364)
19. b (p. 364)
20. a (p. 364)
21. c (pp. 364-365)
22. c (p. 366)
23. a (p. 358)
24. b (p. 359)
25. c (p. 359)
26. b (p. 359)
27. b (p. 359)
28. b (p. 359)
29. a (p. 359)
30. d (p. 358)
31. a (p. 358)
32. b (p. 358)
33. c (p. 358)
34. c (p. 360)
35. d (p. 360)
36. b (p. 361)
37. c (p. 360)
38. b (p. 361)

III. Fill-in and discussion
1. VOCABULARY. Definitions may vary according to reference consulted. (See Glossary or medical dictionary.)
   a. **Embolism:** a clot carried in the bloodstream from one area to another and causing obstruction in a blood vessel
   b. **Intermittent claudication:** pain that occurs only after a certain amount of exercise
   c. **Lymph:** colorless fluid circulating in the lymphatic system
   d. **Lymphedema:** accumulation of tissue fluid due to an obstruction of lymph vessels
   e. **Phlebothrombosis:** presence of clots in the vein with little or no inflammation
   f. **Stasis:** stagnation, stoppage of flow
   j. **Thrombophlebitis:** inflammation of the vein

with clot formation
- h. **Thrombosis:** a blood clot inside a blood vessel
2. Treatment is tedious and sometimes painful; results of treatment are gradual; months of therapy produces concern over employment, finances, family and civic responsibilities (p. 352).
3. (1) **Feet:** keep clean, wash daily; wear clean socks, keep feet dry and avoid moisture
   (2) **Toenails:** trim regularly; cut nails straight
   (3) **Corns, calluses:** don't treat but ask physician's advice
   (4) **Shoes:** wear comfortable shoes that fit, shoes should give good support
   (5) **Socks, stockings:** should be large enough to avoid pressure; avoid bulky darns that could cause pressure
   (6) **Garters:** do not wear circular garters and avoid garments that cause constriction around the thigh
   (7) **Standing:** avoid prolonged standing (pp. 357-358)
4. Pain; redness; swelling; fever; anorexia; malaise; fatigue; mottled blue color to extremities; part is warm to touch (p. 362).
5. Burns; excessive radiation; extensive surgery for malignancy requiring removal of lymphatic vessels; infection; malignancy; phlebitis (pp. 362-363).
6. Check color, temperature of leg; check peripheral pulses in leg (pp. 363-364).

CHAPTER 28

I. True or false

1. true (p. 371)
2. false (pp. 371-372)
3. false (p. 372)
4. true (p. 372)
5. false (p. 372)
6. true (p. 373)
7. true (p. 373)
8. false (p. 373)
9. false (p. 373)
10. false (p. 373)
11. true (p. 375)
12. true (p. 376)
13. false (pp. 376-377)
14. true (p. 378)
15. true (p. 379)
16. true (pp. 379-380)
17. false (p. 380)

II. Multiple choice

1. b (p. 371)
2. a (p. 371)
3. d (p. 371)
4. a (pp. 371-372)
5. a (p. 372)
6. b (p. 372)
7. c (p. 372)
8. b (p. 374)
9. c (p. 376)
10. a (p. 376)
11. b (p. 376)
12. d (p. 376)
13. a (p. 377)
14. d (p. 378)
15. c (p. 378)
16. c (p. 379)
17. d (p. 379)
18. b (p. 380)
19. a (p. 380)
20. d (p. 380)
21. c (p. 380)
22. c (p. 380)
23. a (p. 381)

III. Fill-in and discussion

1. (p. 370, Figure 28-1) 1. *trachea*; 2. *liver*; 3. *gallbladder*; 4. *common duct*; 5. *duodenum*; 6. *ascending colon*; 7. *appendix*; 8. *anus*; 9. *rectum*; 10. *small bowel*; 11. *descending colon*; 12. *transverse colon*; 13. *pancreas*; 14. *spleen*; 15. *stomach*; 16. *diaphragm*; 17. *esophagus*.
2. The gastrointestinal tract is laden with bacteria; food and fluids that are eaten are not sterile (p. 371).
3. Check if the patient is having regular bowel movements; check whether the barium is appearing in the stool (stool will be white) (p. 373).
4. (1) Preparation of the patient: enemas, explaining the procedure, showing the knee-chest position.
   (2) Positioning the patient.
   (3) Draping the patient.
   Also accepted: preparing the equipment, cleansing the region after examination, caring for used equipment; sending specimens to laboratory; discarding waste (pp. 374-375).
5. (1) Withdrawal of specimens of gastric content for diagnostic purposes.
   (2) Prevention and treatment of postoperative distention.
   (3) Removal of accumulated contents of the gastrointestinal tract.
   Also acceptable: emptying the stomach before surgery or after swallowing of poisons (pp. 375-376).

CHAPTER 29

I. True or false

1. false (pp. 382-383)
2. true (p. 383)
3. true (p. 383)
4. true (p. 384)
5. false (p. 384)
6. false (p. 384)
7. true (p. 385)
8. false (p. 385)
9. true (p. 386)
10. true (p. 386)
11. true (p. 387)
12. false (p. 387)
13. false (p. 388)
14. true (p. 389)

II. Multiple choice

1. c (p. 382)	6. b (p. 383)	11. c. (p. 385)	16. c (p. 386)	21. a (p. 387, Table 29-1
2. b (pp. 382-383)	7. d (p. 384)	12. c (pp. 373, 386)	17. b (pp. 386-387)	22. b (p. 388)
3. b (p. 383)	8. c (p. 384)	13. a (p. 386)	18. d (pp. 387-388)	23. d (p. 388)
4. d (p. 383)	9. a (p. 384)	14. d (pp. 386-387)	19. d (p. 387)	
5. a (p. 383)	10. b (p. 384)	15. b (p. 386)	20. c (p. 388)	

III. Fill-in and discussion

1. Diarrhea (15 to 20 or more stools per day); stools contain blood and mucus; weight loss; fever; anorexia; severe electrolyte imbalance; anemia; dehydration; nausea; vomiting; urge to defecate is sudden; may be incontinent of feces (p. 383)
2. The following items should be checked: milk, mashed potato, chicken, asparagus soup (creamed), cooked beets, creamed spinach, butter, cottage cheese, eggs (poached), banana, gelatin dessert, buttermilk (pp. 386, 390).
3. Pallor; weak rapid pulse; thirst; sweating; collapse; faintness (p. 389).
4. Nausea; vomiting; pain; abdominal distention (p. 389).
5. Sudden excruciating pain; profuse perspiration; face ashen and drawn; abdomen "boardlike" and extremely tender and painful; patient may lie with knees flexed to lessen pain; rapid and shallow breathing; temperature normal or subnormal (pp. 389-390).
6. Face flushed; fever; abdomen distended; abdomen less rigid than before perforation; pulse weak and rapid (pp. 389-399).

CHAPTER 30

I. True or false

1. false (p. 393)	5. false (p. 394)	8. true (pp. 397-398)	11. false (pp. 399-400)	
2. true (p. 393)	6. true (p. 396)	9. true (p. 398)	12. false (p. 401)	
3. true (p. 393)	7. true (p. 397)	10. true (p. 399)	13. true (p. 401)	
4. false (p. 393)				

II. Multiple choice

1. c (p. 396)	10. b (p. 395)	19. b (p. 397)	28. a (pp. 399-400)
2. d (p. 398)	11. c (p. 395)	20. d (p. 397)	29. a (pp. 399-400)
3. a (p. 399)	12. b (p. 395)	21. b (p. 397)	30. c (p. 400)
4. a (p. 399)	13. a (p. 395)	22. a (p. 397)	31. a (p. 400)
5. d (pp. 393-394)	14. a (p. 395)	23. c (p. 398)	32. a (p. 400)
6. c (p. 393)	15. b (p. 395, Table 30-1)	24. b (p. 398)	33. c. (pp. 399-401)
7. b (p. 398)	16. c (p. 395)	25. a (p. 398)	34. b (p. 401)
8. d (p. 398)	17. b (p. 396)	26. b (p. 398)	35. b (p. 401)
9. a (p. 399)	18. d (pp. 396-397)	27. c (p. 398)	36. d (p. 401)

III. Discussion question

1. Provide privacy during first attempt to eat and swallow; help minimize problems of drooling by providing plenty of tissues; show him how to tilt his head to aid in swallowing saliva; help him pay extra attention to grooming (pp. 395-396).

CHAPTER 31

I. True or false

1. true (p. 404)	5. false (pp. 406, 408-409)	9. true (p. 412)	13. false (p. 415)	
2. false (p. 404)	6. true (p. 411)	10. false (p. 412)	14. false (p. 415)	
3. false (pp. 405-406)	7. false (p. 412)	11. true (p. 413)		
4. true (p. 406)	8. true (p. 412)	12. true (p. 415)		

II. Multiple choice

1. a (p. 404)
2. d (p. 404)
3. d (p. 405)
4. c (p. 406)
5. a (p. 406)
6. b (pp. 406-408)
7. d (p. 407)
8. b (p. 408)
9. a (pp. 408-409)
10. a (p. 409)
11. c (p. 410)
12. b (p. 410)
13. a (p. 412)
14. b (p. 412)
15. a (p. 415)
16. d (p. 415)
17. a (p. 411)
18. b (p. 411)
19. c (p. 412)
20. a (p. 412)
21. b (p. 412)
22. c (pp. 413-414)
23. a (p. 414)
24. b (p. 414)
25. c (p. 414)
26. a (p. 414)
27. c (p. 414)

III. Fill-in and discussion

1. Ulcerative colitis; cancer; multiple polyposis; diverticulitis; other obstructive lesions (p. 404).
2. Carry out dressing changes quickly and promptly; control odors; be sure dressing changes are done in absolute privacy; keep everything in the area spotless; allow patient to express his feelings. Other answers may also be accepted (p. 405).
3. Answers will vary.

CHAPTER 32

I. True or false

1. true (p. 417)
2. false (p. 418)
3. true (p. 418)
4. true (p. 418)
5. false (p. 420)
6. true (p. 420)
7. false (p. 421)
8. false (p. 420)
9. true (p. 422)
10. true (p. 422)
11. true (p. 423)
12. true (p. 423)
13. false (p. 424)
14. true (p. 424)
15. true (p. 424)
16. false (p. 424)
17. false (pp. 426-427)
18. true (p. 426)
19. true (p. 427)

II. Multiple choice

1. b (p. 418)
2. c (p. 418)
3. a (p. 419)
4. d (p. 419)
5. a (p. 420)
6. d (p. 420)
7. a (p. 420)
8. c (p. 420)
9. d (p. 421)
10. b (p. 422)
11. a (p. 422)
12. b (p. 422)
13. c (p. 422)
14. a (p. 422)
15. c (p. 424)
16. a (p. 425)
17. a (p. 425)
18. d (p. 425)
19. d (p. 426)
20. c (p. 426)
21. b (p. 427)
22. b (p. 427)
23. c. (p. 423)
24. d (p. 423)
25. a (p. 423)
26. c (p. 423)
27. c (p. 424)
28. b (p. 424)
29. a (p. 424)
30. a (p. 424)
31. b (p. 424)

III. Fill-in and discussion

1. VOCABULARY. Definitions may vary slightly according to reference consulted. (See Glossary or medical dictionary.)
   a. **Diverticula**: sacs or pouches caused by herniation of the intestinal mucosa through a weakened portion of the muscular coat of the intestine or other structure
   b. **Diverticulitis**: inflammation or infection of diverticula
   c. **Diverticulosis**: presence of diverticula
   d. **Fecalith**: a hard mass of feces
   e. **Hernia**: protrusion of intestines through a defect in the abdominal wall
   f. **Herniorrhaphy**: an operation performed for the repair of a hernia
   g. **Hirsute**: hairy
   h. **Paralytic ileus**: paralysis of the intestines
   i. **Peritonitis**: inflammation of the peritoneum
   j. **Regional enteritis**: inflammation of the terminal ileum of the small intestine
   k. **Steatorrhea**: a high content of fat in the stool
   l. **Volvulus**: a twisting or kinking of the intestine
2. Both increase peristalsis which may result in perforation of an inflamed appendix (p. 418).
3. Severe abdominal pain and tenderness; nausea; vomiting; fever; pulse rapid and weak; respirations shallow; leukocytosis; abdominal distention; patient avoids moving abdomen when breathing; patient may lie with knees drawn up to lessen pain (p. 419).

CHAPTER 33

I. Correct the false statements

1. false—hepatic (p. 430)
2. true (p. 430)
3. false—increased (p. 431)
4. false—increased (p. 431)
5. true (p. 432)
6. true (p. 432)
7. false—cirrhosis (p. 432)
8. true (p. 433)
9. false—portacaval (p. 436)
10. true (p. 436)
11. false—cholelithiasis (p. 439)
12. false—insulin (p. 441)

II. True or false

1. true (p. 430)
2. false (p. 430)
3. false (p. 430)
4. true (p. 431)
5. true (p. 431)
6. false (p. 432)
7. true (p. 433)
8. false (p. 433)
9. true (p. 436)
10. false (p. 436)
11. true (p. 436)
12. false (p. 437)
13. true (p. 437)
14. false (p. 438)
15. true (p. 438)
16. true (p. 438)
17. true (p. 439)
18. false (p. 439)
19. true (p. 440)
20. true (pp. 441-442)
21. true (p. 442)

III. Multiple choice

1. a (p. 431)
2. d (p. 431)
3. a (p. 431)
4. b (p. 432)
5. b (p. 432)
6. c (p. 432)
7. b (pp. 434-435)
8. a (p. 436)
9. b (p. 436)
10. c (p. 437)
11. b (p. 437)
12. d (p. 437)
13. b (p. 439)
14. a (p. 439)
15. d (p. 439)
16. b (p. 440)
17. d (p. 441)
18. b (p. 441)
19. b (p. 430)
20. b (p. 432)
21. d (p. 432)
22. d (p. 433)
23. c (p. 433)
24. c (p. 433)
25. a (p. 433)
26. b (pp. 433-434)
27. a (pp. 433-434)
28. d (p. 434)
29. c (pp. 434-435)
30. c (p. 434)
31. a (p. 434)
32. b (p. 442)
33. a (p. 442)
34. d (p. 442)
35. c (p. 442)
36. a (pp. 441-442)

IV. Fill-in and discussion

1. VOCABULARY. Definitions may vary slightly according to reference consulted. (See Glossary or medical dictionary.)
   a. **Cholecystectomy:** surgical removal of the gallbladder
   b. **Cholelithiasis:** stones in the gallbladder, gall stones
   c. **Endocrine gland:** a ductless gland which secretes its hormone(s) into the bloodstream
   d. **Endogenous:** originating in an organism or cell
   e. **Exocrine:** a duct gland whose secretion(s) reaches an area by a duct. The pancreas is both an exocrine and endocrine gland.
   f. **Exogenous:** originating outside of an organ or structure. The opposite of endogenous
   g. **Glycogen:** a carbohydrate stored in the body, principally in the liver, for future conversion to sugar
   h. **Hormone:** a substance produced in one part of the body and conveyed by way of the bloodstream to another part of the body stimulating that part(s) to increased function or activity
   i. **Hypercholesterolemia:** excessive amount of cholesterol in the blood
   j. **Icterus (adjective—icteric):** jaundice
   k. **Reticuloendothelial cells:** cells with the ability to ingest bacteria and other cells, such as worn out red blood cells

2. Formation and excretion of bile; utilization, transformation and distribution of vitamins, proteins, fats and carbohydrates; storage of glycogen; synthesis of factors needed for coagulation of blood; detoxification of endogenous and exogenous chemicals and foreign elements that may be harmful; formation of antibody and immunizing substances (p. 430).

3. Vital signs; check for abdominal pain and distention; check dressing for bleeding (p. 431).

4. Give intramuscular injections with a small needle; press injection site for 2 to 3 or more minutes after withdrawal of needle; avoid minor skin trauma; when removing intravenous needle or catheter place prolonged pressure on vein to prevent hematoma (p. 432).

CHAPTER 34

I. True or false

1. true (p. 447)
2. false (p. 447)
3. true (p. 447)
4. true (p. 447)
5. true (p. 446, Figure 34-1)
6. false (p. 446, Figure 34-1)
7. true (p. 448)
8. true (p. 449)
9. true (p. 449)
10. true (p. 450)
11. false (p. 450)
12. true (p. 450)
13. true (p. 451)
14. true (p. 456)
15. false (p. 461)
16. true (p. 462)
17. false (p. 462)
18. true (p. 462)
19. true (p. 464)
20. false (p. 466)
21. true (p. 468)
22. false (p. 468)
23. true (p. 469)
24. false (p. 469)
25. false (p. 469)
26. true (p. 470)
27. true (p. 470)
28. false (p. 471)
29. true (p. 472)

II. Multiple choice

1. b (p. 447)	13. b (p. 451)	25. d (p. 460)	37. a (p. 470)	48. d (p. 470)
2. a (p. 447)	14. b (p. 451)	26. c (p. 462)	38. b (p. 470)	49. a (p. 470)
3. c (p. 448)	15. c (p. 451)	27. c (p. 463)	39. c (p. 472)	50. a (p. 470)
4. a (p. 448)	16. a (p. 454)	28. b (p. 465)	40. a (p. 472)	51. c (p. 471)
5. b (p. 448)	17. a (p. 455)	29. c (p. 464)	41. a (p. 460)	52. a (p. 471)
6. b (p. 449)	18. c (p. 455)	30. d (p. 465)	42. a (p. 460)	53. a (p. 471)
7. a (p. 449)	19. d (p. 456)	31. d (p. 465)	43. b (p. 461)	54. a (p. 471)
8. d (p. 449)	20. c (p. 456)	32. b (p. 466)	44. c (p. 461)	55. b (p. 471)
9. c (p. 450)	21. d (p. 456)	33. c (p. 467)	45. b (p. 461)	56. c (p. 471)
10. a (p. 450)	22. a (p. 457)	34. a (p. 468)	46. b (p. 462)	57. b (p. 471)
11. c (p. 450)	23. b (p. 457)	35. d (p. 469)	47. b (p. 463, Table 34-2)	58. a (p. 471)
12. c (p. 450)	24. a (p. 459)	36. a (p. 469)		59. a (p. 472)

III. Fill-in and discussion

1. 1. *kidney*; 2. *ureter*; 3. *bladder*; 4. *urethra* (p. 446, Fig. 34-1).
2. The following should be checked: pH, glucose, red blood cells (p. 447).
3. Inspection, biopsy, treatment (pp. 449–450).
4. Tea, coffee, cola, gelatin, milk, certain fruit juices, ginger ale, other carbonated beverages, eggnog, ice cream (p. 452).
5. a. **Itching:** anesthetic ointment if ordered, cleanliness, patient may need 2 baths per day
   b. **Odor:** prompt cleaning of the incontinent patient, adequate room ventilation
   c. **Dryness of mouth:** glycerine and lemon swabs or other lubricant to lips, frequent mouth rinses
   d. **Pain or burning:** sitz baths if ordered, force fluids if burning due to cystitis
   e. **Long-term bed rest:** range-of-motion exercises, frequent position change
   f. **Embarrassment and fear:** care in not exposing patient, allow patient to express his feelings (pp. 452–453).
6. Tumor, stone, cyst, kink in ureter, stenosis or spasms of the ureter, diverticuli in bladder, enlarged prostate, congenital stricture (p. 458).
7. Urgency, frequency, dysuria, perineal and suprapubic pain, hematuria, chills, fever (p. 469).

CHAPTER 35

I. True or false

1. true (p. 476)	5. true (p. 478)	9. true (p. 482)	13. true (p. 484)	17. true (p. 487)
2. true (p. 476)	6. false (p. 479)	10. true (p. 482)	14. true (p. 484)	18. true (p. 486)
3. true (p. 476)	7. true (p. 481)	11. false (p. 483)	15. false (p. 485)	19. false (p. 487)
4. false (p. 477)	8. false (p. 481)	12. false (p. 484)	16. true (p. 486)	20. false (p. 488)

II. Multiple choice

1. b (p. 481)	13. c (p. 483)	25. a (p. 488)	36. b (p. 480)	45. a (p. 484)
2. a (p. 481)	14. a (p. 484)	26. c (p. 476)	37. d (p. 481, Table 35-1)	46. b (p. 485)
3. d (p. 481)	15. c (p. 484)	27. d (p. 476)	38. b (pp. 480–481, Table 35-1)	47. d (p. 485)
4. c (p. 481)	16. b (p. 484)	28. b (pp. 476–477)		48. a (p. 485)
5. c (p. 482)	17. a (p. 484)	29. b (p. 478)	39. b (p. 480)	49. b (p. 485)
6. b (p. 482)	18. a (p. 487)	30. b (p. 478)	40. a (pp. 480–481)	50. b (pp. 485–486)
7. c (p. 482)	19. b (p. 487)	31. b (p. 478)	41. a (p. 484)	51. a (p. 486)
8. a (p. 483)	20. d (p. 487)	32. d (p. 479)	42. c (p. 484)	52. d (p. 486)
9. b (p. 483)	21. c (p. 488)	33. a (p. 480)	43. a (p. 485)	53. a (p. 486)
10. a (p. 483)	22. a (p. 488)	34. c (p. 481, Table 35-1)	44. b (p. 485)	54. c (p. 486)
11. a (p. 483)	23. a (p. 488)	35. a (p. 480)		55. c (p. 487)
12. d (p. 483)	24. b (p. 488)			

III. Fill-in and discussion

1. 1. *pituitary*; 2. *adrenal gland*; 3. *pancreas*; 4. *ovary*; 5. *testis*; 6. *thyroid gland*; 7. *parathyroid*; 8. *thymus* (p. 476, Fig. 35-1).
2. Never increase or decrease the dose except by order of the physician; never omit or stop the drug; if ill and unable to take the drug orally go to the hospital (preferably where the personal physician is on staff); carry identification such as Medic Alert; report any signs of illness and infection to the physician immediately (pp. 485–486).

CHAPTER 36

I. True or false

1. true (p. 491)
2. true (p. 491)
3. true (p. 492)
4. false (p. 492)
5. false (p. 491)
6. true (p. 493)
7. true (p. 494)
8. false (p. 494)
9. false (p. 495, Table 36-1)
10. false (pp. 494-495)
11. false (p. 496)
12. true (p. 497)
13. false (p. 498)
14. true (p. 499)

II. Multiple choice

1. b (p. 491)
2. a (p. 491)
3. b (p. 492)
4. d (p. 493)
5. b (p. 496)
6. c (p. 496)
7. a (p. 497)
8. a (p. 498)
9. b (p. 498)
10. d (p. 499)
11. d (p. 499)
12. c (p. 500)
13. a (p. 499)
14. a (pp. 491-492)
15. d (p. 491)
16. b (p. 492)
17. a (p. 497)
18. c (p. 494)
19. c (pp. 495-496)
20. b (p. 495)
21. b (p. 491)
22. b (p. 493)
23. c (p. 493)
24. a (p. 493)
25. a (p. 493)
26. d (p. 493)
27. b (p. 494)
28. a (p. 495, Table 36-1)

III. Fill-in and discussion

1. Fill in the blanks
    1. glycosuria (p. 491)
    2. hyperglycemia (p. 491)
    3. polydipsia (p. 491)
    4. ketone (p. 491)
    5. hypoglycemia (p. 497)
    6. polyphagia (p. 491)
    7. polyuria (p. 491)
    8. pancreas (p. 491)
    9. beta, Langerhans (p. 491)
2. The following should be checked: honey, pie, chewing gum, soft drinks, candy. (*Note:* the physician may allow the use of unsweetened soft drinks and gum) (p. 494).
3. Keep insulin in a cool place; do *not* put insulin near heat such as radiators or on a windowsill; in very hot weather it may be necessary to put insulin in the lower part of the refrigerator. Allow insulin to warm to room temperature before using; when traveling, insulin may be kept in an insulated bag (p. 494).
4. Headache; nausea; drowsiness; malaise; weakness; nervousness; hunger; tremors; excessive perspiration; personality change; confusion; aphasia; vertigo; difficulty in coordination. Other answers may also be acceptable (pp. 497-498, Table 36-3).

CHAPTER 37

I. True or false

1. true (p. 505)
2. true (p. 505)
3. true (p. 505)
4. false (p. 507)
5. true (p. 507)
6. true (p. 507)
7. false (p. 507)
8. true (p. 507)
9. true (pp. 507-509)
10. false (p. 510)
11. true (p. 510)

II. Multiple choice

1. a (p. 505)
2. b (p. 506)
3. d (p. 506)
4. b (p. 506)
5. c (pp. 506-507)
6. b (p. 506)
7. c (p. 509)
8. d (p. 509)
9. a (p. 509)
10. a (p. 509)
11. d (p. 510)
12. c (p. 510)
13. b (p. 511, Table 37-1)

III. Fill-in and discussion

1. VOCABULARY. Definitions may vary slightly according to reference consulted. (See Glossary or medical dictionary.)
    a. **Amenorrhea:** absence of menstrual flow
    b. **Dysmenorrhea:** painful menstruation
    c. **Endometrium:** the lining of the uterus which undergoes changes each month and if pregnancy does not occur, is shed. Shedding of the endometrium is menstruation.
    d. **Menarche:** the start of menstruation
    e. **Menopause:** cessation of menstrual activity
    f. **Menorrhagia:** excessive bleeding at the time of normal menstruation
    g. **Menses:** the menstrual flow
    h. **Metrorrhagia:** bleeding at a time other than the menstrual period
2. 1. *bladder*; 2. *urethra*; 3. *rectum*; 4. *fallopian*

tube; 5. *ovary*; 6. *uterus*; 7. *vagina* (p. 504, Fig. 37-1)
3. Loss of female role; concern for loss of marital relationship; loss of attractiveness and femininity; fear of physical or mental disability all of which are unfounded. Discussions of these may vary (pp. 507-508).

CHAPTER 38

I. True or false

1. false (p. 514)
2. true (p. 514)
3. true (pp. 514-516)
4. false (p. 516)
5. true (p. 516)
6. true (p. 517)
7. false (p. 518)
8. true (p. 518)
9. true (p. 518)
10. true (p. 519)
11. true (p. 519)
12. true (p. 520)
13. false (p. 522)
14. false (p. 523)
15. false (p. 524)
16. true (p. 524)
17. true (p. 527)
18. true (p. 528)
19. false (p. 529)

II. Multiple choice

1. c (p. 516)
2. c (p. 517)
3. a (p. 517)
4. b (p. 518)
5. b (p. 518)
6. d (p. 518)
7. a (p. 519)
8. b (p. 519)
9. d (p. 519)
10. a (p. 519)
11. b (p. 519)
12. a (p. 520)
13. b (p. 521)
14. d (p. 521)
15. c (p. 521)
16. d (pp. 521-522)
17. c (p. 522)
18. b (p. 522)
19. c (p. 523)
20. b (p. 523)
21. a (p. 524)
22. a (p. 525)
23. b (p. 525)
24. d (p. 525)
25. c (p. 526)
26. a (p. 524)
27. b (pp. 527-528)
28. d (p. 528)
29. d (p. 529)
30. b (p. 529)
31. c (p. 530)
32. c (p. 524)
33. c (p. 527)
34. b (p. 527)
35. a (p. 527)
36. b (pp. 526, Table 38-2; 527)
37. b (p. 514)

III. Fill-in and discussion

1. VOCABULARY. Definitions may vary slightly according to reference consulted. (See Glossary or medical dictionary.)
   a. **Curettage:** scraping
   b. **Cystocele:** herniation of the bladder into the vagina
   c. **Exfoliate:** the scaling of dead tissue
   d. **Hysterectomy:** removal of the uterus
   e. **Leukorrhea:** a white or yellowish discharge from the cervix or vagina
   f. **Oophorectomy:** removal of the ovary which may be either unilateral or bilateral
   g. **Oophoritis:** inflammation of the ovaries
   h. **Salpingectomy:** removal of the fallopian tube which may be either unilateral or bilateral
   i. **Salpingitis:** inflammation of the fallopian tubes
   j. **Rectocele:** herniation of the rectum into the vagina
2. Sitz baths; frequent cleansing of the area; waterproof underpants; dusting with cornstarch; perineal pads—which must be changed frequently; wearing an absorbent liner next to the skin (pp. 528-529).

CHAPTER 39

I. True or false

1. true (p. 532)
2. false (p. 532)
3. false (p. 532)
4. false (p. 532, Figure 39-1)
5. true (p. 534)
6. false (p. 534)
7. true (p. 535)
8. true (p. 535)
9. true (p. 536)
10. false (p. 536)
11. false (p. 536)
12. true (p. 537)

II. Multiple choice

1. b (p. 537)
2. b (p. 538)
3. c (p. 538)
4. c (p. 538)
5. a (p. 538)
6. a (p. 539)
7. d (p. 539)
8. d (p. 532)
9. d (pp. 532-533)
10. b (p. 533)
11. a (p. 533)
12. d (p. 533)
13. d (p. 533)
14. b (p. 534, Table 39-1)
15. b (p. 534, Table 39-1)
16. b (p. 534, Table 39-1)
17. a (p. 534)
18. a (pp. 534-535)
19. b (p. 535)
20. d (p. 535)
21. b (p. 535)
22. b (p. 536)
23. d (p. 536)
24. d (p. 536)
25. a (p. 536)
26. a (p. 536)
27. b (pp. 536-537)
28. a (p. 537)
29. b (p. 537)
30. b (p. 537)
31. c (p. 537)
32. a (p. 537)

III. Fill-in and discussion

1. 1. *bladder*; 2. *symphysis pubis*; 3. *prostate*; 4. *penis*; 5. *urethra*; 6. *testis*; 7. *epididymis*; 8. *seminal vesicle*; 9. *rectum* (p. 532, Fig. 39-1).

CHAPTER 40

I. True or false

1. true (p. 541)
2. true (p. 541)
3. false (p. 541)
4. false (p. 543)
5. false (p. 544)
6. true (p. 546)
7. false (p. 545)
8. true (p. 546)
9. true (p. 548)
10. true (p. 550)

II. Multiple choice

1. a (p. 542)
2. c (p. 541)
3. a (p. 543)
4. a (p. 543)
5. d (p. 543)
6. a (p. 543)
7. c (p. 544)
8. d (p. 544)
9. d (p. 545, Table 40-1)
10. c (p. 545, Table 40-1)
11. a (p. 545, Table 40-1)
12. a (p. 544)
13. b (p. 545)
14. a (p. 546)
15. c (p. 546)
16. b (p. 546)
17. a (p. 547)
18. c (p. 548)
19. a (p. 548)
20. d (pp. 548-549)
21. a (p. 550)
22. d (pp. 549-550)
23. c (p. 549)
24. d (p. 549)

III. Fill-in and discussion

1. (a) Any changes in breast size, any signs of puckering or dimpling of the skin, any discharge or change in the nipples
   (b) Lie flat on the back, place a pillow behind or under the left shoulder, place left hand under head
   (c) Fingers held together and flat (p. 542)
2. Treatment usually is surgical drainage and packing of the abscess plus the administration of antibiotics. The patient is usually placed in isolation and the dressings are handled according to isolation techniques (p. 550).

CHAPTER 41

I. True or false

1. false (p. 552)
2. true (p. 552)
3. true (p. 552)
4. false (p. 552)
5. true (p. 554)
6. true (p. 554)
7. true (p. 554)
8. false (p. 554)
9. false (p. 554)
10. true (p. 555)
11. false (p. 555)
12. true (p. 556)

II. Multiple choice

1. a (p. 552)
2. a (p. 552)
3. b (p. 552)
4. d (p. 552)
5. c (p. 552)
6. a (p. 552)
7. a (p. 552)
8. a (p. 553)
9. d (p. 553)
10. c (p. 553)
11. b (p. 553)
12. c (p. 553)
13. c (p. 553)
14. a (p. 554)
15. c (p. 554)
16. a (p. 554)
17. d (p. 554)
18. b (p. 554)
19. c (p. 555)
20. b (p. 553)
21. c (p. 555)
22. b (p. 555)

III. Fill-in and discussion

1. Fill in the blanks
   (1) Syphilis and gonorrhea (p. 551)
   (2) *Neisseria gonorrhoeae* (or gonococcus) (p. 552)
   (3) Locomotor ataxia (or syphilitic posterior spinal sclerosis) (p. 554)
   (4) A large virus (p. 555)
   (5) Chancroid (p. 555)
2. Answers may vary but may include fear of reprisal from spouse, prospect of divorce or separation; shame; fear that this may have been a criminal act if contact was with a prostitute.

CHAPTER 42

I. True or false

1. false (p. 560)
2. true (p. 560)
3. true (p. 560)
4. true (p. 560)
5. false (p. 560)
6. true (p. 560)
7. false (pp. 561-563)
8. true (p. 564)
9. true (p. 565)
10. false (p. 566)
11. true (p. 566)
12. true (pp. 566-567)
13. true (p. 568)
14. true (p. 568)
15. true (p. 569)
16. true (p. 569)
17. false (p. 570)
18. true (p. 570)
19. true (p. 570)
20. true (p. 572)
21. true (p. 563, Table 42-2)
22. true (p. 572)
23. false (p. 573)

II. Multiple choice

1. a (p. 561)	6. c (p. 565)	11. a (p. 567)	15. c (p. 569)	20. c (p. 570)
2. c (p. 561)	7. a (p. 565)	12. c (p. 568)	16. a (p. 569)	21. a (p. 571)
3. a (p. 561)	8. b (p. 566)	13. a (p. 568)	17. b (p. 569)	22. b (p. 572)
4. b (p. 564)	9. a (p. 566)	14. b (p. 568)	18. d (p. 569)	
5. d (p. 564)	10. d (p. 567)		19. c (p. 570)	

III. Fill-in and discussion

1. Matching Column B should read, from top to bottom: 2 (p. 571), 3 (p. 571), 4 (p. 565), 8 (p. 567), 1 (p. 571), 6 (p. 570), 7 (p. 571), 9 (p. 561), 5 (p. 561).
2. Answers may vary (pp. 562-564).
3. The following numbers should be checked: 1, 3, 4, 6 (p. 567).

CHAPTER 43

I. True or false

1. true (p. 576)	3. true (p. 576)	5. false (p. 577)	7. true (p. 577)	9. true (p. 577)
2. true (p. 576)	4. true (p. 577)	6. false (p. 577)	8. false (p. 577)	10. false (p. 577)

II. Multiple choice

1. d (pp. 574-575)	3. b (p. 577)	5. d (p. 577)	7. c (p. 577)	9. d (p. 588)
2. a (p. 576)	4. b (p. 577)	6. a (p. 577)	8. c (p. 577)	

III. Discussion question

1. Answers will vary.

CHAPTER 44 AND CHAPTER 45

I. True or false

1. true (p. 582)	4. true (p. 585)	7. true (p. 587)	9. true (p. 587)	11. true (p. 588)
2. false (p. 583)	5. true (p. 585)	8. true (p. 587)	10. false (p. 588)	12. true (p. 589)
3. true (p. 585)	6. false (p. 586)			

II. Multiple choice

1. a (p. 585)	4. c (p. 585)	7. c (p. 587)	10. a (p. 587)	13. b (p. 588)
2. b (p. 585)	5. b (p. 585)	8. b (p. 587)	11. a (pp. 587-588)	14. c (pp. 588-589)
3. a (p. 585)	6. b (p. 585)	9. c (p. 587)	12. d (p. 588)	

III. Fill-in and discussion

1. Palpate the radial artery. Using a sphygmomanometer, inflate the cuff to obliterate the pulse. Slowly let the air out of the cuff. When the radial pulse can be palpated again this is recorded as the systolic blood pressure (p. 586).
2. a. **Skin:** cold, clammy, pale, may be cyanotic
   b. **Arterial blood pressure:** depends on patient's original blood pressure—consistent, progressive fall in blood pressure with a rapid, thready pulse indicates shock
   c. **Pulse:** compensatory tachycardia, weak and thready
   d. **Pulse pressure:** narrowed
   e. **Respirations:** tachypnea
   f. **Temperature:** subnormal (except in bacteremia shock where it may be elevated) (pp. 586-587).

CHAPTER 46

I. True or false

1. true (p. 592)	4. false (p. 593)	7. false (p. 595)	10. true (p. 596)	13. true (p. 598)
2. true (p. 592)	5. true (p. 593)	8. true (p. 595)	11. true (p. 597)	14. true (p. 598)
3. true (p. 593)	6. true (p. 594)	9. false (p. 595)	12. false (p. 597)	15. false (p. 598)

II. Multiple choice

1. d (p. 593)	6. c (p. 594)	11. b (p. 595)	16. a (p. 597)	21. b (p. 598)
2. d (p. 593)	7. a (p. 594)	12. c (p. 595)	17. d (p. 597)	22. c (p. 598)
3. c (p. 593)	8. a (p. 595)	13. c (p. 596)	18. d (p. 597)	23. c (p. 599)
4. a (p. 593)	9. a (p. 595)	14. b (p. 597)	19. b (p. 598)	
5. c (p. 594)	10. a (p. 595)	15. b (p. 597)	20. a (p. 598)	

III. Fill-in and discussion

1. VOCABULARY. Definitions may vary according to reference consulted. (See Glossary or medical dictionary.)
   a. **Diffusion:** the process whereby oxygen and carbon dioxide are exchanged across the alveolar-capillary membrane
   b. **Hypercapnia:** excess carbon dioxide in body fluids
   c. **Hypocapnia:** decrease in carbon dioxide in body fluids
   d. **Hypoxemia:** reduced oxygen in body fluids
   e. **Hypoxia:** diminished availability of oxygen to cells in the body
   f. **Ventilation:** the movement of air in and out of the lungs

CHAPTER 47

I. True or false

1. true (p. 601)	6. true (p. 604)	11. false (p. 605)	16. false (p. 608, Table 47-1)	20. false (p. 609)
2. true (p. 601)	7. false (p. 603)	12. true (p. 606)	17. false (p. 609)	21. false (pp. 609-610)
3. false (p. 601)	8. true (p. 603)	13. true (p. 606)	18. true (p. 609)	22. false (p. 610)
4. true (p. 601)	9. true (p. 604)	14. true (p. 607)	19. true (p. 609)	23. true (p. 610)
5. false (p. 602)	10. true (p. 605)	15. true (p. 608)		24. true (p. 611)

II. Multiple choice

1. b (p. 601)	7. b (p. 603)	12. b (p. 605)	17. d (p. 609)	22. d (p. 609)
2. c (p. 601)	8. c (p. 604)	13. d (p. 605)	18. a (p. 606)	23. d (p. 609)
3. a (p. 601)	9. b (p. 604)	14. c (p. 605)	19. b (p. 607)	24. b (p. 610)
4. c (p. 601)	10. a (p. 604)	15. d (p. 606)	20. c (p. 607)	25. a (p. 610)
5. d (p. 602)	11. d (p. 604)	16. a (pp. 606-607)	21. d (p. 608)	26. c (p. 611)
6. b (p. 602)				

III. Fill-in and discussion

1. Fill in the blanks
   (1) S-A or sinoatrial (p. 601)
   (2) Third (p. 604)
   (3) Depolarization (p. 601)
   (4) Repolarization (p. 601)
   (5) Sympathetic—parasympathetic (p. 601)
   (6) PVC or premature ventricular contractions (p. 605)
   (7) Purkinje system (p. 601)
2. A **Stands for airway**—airway should be established immediately
   B **Stands for breathing**—use mouth to mouth or an assistive device to breathe for the victim
   C **Stands for circulation**—should be restored by closed chest cardiac compression
   D **Stands for definitive therapy**—ordered by the physician and usually includes drugs such as sodium bicarbonate, vasopressors, etc.
   E **Stands for evaluation**—this is the victim's response to therapy—are the efforts effective? (pp. 609-610)

CHAPTER 48

I. True or false

1. true (p. 614)	5. true (p. 615)	9. true (p. 618)	13. true (p. 618)	17. true (p. 622)
2. true (p. 614)	6. false (p. 615)	10. false (p. 618)	14. true (p. 619)	18. true (p. 622)
3. false (p. 614)	7. true (p. 617)	11. true (p. 618)	15. false (p. 621)	19. true (p. 623)
4. true (p. 615)	8. false (p. 617)	12. true (p. 619)	16. true (p. 622)	

II. Multiple choice

1. c (p. 614)
2. b (p. 614)
3. c (p. 615)
4. d (p. 615)
5. a (p. 617)
6. a (p. 617)
7. b (p. 617)
8. a (p. 617)
9. d (p. 617)
10. d (p. 618)
11. d (p. 618)
12. c (p. 619)
13. b (p. 614)
14. a (p. 619)
15. a (p. 619)
16. c (p. 619)
17. b (p. 620)
18. a (p. 621)
19. d (p. 621)
20. a (p. 621)
21. a (p. 622)
22. c (p. 622)

III. Fill-in and discussion

1. Sudden severe chest pain usually substernal or precordial—pain may radiate to shoulder, arm, teeth, jaw or throat.
   Symptoms of shock: pallor, sweating, faintness, drop in blood pressure, rapid weak pulse—nausea—vomiting—fever—restlessness
   Symptoms of left-sided heart failure: dyspnea, cyanosis cough (p. 614)
2. (1) What allergies does he have?
   (2) What (past) medical problems does he have? Treated? With what?
   (3) Has he had any major surgeries? What were they?
   (4) Does he take *any* drugs? Prescription? Non-prescription? When was last dose taken?
   (5) What drugs does he take that must not be stopped, such as insulin, corticosteroids?
   (6) What symptoms were experienced prior to admission? (pp. 617-618)
3. Answers may vary but may include fear of impending death, fear of living with impending death, financial crisis, loss of employment, restriction of favorite activities, and so on (pp. 620-621).

CHAPTER 49

I. True or false

1. true (p. 626)
2. true (p. 626)
3. true (p. 627)
4. false (p. 627)
5. true (p. 627)
6. true (p. 627)
7. false (p. 627)
8. false (pp. 627-628)
9. true (p. 628)
10. false (p. 630)
11. true (pp. 632-633)

II. Multiple choice

1. a (p. 626)
2. c (p. 627)
3. c (p. 627)
4. b (p. 628)
5. d (p. 629)
6. d (p. 629)
7. d (p. 629)
8. a (p. 630)
9. b (p. 631)
10. c (p. 631)
11. c (p. 632)
12. d (p. 632)
13. a (p. 632)
14. b (p. 633)
15. c (p. 633)
16. b (p. 633)

III. Discussion question

1. (1) Explain the purpose of the intensive care unit.
   (2) Explain the immediate physical preparations before the patient enters the operating room.
   (3) Have the patient practice deep-breathing and coughing exercises.
   (4) Begin preoperative practice with intermittent positive pressure breathing apparatus.
   (5) Teach the exercises to be done after surgery.
   (6) Assure the patient that analgesics will be given for pain.
   (7) Explain the placing of the patient on the serious list to family.
   (8) Plan a visit to the recovery room and intensive care unit.
   (9) Explain tubes, catheters, monitors (any of the above 4) (pp. 630-631).

CHAPTER 50

I. True or false

1. true (p. 636)
2. true (p. 636)
3. false (p. 637)
4. true (p. 637)
5. false (pp. 637-638)
6. true (p. 637)
7. false (p. 638)
8. true (p. 638)
9. true (p. 639)
10. true (p. 640)
11. false (p. 640)
12. true (p. 639)
13. false (p. 641)
14. true (p. 641)
15. false (pp. 641-642)
16. true (p. 642)

II. Multiple choice

1. d (p. 636)
2. a (p. 636)
3. c (p. 636)
4. b (p. 639)
5. a (p. 637)
6. b (p. 638)
7. c (p. 638)
8. d (p. 638)
9. a (p. 638)
10. d (p. 639)
11. d (p. 639)
12. c (p. 640)
13. a (p. 640)
14. b (p. 640)
15. c (p. 641)
16. c (p. 641)
17. b (p. 642)
18. d (p. 642)

III. Discussion question

1. (1) the patient is pale, (2) edema eyes, (3) edema of ankles, (4) pruritus, (5) halitosis, (6) ulceration of oral mucosa, also generalized body odor suggestive of urine, mental processes may be slowed, dizziness, irritability, bleeding from GI tract, hematemesis (pp. 636-637).

CHAPTER 51

I. True or false

1. false (p. 644)
2. true (pp. 644 and Table 51-1; 645)
3. true (p. 644)
4. true (pp. 646, Table 51-1; 647)
5. true (p. 647)
6. false (p. 647)
7. false (p. 648)
8. true (p. 648)
9. false (p. 648)
10. true (p. 649)
11. false (p. 649)
12. true (p. 649)
13. false (pp. 650, Table 51-4; 651)
14. true (p. 651)
15. true (p. 651)

II. Multiple choice

1. a (pp. 645-646)
2. b (p. 646)
3. d (p. 646)
4. c (p. 646)
5. a (p. 646)
6. a (p. 647)
7. b (p. 647)
8. c (p. 647)
9. d (p. 647)
10. c (p. 647)
11. c (p. 648)
12. a (p. 648)
13. d (p. 650, Table 51-4)
14. a (p. 650, Table 51-4)
15. b (p. 648)
16. d (p. 648)
17. b (p. 649)
18. b (p. 649)
19. a (p. 649)
20. d (p. 649)
21. d (p. 649)
22. a (p. 649)
23. b (p. 649)
24. c (p. 649)
25. b (p. 649)
26. d (p. 652)

III. Fill-in and discussion

1. Television (if available in the area); discussion of current events, such as the weather, sports, special news items; radio; allow visitors when possible; newspapers and magazines (p. 650).
2. Infection; Curling's ulcer; kidney failure; anemia; gastrointestinal disturbances; contractures; decubitus ulcers; respiratory problems such as pneumonia and atelectasis (pp. 651-652).

CHAPTER 52

I. True or false

1. true (p. 655)
2. true (p. 655)
3. false (p. 655)
4. false (p. 657)
5. false (p. 657)
6. true (p. 657)
7. true (pp. 657-658)
8. true (p. 658)
9. true (p. 658)
10. true (p. 658)
11. false (p. 659)
12. true (p. 659)
13. true (p. 659)
14. false (p. 659)
15. true (p. 662)

II. Multiple choice

1. b (p. 657)
2. c (p. 657)
3. d (p. 657)
4. c (p. 657)
5. b (p. 658)
6. b (p. 658)
7. a (p. 658)
8. c (p. 658)
9. a (p. 658)
10. b (p. 658)
11. c (pp. 659-660)
12. a (p. 655, Table 52-1)
13. a (p. 655, Table 52-1)
14. b (pp. 656-657)
15. d (p. 656)
16. a (p. 656)
17. b (p. 656)
18. a (pp. 656-657)
19. c (p. 657)
20. d (p. 659)
21. a (p. 659)
22. b (pp. 659-660)
23. d (p. 660)
24. a (p. 661)
25. c (p. 661; Figure 52-1, p. 655)
26. d (p. 662)

III. Fill-in and discussion

1. Fill in the blanks
   (1) Ventricles, dural venous sinuses (pp. 654-655)
   (2) Papilledema (p. 655)
   (3) Epidural (or extradural) (p. 657)
   (4) Subdural (p. 657)
   (5) Craniotomy (p. 659)
2. (a) **Pulse rate:** initially may be increased, later becomes slow, full and bounding
   (b) **Blood pressure:** rises with a widening pulse pressure
   (c) **Respirations:** irregular, with Cheyne-Stokes or Kussmaul's breathing
   (d) **Pupils:** may be unequal and may not react to light
   (e) **Level of consciousness:** progressively deepens; patient ultimately may become comatose (p. 655, Table 52-1)